MW01517976

2007 01 19

PSYCHOLOGY OF STRESS

PSYCHOLOGY OF STRESS

KIMBERLY V. OXINGTON
EDITOR

Nova Biomedical Books
New York

For permission to use material from this book please contact us:
Telephone 631-231-7269; Fax 631-231-8175
Web Site: http://www.novapublishers.com

NOTICE TO THE READER

The Publisher has taken reasonable care in the preparation of this book, but makes no expressed or implied warranty of any kind and assumes no responsibility for any errors or omissions. No liability is assumed for incidental or consequential damages in connection with or arising out of information contained in this book. The Publisher shall not be liable for any special, consequential, or exemplary damages resulting, in whole or in part, from the readers' use of, or reliance upon, this material.

This publication is designed to provide accurate and authoritative information with regard to the subject matter covered herein. It is sold with the clear understanding that the Publisher is not engaged in rendering legal or any other professional services. If legal or any other expert assistance is required, the services of a competent person should be sought. FROM A DECLARATION OF PARTICIPANTS JOINTLY ADOPTED BY A COMMITTEE OF THE AMERICAN BAR ASSOCIATION AND A COMMITTEE OF PUBLISHERS.

Library of Congress Cataloging-in-Publication Data

Psychology of stress / Kimberly V. Oxington, editor.
    p. cm.
Includes index.
ISBN 1-59454-246-5 (hardcover)
1. Stress (Psychology) I. Oxington, Kimberly V.
BF575.S75P82   2005
155.9'042--dc22   2004028384

Published by Nova Science Publishers, Inc. ✤ New York

CONTENTS

PREFACE

Stress is a physical response to an undesirable situation. Mild stress can result from missing the bus, standing in a long line at the store or getting a parking ticket. Stress can also be severe. Divorce, family problems, an assault, or the death of a loved one, for example, can be devastating. One of the most common sources of both mild and severe stress is work. Stress can be short-term (acute) or long-term (chronic). Acute stress is a reaction to an immediate threat — either real or perceived. Chronic stress involves situations that aren't short-lived, such as relationship problems, workplace pressures, and financial or health worries. Stress is an unavoidable consequence of life. As Hans Selye (who coined the term as it is currently used) noted, "Without stress, there would be no life". However, just as distress can cause disease, it seems plausible that there are good stresses that promote wellness. Stress is not always necessarily harmful. Winning a race or an election can be just as stressful as losing, or more so, but may trigger very different biological responses. Increased stress results in increased productivity up to a point. This new book deals with the dazzling complexity of this good-bad phenomenon and presents up-to-date research from throughout the world.

Individuals have been instructed to live life well throughout history, in numerous cultures, and in various works of poetry, philosophy, and religious doctrine. In his conception of life as Eudaimonia, Aristotle suggested a tradeoff between society and the individuals, and he foreshadowed the shift toward modern conceptions of the fruits and seeds of a life lived well. That is, personal happiness is the fruit that comes from a lifetime that has been lived in pursuit of the identification, development, and use of one's talents and abilities. The topic of well-being more generally raises two key questions that will be covered in Chapter I.

The study in Chapter II examines the efficacy of a psychoeducational intervention program relative to a control group in promoting psychological well-being in 70 African American working women. A quasi-experimental repeated measures design was utilized. The psychoeducational program focused on reducing role conflict, enhancing self-esteem, life satisfaction and instrumentality, decreasing depression and facilitating coping through cognitive based problem solving strategies. This study has advanced knowledge on stressors that African American working women experience and identified stress-reduction strategies that enhanced psychological well-being in regards to increasing self-esteem scores and decreasing depression and role conflict scores.

In Chapter III, we will review the empirical support for stress management (SM) interventions developed for various medical patient populations, focusing on those applied to patients with human immunodeficiency virus (HIV) infection/acquired immune deficiency syndrome (AIDS) and cancer. SM interventions for other patient populations will also be briefly discussed. Additionally, we will briefly discuss the implications of these findings and suggest directions for future research.

Bereavement represents a specific type of stressful life events. It could be detrimental to health both in the short-term and in the long run. The aim of the study in Chapter IV is to examine the possible health effects of parental bereavement. Only severe health consequences that may lead to death or hospitalization were studied. We observed an increased mortality in bereaved mothers. The death of a child may lead to an increased risk of MI, MS, and a mildly increased risk of cancer as well as worse cancer survival in bereaved parents.

As discussed in Chapter V, mankind since the dawn of history has been afflicted with various forms of diseases. Communicable diseases that took a heavy toll of human life in medieval and prehistoric times, have been replaced by non- communicable diseases and conditions in the recent times. Among the six factors which are responsible for the major share of these diseases, stress occupies an important place. The Oxford English dictionary defines stress as pressure, tension or worry resulting from the problems in one's life. It is thus a condition of the mind, in which a person loses his calm tranquility and equanimity and experiences extreme discomfiture.

The research reported in Chapter VI compared patterns of moderating factors explaining stress reactions during two kinds of states: chronic without acute versus chronic plus acute stress. We examined the hypothesis that during a prolonged stress state, personal dispositions would have more explanatory power to understand stress reactions than in an acute situation. Five variables were examined as moderating factors: trait anxiety, sense of coherence, cognitive appraisal of the political situation, family sense of coherence, and sense of community. These data support the value of developing a model that would recognize the different types of stress situations in the study of moderating effects of stress.

The purpose of Chapter VII was to compare the predictive validity of the demand/control and reward/imbalance models, alone and in combination with each other, for self-reported health status and the self-reported presence of any chronic disease condition. Self-reports for psychosocial work conditions were obtained in a sample of sawmill workers using the demand/control and effort/reward imbalance models. The demand/control and effort/reward imbalance models independently predicted poor self-reported health status. The effort-reward imbalance model predicted the presence of a chronic disease while the demand/control model did not. Future work should explore the combined effects of these two models of psychosocial stress at work on health more thoroughly.

Somatization is the translation of emotional distress into physical symptoms that have no identifiable physical cause. Somatization is widespread: clinical, historical, and anthropological studies have demonstrated its prevalence in different historical periods and across cultures. The majority of literature on somatization conceptualizes it as maladaptive, effectively complicating diagnosis and treatment. Chapter VIII reviews research literature on somatization and summarizes the findings from an empirical study of somatization in the United States and South Korea.

Each year millions of children are exposed to traumatic experiences. The body of literature related to children and their responses to disasters and trauma is growing. Mental health professionals are increasing their understanding about what factors are associated with increased risk (vulnerability) or decreased risk (resilience) for developing psychopathology after exposure to traumatic experiences. Research on resilience in development reveals that extraordinary resilience and recovery power of children depend on basic human protective systems operating in their favour. Chapter IX reviews some strategies fostering resilience and describes the main characteristics and technical features of a novel psychotherapeutic strategy, Well-Being Therapy.

In Chapter X, the authors summarize the research on psychological effects of providing care for an older family member. After a brief overview of sources of caregiver stress, we compare psychological and physical health of caregivers and noncaregivers. Then we explore which aspects of caregiving are most stressful to caregivers. The chapter also reviews the effects of interventions with caregivers. On average, interventions show statistical significant improvements of caregiver knowledge and perceived abilities, caregiver burden, depressive symptoms, and positive well-being.

The aim of Chapter XI is to illuminate pain and distress and quality of care in relation to elderly people, family member, and caregiver perspectives. This chapter is mainly based on previously published studies within the following two areas: pain and distress and quality of care.

In: Psychology of Stress
Editor: Kimberly V. Oxington, pp. 1-15

ISBN 1-59454-246-5
©2005 Nova Science Publishers, Inc.

Chapter I

GENDER AND SUBJECTIVE WELL-BEING IN THE UNITED STATES: FROM SUBJECTIVE WELL-BEING TO COMPLETE MENTAL HEALTH

Corey L. M. Keyes

Department of Sociology of Emory University and the Department of Behavioral Sciences and Health Education of the Rollins School of Public Health USA

Nor love thy life, nor hate; but what thou liv'st Live well:
how long or short permit to heaven

John Milton (*Paradise Lost*, Book XI, Line 553)

ABSTRACT

Individuals have been instructed to live life well throughout history, in numerous cultures, and in various works of poetry, philosophy, and religious doctrine. In his conception of life as Eudaimonia, Aristotle suggested a tradeoff between society and the individuals, and he foreshadowed the shift toward modern conceptions of the fruits and seeds of a life lived well. That is, personal happiness is the fruit that comes from a lifetime that has been lived in pursuit of the identification, development, and use of one's talents and abilities (see e.g., Waterman, 1984). The topic of well-being more generally raises two key questions that will be covered in this chapter. First, who decides whether one's life is being lived well? Second, is the ability to engage in eudaimonia distributed equally in society? Do people of various ethnicities, creeds, and colors have an equal chance to develop and to employ their talents and abilities?

WELL-BEING AND SOCIAL STRUCTURE

The quality of an individual's life can be assessed externally and objectively or internally and subjectively. From an objective standpoint, other people measure and judge another's life according to criteria such as wealth or income, educational attainment, occupational prestige, and health status or longevity. Individuals who are wealthier, have more education, and live longer are considered to have higher quality of life or personal well-being. From the subjective standpoint, an individual evaluates his or her own life and subjective well-being is the feeling toward and thoughts about how well he or she is living life. Subjective well-being is unveiled through evaluations that people make about their lives after reviewing, summing, and weighing the "substance" of their lives. Life and its substance consist of activities of work (i.e., maintenance and productivity), love (i.e., relationships and intimacy), and play (i.e., socializing and leisure). Individuals evaluate their lives overall, and they judge the quality of their functioning in life.

Two central questions guiding sociological research are whether the quality of individuals' lives is distributed equally in society, and the origins of social orders that generate social inequalities (see e.g., Wrong, 1994). In the U. S., research has shown an abundance of social inequality in the quality of individual's lives, and gender has been shown to be a consistent source of social order that is implicated in the causes of social inequalities. Findings relevant to the topic of subjective well-being and gender focus on the consistent finding of gender differences in major depressive disorder. The rate of major depression in the U. S. population reveals that women are at a twofold risk for depression than men (see e.g., Kessler & Zhao, 1999). Starting around the onset of puberty and persisting throughout adulthood, females in the U. S. are more likely than males to report more symptoms of depression and to fit the criteria for a major episode of depression.

There is now a corpus of research that reveals that the etiology of gender differences in depression reflect biological, psychological, and social causes. Thus, while neurohormonal differences may predispose women to become depressed, biological differences between men and women cannot explain the gender gap in depression. Rather, research also shows that women may place greater importance on the social relationships at the same time that they are exposed to more social stressors and bear the unequal burden of responsibility for maintaining social relationships (Turner, Wheaton, & Lloyd, 1995; Cyranowski, Frank, Young, & Shear, 2000).

While there a substantiated explanations for why women have lower quality of life than men in terms of depression, most epidemiological studies show that about 1 in 10 adults in the U.S. population of adults above the ages of 18 fit the criteria for major depression in any year and about half of the adult population will not experience any mental illness over the lifespan (U.S. Department of Health and Human Services, 1999). In other words, a very large portion of the adult population in the U.S. remains free of mental illness annually and over a lifetime. This, then, begs the question whether individuals who are free from mental illness are truly mentally healthy. This has been the driving question behind the study of subjective well-being in adulthood: "Are most adults in the U.S., who tend to be free of mental illness, mentally health with high levels of subjective well-being?"

SUBJECTIVE WELL-BEING: CRITERIA OF A LIFE WELL-LIVED

Psychologists have traditionally equated subjective well-being with the degree of positive feelings (e.g., happiness) and perceptions (e.g., satisfaction) toward one's life overall (Diener, Suh, Lucas, & Smith, 1999; Gurin, Veroff, & Feld, 1960). However, a second stream of well-being research has elaborated manifold dimensions of positive functioning that reflect psychological well-being (Jahoda, 1958; Keyes, 1998; Ryff, 1989a, 1989b, Ryff & Keyes, 1995) and social well-being (Keyes, 1998; Keyes & Shapiro, 2004). Together, subjective well-being consists of the two broad domains of emotional well-being and positive functioning. These domains, their conceptions, and the quality of their measures are reviewed next. Because most research on subjective well-being focuses on individuals aged 18 or older and therefore this chapter focuses on well-being in adults.

Emotional Well-Being

Emotional well-being consists of perceptions of avowed happiness and satisfaction with life, and the experience of the balance of symptoms of positive to negative affect. According to Bradburn (1969), well-being is the balance between two independent affects: positive and negative. In addition to these affects, Andrews and Withey (1976) delineated the cognitive basis of life satisfaction. While life satisfaction is a judgmental and more long-term assessment of life, happiness and positive affect are more spontaneous reflections of one's immediate experience.

Single-items measures of life satisfaction are based on Cantril's (1965) Self-Anchoring Scale, which asks respondents to "rate their life overall these days" on a scale from 0 to 10, where 0 meant the "worst possible life overall" and 10 meant "the best possible life overall." Variations on Cantril's measure have been employed widely in numerous studies worldwide, and have been applied to the measurement of avowed happiness with life (Andrews & Withey, 1976; Andrews & Robinson, 1991). Valid and reliable multi-item scales of life satisfaction and happiness have also been developed and employed extensively (see Diener, 1984, p. 546).

Most measures of positive and negative affect investigate the frequency of time a respondent reports the experience of symptoms of positive and negative affect. For example, individuals are often asked to indicate how much of the time during the past month (i.e., or 30) days they have felt six types of negative and six types of positive indicators of affect: "all," "most," "some," "a little," or "none of the time." The indicators of negative affect routinely include (1) so sad nothing could cheer you up, (2) nervous, (3) restless or fidgety, (4) hopeless, (5) that everything was an effort, and (6) worthless. The indicators of positive affect usually include the feelings of being (1) cheerful, (2) in good spirits, (3) extremely happy, (4) calm and peaceful, (5) satisfied, and (6) full of life. The internal reliability of the multi-item scales of life satisfaction (Diener, 1993; Diener, Emmons, Larson, & Griffin, 1985; Pavot & Diener, 1993) and positive and negative affect (see e.g., Mroczek & Kolarz, 1998) are usually excellent and above .80.

Psychological Well-Being

Psychological theory consists of a variety of concepts of personality and development that have been synthesized as criteria of mental health (Jahoda, 1958) and psychological well-being (Ryff, 1989a). Elements of psychological well-being are descended from the Aristotelian theme of *eudaimonia* (Waterman, 1984), and personified in concepts of self actualization (Maslow, 1968), full functioning (Rogers, 1961), individuation (Jung, 1933), maturity (Allport, 1961), and successful adult developmental stages and tasks (Erikson, 1959; Neugarten, 1968, 1973). Each dimension of psychological well-being (see Ryff, 1989a, 1989b; Ryff & Keyes, 1995) indicates the challenges individuals encounter as they strive to function fully and realize their unique talents.

Environmental mastery is the active engagement of the environment to mold it to meet one's needs and wants. Healthy individuals recognize personal needs and desires and also feel capable of, and permitted to, take an active role in getting what they need from their environments. *Purpose in life* is the criterion that adults also endeavor for a direction in life, when the world offers none or provides unsavory alternatives. Healthy individuals see their daily lives as fulfilling a direction and purpose, and therefore they view their personal lives as meaningful. Last, *personal growth* is the ability and desire to seek to develop existing skills and talents, and to seek opportunities for personal development. In addition, healthy individuals are open to experience and have the capacity to identify challenges in a variety of circumstances.

Self-acceptance is the criterion that adults must strive to feel good about themselves, while facing complex and sometimes unpleasant personal aspects. In addition, individuals accumulate a past and have the capacity to recall and remember themselves through time. Healthy individuals hold a positive attitudes toward themselves and accept all parts of themselves. *Positive relations with others* consist of the ability to cultivate warm, intimate relationships with others. It also includes the presence of satisfying social contacts and relations. *Autonomy* is the criterion that people also seek some degree of self-determination and personal authority, in a society that sometimes compels obedience and compliance. However, healthy individuals seek to understand their own values and ideals. In addition, healthy individuals see themselves guiding their own behavior and conduct from internalized standards and values.

Social Well-Being

Social well-being consists of five elements that, together, indicate whether and to what degree an individuals is functioning well in their social lives -- e.g., as neighbors, as coworkers, and as citizens (Keyes, 1998). Social well-being emerges from classic sociological themes of anomie and alienation. Drawing on these theoretical roots, Keyes (1998) developed multiple operational dimensions of social well-being. Each dimension of social wellness represents challenges that people face as social beings. As with the measures of psychological well-being, the social well-being items are evaluated from respondents' own viewpoints, indicating how well they see themselves rising to life's challenges.

Social actualization is the evaluation of the potential and the trajectory of society. This is the belief in the evolution of society and the sense that society has potential that is being realized through its institutions and citizens. *Social acceptance* is the construal of society through the character and qualities of other people as a generalized category. Individuals must function in a public arena that consists primarily of strangers. Individuals who illustrate social acceptance trust others, think that others are capable of kindness, and believe that people can be industrious. Socially accepting people hold favorable views of human nature and feel comfortable with others.[1]

Social integration is the evaluation of the quality of one's relationship to society and community. Integration is therefore the extent to which people feel they have something in common with others who constitute their social reality (e.g., their neighborhood), as well as the degree to which they feel that they belong to their communities and society. *Social contribution* is the evaluation of one's value to society. It includes the belief that one is a vital member of society, with something of value to give to the world. *Social coherence* is the perception of the quality, organization, and operation of the social world, and it includes a concern for knowing about the world. Social coherence is analogous to meaninglessness in life (Mirowsky and Ross 1989; Seeman 1959), and involves appraisals that society is discernable, sensible, and predictable.

THE STRUCTURE OF SUBJECTIVE WELL-BEING

Is subjective well-being a multidimensional construct? The threefold structure of life satisfaction, positive affect, and negative affect has been repeatedly confirmed in numerous studies (Bryant & Veroff, 1982; Lucas, Diener, & Suh, 1996; Shmotkin, 1998). However, the debate over the structure of positive and negative affect continues to this day. Are positive and negative affect opposing ends of a single continuum (i.e., highly correlated), or are positive and negative feelings relatively independent (i.e., modestly correlated) dimensions of well-being? Evidence supports the unidimensional (Feldman-Barrett & Russell, 1998; Keyes, 2000) *and* the bidimensional (Diener & Emmons, 1984; Watson & Tellegen, 1985) model.

Artifacts of measurement have been implicated as an explanation for the inconclusiveness of the dimensional structure of emotional well-being measures. Prior to the demonstrated validity of frequency as a response choice (see Diener, Sandvik, & Pavot, 1991), measures of emotional well-being tended to confound frequency and intensity of emotional experience. Measures of the intensity of positive affect and of negative affect are strong and positive; measures of the frequency of the experience of symptoms of positive and negative affect are negative and tend to be modest (Diener, Larson, Levine, & Emmons, 1985). Nonrandom measurement errors between indicators of positive and negative affect may also suppress the negative correlation between the latent constructs of positive and negative affect (Green, Goldman, & Salovey, 1993).

According to the context-dependence theory of affects (Zautra, Potter, & Reich, 1997), evidence for unidimensional and bidimensional models of affect depends on the state of the

---

[1] See Keyes and Waterman (2003) for a review of the items used to measure emotional, psychological, and social well-being in the MacArthur Foundation Midlife in the United States survey conducted in 1995.

individual. When individuals are experiencing high levels of demands or are distressed, the structure of affect becomes unidimensional. The correlation of positive and negative affect is highly correlated among individuals who are stressed, while this correlation should be modest among individuals who are not stressed. Zautra et al. (1997) found a significantly larger negative correlation of positive and negative affect among individuals who had experience a high number of life events in the past week, compared with those who had experience few life events in the past week. In addition, the self-theory of subjective change and mental health (Keyes & Ryff, 2000) suggests that perceived personal changes are distressing while the perception of remaining the same person is conducive to mental health.

Drawing together the theory of subjective change (Keyes & Ryff, 2000) with the context-dependence of affects, Keyes (2000) hypothesized and found that the correlation of positive and negative affect was substantially higher at high levels of perceived improvement ($r = -.78$) and high levels of perceived declines ($r = -.75$), compared with low levels of perceived change ($r = -.59$). As such, the structure of positive and negative affect may reflect states of the organism such as levels of demands, life events, and distress. Although certain measurement artifacts and the state of the organism partially affect the correlation between the two affects, evidence confirms the functional separation of positive and negative affect.

Several studies employing community and nationally representative samples have supported the theories of the factor structure of social and psychological well-being. Confirmatory factor models have revealed that the proposed five-factor theory of social well-being is the best-fitting model (Keyes, 1998), and the proposed six-factor theory of psychological well-being is the best-fitting model (Ryff & Keyes, 1995). Moreover, elements of social and psychological well-being are empirically distinct. The scales of social and psychological well-being correlated as high as .44, and exploratory factor analysis revealed two correlated ($r = .34$) factors with the scales of social well-being loading on a separate factor from the items measuring happiness, satisfaction, and the overall scale of psychological well-being (Keyes, 1996).

Measures of social well-being also are factorially distinct from traditional measures (happiness and satisfaction) of emotional well-being (Keyes, 1996). Measures of emotional well-being (positive and negative affect, life satisfaction) are factorially distinct from the measures of psychological well-being (Keyes, Shmotkin, & Ryff, 2002). McGregor and Little's (1998) factor analysis also yielded two distinct factors that reveal an underlying emotional factor (including depression, positive affect, and life satisfaction) and an underlying psychological functioning factor (including four of the psychological well-being scales: Personal growth, purpose in life, positive relations with others, and autonomy).

Measures of subjective well-being also are modestly correlated with measures of symptoms of mental illness (viz. depression). The scales of social well-being correlated around -.30 with a measure of dysphoric symptoms (Keyes, 1998). Keyes and Lopez's (2002) review also reported an average correlation of the scales of psychological well-being with standard measures of depression (i.e., CESD and the Zung Scale) around -.50, while measures of life satisfaction and quality of life correlated on average around -.40. Confirmatory factor analyses of the CESD subscales and the psychological well-being scales in the U.S. (as well as South Korea) have shown that a two-factor model consisting of a mental illness and a mental health latent factor provided the best fit to the data (Keyes &

Ryff, 2003). In that same study, the overall CESD and psychological well-being scales correlated -.68 in the U.S.

GENDER DIFFERENCE

Dimensions of Subjective Well-Being

Though women are more prone to depression than men, men and women report happiness and life satisfaction in equal proportions (Lykken, 1999; Myers, 2000). There is little difference found between the genders for global happiness or satisfaction. However, two studies did find that ". . . younger women are happier than younger men, and older women are less happy than older men" (Diener, 1984 p. 555). More recently, Mroczek and Kolarz (1998) found that negative affect was unrelated with age among women while it decreased with age among married men.

In terms of psychological well-being, studies have shown that there are more similarities than differences in levels between women and men (Keyes & Ryff, 1999). Women are as self accepting and autonomous as men, and females report similar amounts of personal growth, purpose in life, and environmental mastery as males. However, a striking and very consistent finding over numerous studies is that women report markedly higher levels of positive relationships with others than men. That is, the only gender difference in psychological well-being favors women over men, with females having more warm, trusting, and meaningful interpersonal relationships than men (Keyes & Ryff, 1999).

There has been one large-scale national study of gender differences in social well-being. In the MacArthur Midlife in the United States national study of adults between the ages of 25 and 74, finds reveal greater disadvantage for women than men in terms of social well-being. With controls for socioeconomic status, marital status, and age, women report lower levels of social coherence, social actualization, and social contribution than men (Keyes & Shapiro, 2004). Compared to men, women find the social world to be more meaningless, to have less potential for growth, and feel that they do not contribute much of value to society. On the other hand, women reported the same level of social integration as men, and women reported a higher level of social acceptance than men (Keyes & Shapiro, 2004). Thus, women feel as socially integrated into society as men, and they are better able than men to accept the diversity of individuals in society.

Complete Mental Health

While studies of the distribution of specific dimensions of subjective well-being by gender are informative, they do not permit generalizing to women's overall subjective well-being. Moreover, when the research findings of gender differences in depression and in subjective well-being are juxtaposed, inconsistencies and puzzles emerge. While women have higher rates of depression and men, women also report equivalent levels (e.g., social integration, emotional well-being, and 5 of the 6 psychological well-being scales) and, in other dimensions, higher levels (e.g., social acceptance and positive relations) of subjective well-being. One way to view this situation is that depression and subjective well-being measures separate dimensions of an individual's overall state of mental health. That is, information about an individual's state of mental illness such as depression should be combined with measurement of an individual's subjective well-being to provide a more complete picture of his or her overall mental health. From this perspective, researchers can view gender differences from another level that could provide greater research insights.

Studies show that mental health and mental illness are correlated but separate dimensions rather than opposite ends of a single continuum. About 25% of variance is shared in common between standard scales of depression and sales of subjective well-being. The measures of psychological well-being correlated an average of −.51 with the Zung depression inventory and −.55 with the Center for Epidemiological Studies depression (CESD) scale (see Keyes & Lopez, 2002). Measures of satisfaction with life satisfaction and avowed happiness have been shown to correlate between −.40 to −.50 with scales of depressive symptoms. Confirmatory factor analyses also confirm the theory that measures of subjective well-being and depression are distinct but correlated dimensions (see e.g., Headey, Kelley, & Wearing, 1993; Keyes & Ryff, 2003).

The majority of research on gender and mental health has compared mentally ill men and women against individuals who do not meet Diagnostic and Statistical Manual (DSM— American Psychiatric Association, 1994) criteria for major depressive disorder. This approach treats individuals free of depression as having been mentally healthy over a chosen time period (e.g., past 12 months). However, and using the diagnosis of complete mental health that combines information about depression and subjective well-being, Keyes (2002) has shown that only 22% of the 85.5% of individuals who had not suffered an episode of major depression during the past year fit the criteria for mental health. Put differently, only about one-quarter of the non-depressed adults were actually mentally healthy. Rather, a large portion of the adult population who had been free of major depression actually had moderate-to-low levels of subjective well-being, and their psychosocial functioning in terms of workplace productivity was markedly lower than those adults who were free of depression and had high levels of subjective well-being.

The diagnosis of complete mental health mirrors the diagnosis of major depression. Conceptually as well as empirically, scales of subjective well-being fall into two clusters of symptoms. The measures of emotional well-being comprise a cluster that reflects emotional vitality. In turn, the measures of psychological well-being and social well-being reflect a cluster of symptoms of positive functioning. The emotional vitality and positive functioning clusters of symptoms mirror the symptom clusters used in the DSM-III-R (American Psychiatric Association, 1987) to diagnose major depression episode (MDE). That is, depression consists of symptoms of depressed mood or anhedonia (e.g., loss of pleasure derived from activities) and symptoms of malfunctioning (e.g., insomnia or hypersomnia). Of the nine symptoms of MDE, a diagnosis of depression is made when a patient or respondent reports the presence of five or more symptoms (at least one symptom must be from the affective cluster). Similarly, mental health is best operationalized as syndrome that combines levels of symptoms of emotional well-being, psychological well-being, and social well-being.

In the MacArthur Foundation's Midlife in the United States study, respondents completed measures of positive affect and life satisfaction (i.e., emotional well-being).

Respondents also completed the scales of psychological well-being (i.e., six dimensions = self acceptance, purpose in life, personal growth, environmental mastery, autonomy, positive relations) and social well-being (i.e., five dimensions = social coherence, social integration, social acceptance, social actualization, and social contribution). When combined, the MIDUS includes 2 symptom scales of emotional vitality and 11 symptom scales of positive functioning (i.e., 6 scales of psychological and 5 scales of social well-being).

The diagnostic scheme for mental health parallels the scheme employed to diagnose major depression disorder wherein individuals must exhibit 5 or more symptoms of anhedonia (at least 1) and malfunctioning. To have incomplete mental health – a condition labeled *languishing in life* – an individual must exhibit low levels (low = lower tertile) on 2 of the 3 scales of emotional well-being and low levels on 5 of the 11 scales of positive functioning. To have complete mental health – a condition labeled *flourishing in life* – individuals must exhibit high levels (high = upper tertile) on 2 of the 3 scales of emotional well-being and high levels on 5 of the 11 scales of positive functioning. Adults who are *moderately mentally healthy* are neither flourishing nor languishing in life.

Using the complete mental health diagnosis, Keyes (2002) has shown that 22% of adults in 1995 were mentally healthy (i.e., flourishing), 9.0% were languishing, 4.9% had major depression on top of languishing, and 9.6% were depressed only. Just over one-half (54.5%) of the adult population was moderately mentally healthy. Descriptive findings revealed a statistically significant gender gap in the prevalence of complete mental health categories. Whereas 20% of men were flourishing, only 14.9% of women women fit the criteria of mental health. While, an equal proportion of men and women had a pure case of languishing in life, more women (11.3%) than men (7.1%) had a pure episode of major depression. Moreover, women were twice as likely as men to have complete mental illness; that is, 6.1% of women, compared with 3.0% of men, had an episode of major depression on top of languishing in life. From the perspective of complete mental health, women exhibit a clear disadvantage to men, because they are less likely to be completely mentally healthy (i.e., flourishing) and more likely to be completely mentally ill (i.e., depressed and languishing).

CONCLUSION

Mental illnesses such as depression cause emotional suffering and psychosocial impairment. The economic burden of major depression alone was estimated to be $43.7 billion in 1990 due to work absenteeism, diminished productivity, and treatment (Greenberg, Stiglin, Finkelstein & Berndt, 1993). Globally, depression in 1996 was ranked among the top five causes of disability and premature mortality, and it is projected to become the second leading cause of disability and premature mortality by the year 2020 (Murray & Lopez, 1996).

While the focus on major depression in women's lives is paramount, it is also only one half of the story of women's mental well-being. Indeed, the study of subjective well-being in general, and in women's lives more specifically, can provide another crucial lens through which to understand the quality and burden of women's lives. Compared to knowledge about the burden of major depression, it is not well know that measures of subjective well-being bear strong relationships with premature mortality and the onset of complicating diseases. In studies of aging populations of various ethnicities, research has shown that low emotional well-being (e.g., happiness, positive affect, life satisfaction) has been linked as a risk factor for premature death (Danner, Snowdon, & Friesen, 2001), a rise in physical limitations of daily living (Ostir, Markides, Black, & Goodwin, 2000; Ostir, Markides, Peek, & Goodwin, 2001; Penninx, Guralnik, Bandeen-Roche, Kasper, Simonsick, Ferrucci, & Fried, 2000), and incidence of stroke (Ostir, Markides, Peek, & Goodwin, 2001). Similarly, and independent of controls for dietary and lifestyle factors, low levels of life satisfaction increased the risk of suicide over the 20-year period of the Finnish cohort study (Koivumaa-Honkanen, Honkanen, Viinamäki, Heikkilä, Kaprio, & Koskenvuo, 2001). Here, life satisfaction was operationalized as a composite of an individual's perceived interest in life, happiness with life, perceived ease of living, and feeling of loneliness. Even among older populations with severe chronic physical disabilities, studies have shown that as much as one-third has a high level of subjective well-being, levels of which are associated with modifiable factors such as maintenance of cognitive and visual abilities, frequent face-to-face contact, and emotional support (Penninx, Guralnik, Simonsick, Kasper, Ferrucci, and Fried, 1998).

While subjective well-being may be as instrumental to psychosocial functioning as whether an individual is depressed, studies of the distribution of dimensions of subjective well-being by gender reveal a complicated story. While women, from puberty on, are at a greater risk for depression than men, women also tend to have comparable levels of emotional well-being and psychological well-being as men. There are noteworthy differences in subjective well-being between men and women that reflect the longstanding proposition that women are more communal and interpersonal than men. That is, women report higher levels of positive relationships with others, are more socially accepting, and have comparable levels of social integration as men in the U.S.

However, when the measurement of major depression and subjective well-being are brought together under the rubric of complete mental health, a strikingly clear pattern emerges. Men are much more likely than women to be flourishing in life, free of depression and possessing high levels of most dimensions of subjective well-being. In short, men are more likely than women to be completely mentally healthy. On the other hand, women are twice a likely as men to have had an episode of major depression on top of languishing in life. That is, women are more likely than men to be completely mentally ill, i.e., to be depressed (i.e., have a mental illness) and to be languishing (i.e., to be devoid of mental health). In addition, if they are not completely mentally ill, women are more likely than men to have had a pure episode of major depression over the past year.

Studies show that the psychosocial impairments associated with the absence of mental health (i.e., languishing) is comparable to the impairment associated with the presence of major depressive disorder (Keyes, 2002). Languishing is associated with poor emotional health, with high limitations of daily living, and with a high likelihood of a severe number (i.e., 6 or more) of lost days of work (i.e., due to mental health). Although it was not associated with severe work cutback, languishing was associated with more days of work cutback compared with moderately well adults. A pure episode of depression (i.e., without languishing) was also associated with substantial impairment. A major depressive episode was associated with poor emotional health, high limitations of activities of daily living, and a high likelihood of severe work cutback. However, relative to moderately well adults, adults depressed during the past year were not more likely to have a severe number of days lost of work.

Even more striking is the finding that psychosocial impairment is considerably worse when languishing is comorbid with a major depressive episode. Languishing adults who had a major depressive episode in the past year reported the worst emotional health, the most limitations of activities of daily living, the most days of work lost, and the greatest cutback of productivity. In contrast, functioning is markedly improved among moderately well and flourishing adults. These adults reported the best emotional health, the fewest days of work loss, and the fewest days of work productivity cutbacks. Moreover, flourishing adults reported even fewer limitations of activities of daily living than adults who were moderately well.

Relative to the study of depression, research on subjective well-being in women's lives has been almost non-existent (cf. Barnett, 1997). Moreover, when national health objectives are set for the U.S., it is common to read about objectives to reduce the rates of major depression, but uncommon to ever see any mention of an objective to increase the rates of subjective well-being (see, e.g., *Healthy People 2010 Objectives* for the United States). As such, it would appear that most researchers and policy makers do not view the study and promotion of subjective well-being as essential to the objective of improving women's lives. Rather, the presumption appears to be that if this country can make fewer women depressed, more women will be healthy and lead productive and meaningful lives. This, however, is a false assumption, and the objective of improving women's lives solely by focusing on mental illness is, I believe, doomed to fail. Why? Because research is not clearly showing that the absence of mental health—which is the relatively absence of subjective well-being—is just as impairing as the presence of depression. If the objective is to improve women's well-being, the modus operandi must consistent of promoting higher levels of more facets of subjective well-being as well as reducing the rates of depression. When more women are flourishing in the U.S., only then can we be assured that more women are leading productive, meaningful, and fulfilling lives.

Is the goal of promoting flourishing an objective more suited to the U.S. and more economically developed nations than developing nations? This, too, could be a common assumption, but is it correct? On the one hand, it is intuitive to believe that the conditions that cause impairment and premature death among women in developing nations are primarily physical diseases and social conditions. The Global Burden of Disease study (Murray & Lopez, 1996) has shown that 4 of the 5 leading causes of premature death and disability among women of prime child bearing and child rearing age (i.e., ages 15-44) in developing nations are tuberculosis, iron deficiency anemia, self-inflicted injury, and complications with obstructed labour (childbirth). Yet, the leading cause of premature death and disability among women ages 15 to 44 in developing nations of was major depressive (unipolar) disorder. It accounted for over 12% of the burden of disease, compared with tuberculosis, which was the second leading cause of disease burden that accounted for about 5%. Moreover, major depressive disorder was also the leading cause of premature death and disability among women between the ages of 15 and 44 in developed nations (Murray & Lopez, 1996).

In short, the study of gender and subjective well-being provides two objectives for the improvement of women's well-being. First, improvement of women's mental well-being must be an objective in developed and developing nations. Second, focusing on the promotion of subjective well-being as well as the reduction of depression must be a central objective.

REFERENCES

Allport, G. W. (1961). *Pattern and growth in personality.* New York: Holt, Rinehart & Winston.

American Psychiatric Association. (1987). *Diagnostic and statistical manual of mental disorders (3rd ed.).* Washington, DC: Author.

American Psychiatric Association (1994). *Diagnostic and statistical manual (4th ed.).* Washington, D. C.: Author.

Andrews, F. M., & Robinson, J. P. (1991). Measures of subjective well-being. In J. P. Robinson, P. R. Shaver, & L. S. Wrightsman (Eds.), *Measures of personality and social psychological attitudes* (Vol. 1, pp. 61-114). San Diego, CA: Academic Press.

Andrews, F. M., & Withey, S. B. (1976). *Social indicators of well-being: Americans' perceptions of life quality.* New York: Plenum.

Barnett, R. C. (1997). Gender, employment, and psychological well-being: Historical and life course perspectives. In M. E. Lachman & J. B. James (Eds.), *Multiple paths of midlife development* (pp. 323-343). Chicago: University of Chicago Press.

Bradburn, N. M. (1969). *The structure of psychological well-being.* Chicago: Aldine.

Bryant, F. B., & Veroff, J. (1982). The structure of psychological well-being: A sociohistorical analysis. *Journal of Personality and Social Psychology, 43*, 653-673.

Cantril, H. (1965). *The pattern of human concerns.* New Brunswick, NJ: Rutgers University Press.

Cyranowski, J. M., Frank, E., Young, E. & Shear, K. (2000). Adolescent onset of the gender difference in lifetime rates of major depression. *Archives of General Psychiatry, 57*, 21-27.

Danner, D. D., Snowdon, D. A., & Friesen, W. V. (2001). Positive emotions in early life and longevity: findings from the nun study. *Journal of Personality and Social Psychology, 80*, 804-13.

Diener, E. (1984). Subjective well-being. *Psychological Bulletin, 95*, 542-575.

Diener, E. (1993). Assessing subjective well-being: Progress and opportunities. *Social Indicators Research, 31*, 103-157.

Diener, E., & Emmons, R. A. (1985). The independence of positive and negative affect. *Journal of Personality and Social Psychology, 47*, 1105-1117.

Diener, E., Emmons, R. A., Larsen, R. J., & Griffin, S. (1985). The satisfaction with life scale. *Journal of Personality Assessment, 49*, 71-75.

Diener, E., Larsen, R. J., Levine, S., & Emmons, R. A. (1985). Intensity and frequency: Dimensions underlying positive and negative affect. *Journal of Personality and Social Psychology, 48*, 1253-1265.

Diener, E., Sandvik, E., & Pavot, W. (1991). Happiness is the frequency, not the intensity, of positive versus negative affect. In F. Strack, M. Argyle, & N. Schwarz (Eds.), *Subjective well-being: An interdisciplinary perspective* (pp. 119-139). Oxford, England: Pergamon.

Diener, E., Suh, E. M., Lucas, R. E., & Smith, H. L. (1999). Subjective well-being: Three decades of progress. *Psychological Bulletin, 125,* 276-302.

Erikson, E. (1959). Identity and the life cycle. *Psychological Issues, 1,* 18-164.

Feldman-Barrett, L., & Russell, J. A. (1998). Independence and bipolarity in the structure of current affect. *Journal of Personality and Social Psychology, 74,* 967-984.

Green, D. P., Goldman, S. L., & Salovey, P. (1993). Measurement error masks bipolarity in affect ratings. *Journal of Personality and Social Psychology, 64,* 1029-1041.

Greenberg, P. E., Stiglin, L. E., Finkelstein, S. N., & Berndt, E. R. (1993). The economic burden of depression in 1990. *Journal of Clinical Psychiatry, 54,* 405–418.

Gurin, G., Veroff, J., & Feld, S. (1960). *Americans view their mental health.* New York: Basic Books.

Headey, B. W., Kelley, J., & Wearing, A. J. (1993). Dimensions of mental health: Life satisfaction, positive affect, anxiety, and depression. *Social Indicators Research 29,* 63–82.

Jahoda, M. (1958). *Current concepts of positive mental health.* New York: Basic Books.

Jung, C. G. (1933). *Modern man in search of a soul* (W. S. Dell & C. F. Baynes, Trans.). New York; Hartcourt, Brace & World.

Kessler, R. C., & Zhao, S. (1999). The prevalence of mental illness. In A. V. Horwitz, & T. L. Scheid (Eds.), *A handbook for the study of mental health: Social contexts, theories, and systems* (pp. 58-78). New York: Cambridge University Press.

Keyes, C. L. M. (1996). Social functioning and social well-being: Studies of the social nature of personal wellness. *Dissertation Abstracts International: Section B: the Sciences & Engineering. Vol 56(12-B).*

Keyes, C. L. M. (1998). Social well-being. *Social Psychology Quarterly, 61,* 121-140.

Keyes, C. L. M. (2000). Subjective change and its consequences for emotional well-being. *Motivation and Emotion, 24,* 67-84.

Keyes, C. L. M. (2002). The mental health continuum: From languishing to flourishing in life. *Journal of Health and Social Behavior, 43,* 207-222.

Keyes, C. L. M., & Lopez, S. J. (2002). Toward a science of mental health: Positive directions in diagnosis and intervention. In C. R. Snyder & S. J. Lopez (Eds.), *Handbook of positive psychology* (pp. 45-59). New York: Oxford University Press.

Keyes, C. L. M., & Ryff, C. D. (1998). Generativity in adult lives: Social structural contours and quality of life consequences. In D. McAdams & E. de St. Aubin (Eds.), *Generativity and adult development: Perspectives on caring for and contributing to the next generation* (pp. 227-263). Washington, DC: American Psychological Association.

Keyes, C. L. M., & Ryff, C. D. (1999). Psychological well-being in midlife. In S. L. Willis & J. D. Reid (Eds.), *Middle aging: Development in the third quarter of life* (pp. 161-180). Orlando, FL: Academic Press.

Keyes, C. L. M., & Ryff, C. D. (2000). Subjective change and mental health: A self concept theory. *Social Psychology Quarterly, 63,* 264-279.

Keyes, C. L. M., & Ryff, C. D. (2003). Somatization and mental health: A comparative study of the idiom of distress hypothesis. *Social Science and Medicine, 57,* 1833-1845.

Keyes, C. L. M., & Shapiro, A. (2004). Social well-being in the United States: A descriptive epidemiology. In C. D. Ryff, R. C. Kessler, R. C., & O. G. Brim (Eds.), *How Healthy Are We? A National Study of Well-Being at Midlife* (pp. 350-372). Chicago, IL: University of Chicago Press.

Keyes, C. L. M., Shmotkin, D., & Ryff, C. D. (2002). Optimizing well-being: The empirical encounter of two traditions. *Journal of Personality and Social Psychology, 82,* 1007-1022.

Keyes, C. L. M., & Waterman, M. B. (2003). Dimensions of well-being and mental health in adulthood, in M. Bornstein, L. Davidson, C. L. M. Keyes, & K. A. Moore (Eds.), *Well-being: Positive development throughout the life course* (pp. 481-501). Mahwah, NJ: Erlbaum.

Koivumaa-Honkanen, H., Honkanen, R., Viinamäki, H., Heikkilä, K., Kaprio, J., & Koskenvuo, M. (2001). Life satisfaction and suicide: A 20-year follow-up study. *American Journal of Psychiatry, 158,* 433-39.

Lucas, R. E., Diener, E., & Suh, E. (1996). Discriminant validity of well-being measures. *Journal of Personality and Social Psychology, 71,*616-628.

Lykken, D. (1999). *Happiness: The nature and nurture of joy and contentment.* New York: St. Martin's Griffin.

Maslow, A. (1968). *Toward a psychology of being* (2nd ed.). New York: Van Nostrand.

McGregor, I., & Little, B. R. (1998). Personal projects, happiness, and meaning: On doing well and being yourself. *Journal of personality and Social Psychology, 74,* 494-512.

Mirowsky, J. & Ross, C. E. (1989). *Social causes of psychological distress.* New York: Aldine.

Mroczek, D. K., & Kolarz, C. M. (1998). The effect of age on positive and negative affect: A developmental perspective on happiness. *Journal of Personality and Social Psychology, 75,* 1333-1349.

Murray, C. J. L., & Lopez, A. D. (Eds.) (1996). *The global burden of disease: Acomprehensive assessment of mortality and disability from diseases, injuries, and risk factors in 1990 and projected to 2020.* Cambridge, MA: Harvard School of Public Health.

Myers, D. (2000). The funds, friends, and faith of happy people. *American Psychologist, 55,* 56-67.

Neugarten, B.L. (1968). The awareness of middle age. In B.L. Neugarten (Ed.), *Middle age and aging* (pp. 93-98). Chicago: University of Chicago Press.

Neugarten, B.L. (1973). Personality change in late life: A developmental perspective. In C. Eisdorfer & M.P. Lawton (Eds.), *The psychology of adult development and aging* (pp. 311-335). Washington, D.C.: American Psychological Association.

Ostir, G. V., Markides, K. S., Black, S.A., & Goodwin, J. S. (2000). Emotional well-being predicts subsequent functional independence and survival. *Journal of the American Geriatrics Society, 48,* 473-478.

Ostir, G. V., Markides, K. S., Peek, M. K., & Goodwin, J. S. (2001). The association between emotional well-being and the incidence of stroke in older adults. *Psychosomatic Medicine, 63*, 210-15.

Pavot, W., & Diener, E. (1993). Review of the satisfaction with life scale. *Psychological Assessment, 5*,164-172.

Penninx, B. W. J. H, Guralnik, J. M., Simonsick, E. M. Kasper, J. D., Ferrucci, L., & Fried, L. P. (1998). Emotional vitality among disabled older women: The Women's Health and Aging Study. *Journal of the American Geriatrics Society, 46*, 807–15.

Penninx, B. W. J. H., Guralnik, J. M., Bandeen-Roche, K., Kasper, J. D., Simonsick, E. M., Ferrucci, L., & Fried, L. P. (2000). The protective effect of emotional vitality on adverse health outcomes in disabled older women. *Journal of the American Geriatrics Society, 48*, 1359-66.

Rogers, C. R. (1961). *On becoming a person.* Boston: Houghton Mifflin.

Russell, J. A., & Carroll, J. M. (1999a). On the bipolarity of positive and negative affect. *Psychological Bulletin, 125*, 3-30.

Ryff, C. D. (1989a). Beyond Ponce de Leon and life satisfaction: New directions in quest of successful ageing. *International Journal of Behavioral Development, 12*, 35-55.

Ryff, C. D. (1989b). Happiness is everything, or is it? Explorations on the meaning of psychological well-being. *Journal of Personality and Social Psychology, 57*, 1069-1081.

Ryff, C. D., & Keyes, C. L. M. (1995). The structure of psychological well-being revisited. *Journal of Personality and Social Psychology, 69*, 719-727.

Seeman, M. (1959). On the meaning of alienation. *American Sociological Review, 24*, 783-791.

Shmotkin, D. (1998). Declarative and differential aspects of subjective well-being and implications for mental health in later life. In J. Lomranz (Ed.), *Handbook of aging and mental health: An integrative approach* (pp. 15-43). New York: Plenum.

Turner, R. J., Wheaton, B., & Lloyd, D. A. (1995). The epidemiology of social stress. *American Sociological Review, 60*, 104-125.

U.S. Department of Health and Human Services. (1999). *Mental health: A report of the Surgeon General.* Rockville, MD: Author.

Waterman, A. S. (1984). *The psychology of individualism.* New York: Praeger.

Watson, D., & Tellegen, A. (1985). Toward a consensual structure of mood. *Psychological Bulletin, 98*, 219-235.

Wrong, D. H. (1994). *The problem of social order: What unites and divides society.* New York: The Free Press.

Zautra, A. J., Potter, P. T., & Reich, J. W. (1997). The independence of affects is context-dependent: An integrative model of the relationship of positive and negative affect. In K. W. Schaie & M. P. Lawton (Eds.), *Annual review of gerontology and geriatrics (Vol. 17)* (pp. 75-103). New York: Springer.

In: Psychology of Stress
Editor: Kimberly V. Oxington, pp. 17-33
ISBN 1-59454-246-5
©2005 Nova Science Publishers, Inc.

Chapter II

AN EFFECTIVENESS TRIAL TO INCREASE PSYCHOLOGICAL WELL-BEING AND REDUCE STRESS AMONG AFRICAN AMERICAN BLUE-COLLAR WORKING WOMEN

Linda Napholz
Napa Valley College

ABSTRACT

This study examined the efficacy of a psychoeducational intervention program relative to a control group in promoting psychological well-being in 70 African American working women. A quasi-experimental repeated measures design was utilized. The psychoeducational program focused on reducing role conflict, enhancing self-esteem, life satisfaction and instrumentality, decreasing depression and facilitating coping through cognitive based problem solving strategies. Between the pre to 6-month follow-ups, there was a greater increase in self-esteem scores and a greater decrease in depression scores for treatment participants than for controls. Role conflict and life event scores were different over time for each group, but there was no significant treatment effect. There were no significant differences in satisfaction with life, female or male scores for the entire group over time. This community based psychoeducational program was a viable intervention that reduced multiple stresses through an increase in support networks, knowledge, and awareness. This study has advanced knowledge on stressors that African American working women experience and identified stress-reduction strategies that enhanced psychological well-being in regards to increasing self-esteem scores and decreasing depression and role conflict scores. These findings are important in that, despite the increasing levels of emotional distress reported by African American women, there are few reports of clinical interventions designed to address this issue among at-risk segments of employed African American women who carry our multiple roles.

WORK AND AFRICAN AMERICAN WOMEN

African American women participate at higher rates in the labor market than Euro-American women, yet they have the lowest pay and occupational status jobs of any race/gender groups (Blau & Ferber, 1986; Bowman, 1991; Harris, 1989; Hatchett et al., 1991, Sanchez-Hucles, 1997). The latest projections indicate that 9 million African American women will be labor force participants by the year 2005 (Hughes, 1997). Despite evidence that work constitutes a major life domain among African American women, researchers know relatively little about the work role experiences of this group (Cox & Nkomo, 1990). It is known that African American women encounter prejudicial racial attitudes and other noxious stimuli during every day workplace interactions with Euro-Americans (Hughes & Dodge, 1997).

Job conditions such as high psychological workload, low task variety, and low decision-making authority, are well established occupational stressors (Hughes, 1997). The jobs that African American women hold tend to be intrinsically less rewarding, offer less opportunity for control and skill utilization, and are less secure than those held by men (Mortimer & Sorenson, 1984). African American women experience exclusion from informal social networks, exaggerated performance expectations, assumptions of incompetence on the part of Euro-Americans coworkers, supervisors, and clients, and other forms of racial bias (Feagin & Sikes, 1994).

AFRICAN AMERICAN WOMEN AND MULTIPLE ROLES

African American men have faced overwhelming pressure to meet Euro-American standards of provider, protector, and disciplinarian within the family – while living in a society that has systematically denied them equal access to the ways and means of fulfilling such role obligations. Green (1994) explained that, historically, racism in the workplace has made it difficult/impossible for African American men to find suitable employment. Consequently, African American females have been the ones required to socialize the children and provide essential income for their families. Inasmuch as the role of motherhood is considered important for African American women, they have been blamed for family problems that may really result from institutionalized racism, and they have been charged with perpetuating the negative "matriarchal stereotype of the African American family structure" (Marsh, 1993, p.151)

The management of multiple roles, including work and family responsibilities can be exhausting. National Health Survey statistics indicate an unusually high level of emotional distress and depression among African American women as compared to Euro-American and other ethnic group women (Concran & Mays, 1994) Despite the increasing levels of emotional distress reported by African American women (Austin, 1992), there are few reports of clinical interventions designed to address this distress and increase well-being among the at-risk segments of multiple role African American women in the labor force market (Mays, 1995).

The few studies available have revealed that race and gender have interactive, interlocking, additive, and even multiplicative effects that were previously unknown and unexplained (Johnson, 2001, King, 1988). James, Lovato, and Khoo (1994) have identified significant associations between exposure to discrimination and physiological indicators of adverse effects on well-being such as increased heart rate and blood.

Relative to Euro-Americans, African American women report exposure to more stressors (Williams, Yu, Jackson, & Anderson, 1997). As a consequence, African American women may have to utilize coping responses more frequently to deal with these added stressors than do Euro-Americans, thereby increasing the likelihood of resource strain, behavioral exhaustion, and psychological and physiological distress. Additionally, blue collar African American women are not only exposed to more chronic stressors than white collar African American women, but they may also have fewer resources with which to cope with these stressors, leading to more deleterious mental health outcomes (Feagin, 1991).

THE PROGRAM

A six session psychoeducational intervention was developed to advance knowledge on stressors that African American working women experience and to further identify stress reduction strategies that reduce role conflict and enhance psychological well-being. The intervention was also an attempt to examine the effectiveness of a community-based intervention under real-world conditions. The specific goals of the intervention were: (a) to alleviate or buffer the effects of stress through the provision of positive support networks and increased knowledge of interpersonal and psychosocial variables that may be significant sources of role conflict and resulting stress, and (b) to change patterns of coping through increased awareness of stress reactions, maladaptive responses and adaptive response options (Austin, 1992). The six-session psychoeducational program was conceptualized as both an intervention and a prevention strategy.

Theoretical Underpinning

This research builds on the more general stress-coping model proposed by Lazarus and Folkman (1984). The principal tenet of this psychoeducational program is that the perception of an environmental stimulus such as role conflict results in psychological and physiological stress responses. Over time, these stress responses are posited to influence mental health outcomes. Furthermore, role conflict and ensuing coping responses are postulated to be a function of a complex interplay between an array of psychological behavioral, constitutional, and sociodemographic factors. Coping responses that do not attend stress responses are considered maladaptive and may negatively affect health (Burchfield, 1985). When maladaptive coping responses are used, the perception of an environmental event as role conflict will trigger psychological and physiological stress responses. If an individual fails to replace these maladaptive coping responses with more adaptive ones, a continued state of heightened psychological and physiological activity is predicted (Selye, 1976). Examples of maladaptive responses include chronic feelings of frustration, depression, resentment, distrust, or paranoia (Fernando, 1984; Peterson, Maier, & Seligman, 1993) that lead to passivity, overeating, avoidance, or efforts to gain control (Bullock & Huston, 1987).

Adaptive coping responses, on the other hand, are postulated to mitigate enduring psychological and physiological stress responses, thereby reducing the potential untoward effects of role conflict on psychological well-being. Research has suggested that the effects of more general coping responses such as social support (McNeilly, Anderson, Robinson, et al., 1996), and religious participation (Jones, 1997) may be particularly relevant for African Americans to modify risks for negative mental health outcomes (Clark et al, 1999). It was believed that by promoting adaptive coping skills via a psychoeducational intervention that stress symptoms would be moderated or buffered (Holanhan & Moos, 1987; Holt, 1982, Urban, 2001).

DESCRIPTION OF ACTIVITY

The intervention was developed from previous research by Napholz (1994, 1999, 2001, 2002). An ongoing study builds from the previous study and is designed to capitalize on the participants reported strengths, reduce the effects of stressful life conditions and experiences, and to decrease their reported problems, including negative psychological symptoms. A triangulated method, combining both qualitative and quantitative methods, was used. The quantitative portion of the study was based on a quasi-experimental repeated measures design. The treatment group was compared to the control group in order to assess the effects of the intervention to reduce role conflict and increase psychological well-being. Both groups were measured pre-treatment, at week six of the intervention and six months after the intervention.

A structured format provided the guide for the six one-and-a-half hour intervention sessions. Each week's content built on the previous week with increasing levels of complexity. Table 1 illustrates the weekly content of the intervention.

The purpose of this study was to determine the effectiveness of a six-session psychoeducational intervention on reducing role conflict and depression, and increasing instrumentality, self-esteem, and life satisfaction among African American blue collar working women. The short-term desired outcome was to reduce role conflict and increase instrumentality. The longer-term outcome was to decrease depression and increase life satisfaction and self-esteem six months post intervention.

Table I. Six-Week Stress Reduction Intervention

Intervention Topic by Week	Intervention Format Included Lecture/Discussion/Experiential	Informational Packets for Participants
Week 1 Well-Being and Stress	Lecture: Stress and Stress Management Lecture: Well-Being and Stress Among African American Women. Lecture: How to Develop Goals that Are Reachable	*Physical Manifestations of Stress Checklist *Stressful Life Events Checklist *Strategies for Managing Stress *Realty Check *How to Develop Goals that Are Reachable *Life Checkup *Signs of Discontent Checklist
Week 2 Understanding Depression, Guilt and Regret "Isms"	Lecture: Understanding Depression Lecture: Dealing with Guilt and Regret Lecture: Issues Related to Oppression, Discrimination, Racism and Sexism on Well-Being encountered by African American women in the labor market.	*Depression Symptoms *How to Prevent/Manage Depression *Guilt and Regret Checklist *Antidotes to Regret *Antiguilt Exercise *Manage Your Guilt *What Do you Value?
Week 3 Balancing Multiple Roles	Lecture: Balancing Work and Family Life. Lecture: Ways to Change How You Feel Lecture: Twisted Thinking That Lead to Negative Moods	*Ways to Change How You Feel *Ten Forms of Twisted Thinking That Lead to Negative Moods
Week 4 Understanding Anger and How to Make Your Opinion Count	Lecture: Understanding Anger Lecture: Assertive Behavior Lecture: Conflict/Stress -Self-Assertion in Conflict Lecture: How to Say "No"	*Blocks to Expressing Anger *Effective Ways to Manage Anger *The Ten Commandments of How to Fight Fair *How to Say "No" *Assertive, Aggressive or Passive?
Week 5 How to Build Your Self-Esteem and Self-Confidence	Lecture: Self-Esteem and Self-Esteem Builders Lecture: Self-Confidence	*Self-Esteem Checklist *Self-Esteem Exercise *Self-Esteem Rights *My Declaration of Self-Esteem

Week 6 Feeling Good About Yourself Through Empowerment and Coping	Lecture: Empowerment and Coping
	  The Coping Process
	  What to do to Cope with it All
	  Guide to Self-Empowerment
	  Personal Support Networks
	  Summary and Closure
		*Coping Worksheet
		*The Coping Process
		*What to do to Cope with it All
		*Guide to Self-Empowerment
		*Feeling Good About Yourself
		*Living Purposefully
		*How to Love Yourself
		*Letting Go
		*Your Rights
		*Affirmations
		*Recommended Readings

METHOD

Participants

Ninety-five African American working women volunteered to participate in the research project. Purposive sampling was utilized to obtain participants that met the selection criteria. Participants were paid for their participation and were treated in accordance with ethical principles. Controls were those participants who met selection criteria and agreed to complete the questionnaires three times. Twenty-five (26.3%, n = 95) participants dropped out of the study and did not complete all three data gathering times. Seventy African American working women (38 Treatment and 32 Control) completed all three data gathering times. The only significant difference between the two groups of completers was that the treatment group was significantly older than the control group, $t(66)$ = 2.02, $p<.05$ (see Table 2). Participants completing were compared to the "drop-outs" and there were no significant differences in the demographic characteristics of marital status, living arrangements, age, presence of children, level of education, hours worked, income, family income, and social class (see Table 3).

MEASURES

Procedures

Table 2. Description of Sample and Comparison of Treatment to Control Group

Participants Completing Study	Demographics	Treatment N=38	Control N=32	Total N=70	Statistic (p)
Marital Status	Single/Widowed	52.6%	54.8%	53.9%	Chi-square=.794
	Married	21.1%	25.8%	24.3%	df=2 (.672)
	Divorced	26.3%	19.4%	22.9%	
Occupation Based on Hollingshead	Blue Collar	73.7%	53.1%	64.3%	Chi-square=3.19
	Pink Collar	26.3%	46.9%	35.7%	df=1 (.074)
Work/Family Role Commitment	Work First	35.3%	33.3%	34.4%	Chi-square=.057
	Work/Family Equal	50.0%	50.0%	50%	df=2 (.972)
	Family First	14.7%	16.7%	15.6%	
Living Arrangement	Alone/parents/roommate	26.3%	34.4%	30.0%	Chi-square=1.50
	Husband/Lover/Children	31.6%	37.5%	34.3%	df=2 (.471)
	Children Only	42.1%	28.1%	35.7%	
Mean Age		36.34 (9.81)	31.40 (10.23)	34.09 (10.17)	t=2.02 df=66 (.047)
Children	No Children	19.4%	17.2%	18.5%	Chi-square=.052
	Children	80.6%	82.8%	81.5%	df=1 (.820)
Education	< High School	44.7%	33.3%	39.7%	Chi-square=1.12
	Some College	34.2%	36.7%	35.3%	df=2 (.573)
	> College	21.1%	30.0%	25.0%	
Employment status	Part Time	19.4%	26.7%	22.7%	Chi-square=.486
	Full Time	80.6%	73.3%	77.3%	df=1 (.486)

Table 2. Continued

Income	0-9999 K	21.6%	15.6%	18.8%	Chi-square=1.10
	10000-19999 K	27.0%	25.0%	26.1%	df=3 (.777)
	20000-29999 K	40.5%	40.6%	40.6%	
	> 30000 K	10.8%	18.8%	14.5%	
Family Income	0-9999 K	15.6%	10.0%	12.9%	Chi- square=1.97
	10000-19999 K	25.0%	16.7%	21.0%	df=3 (.577)
	20000-29999 K	34.4%	33.3%	33.9%	
	> 30000 K	25.0%	40.0%	32.3%	
Social Class	Working Class	45.9%	54.8%	50%	Chi-square=2.49
	Lower Middle Class	24.3%	9.7%	17.6%	df=2 (.288)
	Middle/Upper Mid/Upper	29.7%	35.5%	32.4%	
Religion	Protestant	91.2%	87.5%	89.4%	Chi- square= .23
	Other	8.8%	12.5%	10.6%	df=1 (.628)

Table 3. A Comparison of Participants who Dropped Out of the Study Combined with those that Completed the Study

All Participants	Demographics	Treatment N=59	Control N=36	Statistic (p)
Marital Status	Single/Widowed	576%	52.%	Chi-square=1.12 df=2 (.570)
	Married	18.6%	27.8%	
	Divorced	23.7%	19.4%	
Role Commitment Q27	Work	34.6%	33.3%	Chi-square=.051 df=2 (.975)
	Equal	51.9%	51.5%	
	Significant other	13.5%	15.5%	
Living Arrangement	Alone/parents/roommate	25.4%	33.3%	Chi-square=2.07 df=2 (.355)
	Husband/lover/children	32.2%	38.9%	
	Children	42.4%	27.8%	
Age		34.75 (.979)	31.37 (.995)	t=1.60 (.11)
Children	No Children	16.4%	18.2%	Chi-square=2.07 df=1 (.355)
	Children	83.6%	81.1%	
Education	<+ High school	42.4%	32.4%	Chi-square=1.07 df=2 (.584)
	Some col. Or tech	35.6%	38.2%	
	Completed additional ed.	22.0%	29.4%	
Employment status	Part time	20.4%	25.5%	Chi-square=.123 df=1 (.726)
	Full time	79.6%	76.5%	
Income	0-9999	22.8%	13.9%	Chi-square=1.69 df=3 (.639)
	10000-19999	22.8%	22.2%	
	20000-29999	42.1%	44.4%	
	30000+	12.3%	19.4%	
Family Income	0-9999	17.0%	8.8%	Chi-square=3.17 df=3 (.366)
	10000-19999	22.6%	14.7%	
	20000-29999	32.1%	32.4%	
	30000+	28.3%	44.1%	
Social Class	Upper /upper mid/mid	27.6%	35.3%	Chis-square=4.37 df=2 (.112)
	Lower mid	31.0%	11.8%	
	Working	41.4%	52.9%	

RESULTS

Descriptive Statistics

At pretest, sample means and standard deviations on self-report measures were obtained for the study completers *(N* = 70) (see Table 4). Correlation coefficients are reported for the study completers *(N* = 70) (see Table 5) as well as for all study participants *(N* = 95) (see Table 6).

Table 4. Pretest Sample Means and Standard Deviations on Self-Report Measures

Measures	Mean	SD	Alpha
Female Score	23.90	5.54	.83
Male Score	21.53	5.68	.79
Role Conflict	36.21	14.09	.85
Self-Esteem	30.95	4.85	.83
Life Satisfaction	19.10	6.27	.78
Depression	10.52	9.08	.91
Social Support	19.55	3.22	.87
Life Events	15.31	8.65	.88
Plan	6.15	3.41	.92
Helpful Info	5.29	3.22	.90
Help meet	6.08	4.28	.96
No Help	1.45	2.00	.92
Influence	2.17	2.43	.93
Support/help	3.33	2.08	.86

Table 5. Correlations for Completing Participants (*N*=70) at Time 1

	Social Support	Role Conflict	Life Satis'n	Depres'n	RSES	Male	Female
Social Sup	-						
Role Conflict	.153	-					
Life Satisfa'n	.013	.039	-				
Depression	.280*	.229	-.240*	-			
Self-Esteem	-.433**	-.331**	.266*	-.521**	-		
Male	-.089	.037	.207	-.282*	.380**	-	
Female	-.047	.179	.310**	-.248*	.359**	.535**	-
Life Events	-.182	.452**	-.080	-.169	..071	-.096	.160

* Correlation is significant at the 0.05 level (2-tailed)
** Correlation is significant at the 0.01 level (2-tailed)

Table 6. Correlations at Time 1 for All Participants (*N*=95)

	Social Support	Role Conflict	Life Satis'n	Depres'n	RSES	Male	Female
Social Sup.	-						
Role Conf't	.158	-					
Life Satis'n	-.044	-.001	-				
Depression	.297**	.346**	-.252*	-			
Self-Esteem	-.329**	-.320**	.332**	-.579**	-		
Male	-.066	.150	.215*	-.186	.422**	-	
Female	-.026	.228*	.232*	-.189	.332**	.636**	-
Life Events	.009	.415**	-.177	-.381**	-.092	-.012	.148

* Correlation is significant at the 0.05 level (2-tailed)
** Correlation is significant at the 0.01 level (2-tailed)

EFFECTS ON SELF-REPORT MEASURES

Repeated measures analyses of variance evaluated group differences on self-report measures from pretest to posttest and 6-month follow-up (see Table 7). There was a significant interaction between self-esteem and treatment group over time. The treatment group self-esteem scores increased from 30.59 at Time 1 to 32.00 at Time 3, while the control group scores decreased from 31.41 at Time 1 to 29.39 at Time 3. There were significant linear trends for each group. Repeated measures ANOVA, for each group, reveled a significant differences over time for each group (Treatment F=4.55, p=.04; Control F=4.78, p=.037).

Table 7. Mean and Standard Deviations and Analysis of Variance (MANOVA) Results for Measures of Self-Esteem as a Function of Treatment Group

Self-Esteem	n	Time 1	Time 2	Time 3	ANOVA F	
		M SD	M SD	M SD	Time	Time X Group
					.229	5.63**
Treatment	37	30.59 (4.56)	31.31 (4.40)	32.00 (4.64)		
Control	29	31.41(4.49)	30.67 (4.66)	29.39 (4.65)		
Total	66	30.95 (4.52)	31.03 (4.50)	30.85 (4.79)		

* p.≤.05 ** p≤ 01

There was a significant interaction between depression and treatment group over time (see Table 8). The treatment group depression scores decreased from 10.56 at Time 1 to 7.66 at Time 3; while the control group scores increased from 7.70 at Time 1 to 10.16 at Time 3.

Repeated measures ANOVA, for each group, reveled a significant difference over time for each group (Treatment F=4.98 p=.009; Control F=4.25 p=.012).

Table 8. Mean and Standard Deviations and Analysis of Variance (MANOVA) Results for Measures of Depression as a Function of Treatment Group

Depression	n	Time 1	Time 2	Time 3	ANOVA F	
		M SD	M SD	M SD	Time	Time X Group
					2.32	7.04**
Treatment	38	10.56 (8.48)	7.85 (8.22)	7.66 (7.02)		
Control	30	7.70 (6.73)	7.55(7.87)	10.16 (8.23)		
Total	68	9.30 (7.84)	7.72(8.01)	8.76 (7.61)		

* $p \leq 05$ ** $p \leq 01$

There was a significant interaction between role conflict and group over time (see Table 9). The treatment group role conflict decreased from 36.73 at Time 1 to 32.69 at Time 3, while the control group increased from 33.65 at Time 1 to 38.23 at Time 3. Repeated measures ANOVA, for each group indicated that role conflict scores were significantly different over time. (Treatment F=3.49 df=1,35 p=.036) (Control F=5.31 df=1,29, p=.008).

Table 9. Mean and Standard Deviations and Analysis of Variance (MANOVA) Results for Measures of Role Conflict as a Function of Treatment Group

Role Conflict	n	Time 1	Time 2	Time 3	ANOVA F	
		M SD	M SD	M SD	Time	Time X Group
					3.61*	5.55**
Treatment	36	36.73(13.02)	32.67 (14.19)	32.69 (11.85)		
Control	30	33.65(13.82)	31.74(16.11)	38.23 (18.28)		
Total	66	35.33(13.38)	32.25(14.98)	35.21(15.25)		

* $p \leq 05$ ** $p \leq 01$

There was a significant difference in the number of life events for the entire group over time (see Table 10). Both the treatment group and control group's number of life events decreased over time, however there was a greater reduction in the number of life events for the treatment group than the control group. There was no significant treatment effect.

Table 10. Mean and Standard Deviations and Analysis of Variance (MANOVA) Results for Measures of Number of Life Events as a Function of Treatment Group

Life Events	n	Time 1	Time 2	Time 3	ANOVA F	
		M SD	M SD	M SD	Time	Time X Group
					6.65**	1.64
Treatment	38	13.34 (7.36)	10.39 (7.71)	9.52 (6.88)		
Control	32	15.40 (7.99)	13.81(9.29)	14.31 (9.02)		
Total	70	14.28 (7.67)	11.95(8.58)	11.71(8.23)		

* $p \leq 05$ ** $p \leq 01$

There was no significant difference in satisfaction with life scores for the entire group over time. There was no significant treatment effect (see Table 11).

Table 11. Mean and Standard Deviations and Analysis of Variance (MANOVA) Results for Measures Satisfaction with Life as Function of Treatment Group

Satisfaction With Life	n	Time 1 M SD	Time 2 M SD	Time 3 M SD	ANOVA F Time	Time X Group
					.884	.697
Treatment	38	19.78(5.76)	21.53 (6.93)	20.60 (6.21)		
Control	30	19.67 (5.88)	19.76(7.01)	19.06 (5.91)		
Total	68	19.72 (5.77)	20.75(6.96)	19.92(6.08)		

* $p \leq 05$ ** $p \leq .01$

There was a no significant difference in the Female score for the entire group over time. There was no significant treatment effect (see Table 12).

Table 12. Mean and Standard Deviations and Analysis of Variance (MANOVA) Results for Measures Female as Function of Treatment Group

Female	n	Time 1 M SD	Time 2 M SD	Time 3 M SD	ANOVA F Time	Time X Group
					2.05	2.46
Treatment	37	24.40 (4.61)	24.27 (4.90)	24.44 (4.96)		
Control	31	24.31 (4.93)	23.91(4.74)	22.32 (5.44)		
Total	68	24.36 (4.72)	24.10(4.80)	23.47(5.25)		

* $p \leq .05$ ** $p \leq .01$

There was a no significant difference in the Male score for the entire group over time. There was no significant treatment effect (see Table 13).

Table 13. Mean and Standard Deviations and Analysis of Variance (MANOVA) Results for Measures Male as Function of Treatment Group

Female	n	Time 1 M SD	Time 2 M SD	Time 3 M SD	ANOVA F Time	Time X Group
					.554	2.30
Treatment	37	21.78 (4.83)	21.69 (4.43)	22.28 (4.03)		
Control	31	21.09 (6.15)	20.53(5.11)	19.56 (5.57)		
Total	68	21.46 (5.44)	21.16(4.75)	21.04(4.95)		

* $p \leq 05$ ** $p \leq .01$

The treatment only group was assessed about the helpfulness of the group (see Table 14). There was a significant difference in the category "helpful information" that increased over time. The treatment group found the information received during the intervention more helpful over time.

Table 14. Analysis of Variance for Helpfulness of Group

Helpfulness (Rx *n*=38)	Time 1	Time 2	Time 3	F (p)
Plan	6.82 (2.99)	7.13 (2.58)	6.74 (2.84)	1.66 (.712)
Helpful info	5.84 (3.01)	6.34 (2.54)	8.42 (2.46)	14.35 (<.001)
Help meet	7.32 (3.94)	8.42 (2.47)	8.21 (2.80)	1.25 (.271)
No help	1.58 (2.05)	1.97 (2.37)	1.58 (1.85)	.740 (.481)
Influence	2.11 (2.40)	2.24 (2.24)	1.89 (2.05)	.443 (.644)
Sup help	3.89(1.83)	3.92 (1.57)	4.11 (1.18)	.266 (.767)

QUALITATIVE FINDINGS

Qualitative data was collected by audiotaping discussion during each of the six treatment group sessions. Content analysis of transcriptions of the six 1 1/2-hr sessions were coded into themes that emerged from the data. These themes were categorized as: "viewing and being viewed through the lens of race", "searching for external rewards", "marginality", "juggling role obligations", "coping through spirituality", "role conflict with the oppressor and by other oppressed", "isolation and difference", "fears of self-revelation", "testimony", "tests of strength", and "validating experience". Based on the study results, the intervention was modified to strengthen it. Modifications include further refinement of the intervention and additional testing on a larger scale to provide a more adequate test of the study results.

It was found that narrative descriptions of the experience of role conflict and psychological well-being were similar to items on the questionnaires used. This provided some evidence of the appropriateness for these instruments with African American working women. Anecdotally, the participants reported they were excited about the chance to increase their skills and strengths and to be more connected to women like themselves. The treatment group was assessed about the "helpfulness" of the group. There was a significant difference over time in how helpful they found the information provided. During the six-session intervention, participants learned methods to reduce role conflict through establishing priorities, partitioning and separating roles, overlooking role demands, and changing attitudes toward roles in order to maximize satisfaction in a specific role (see Figure 1). Participants described a syndrome of emotional exhaustion, difficulties coping, and conflicts managing multiple roles. Learning and incorporating new coping and problem solving skills helped participants handle (i.e. master, tolerate, or reduce) the role conflicts that emerged in their paid work and non-remunerative environments.

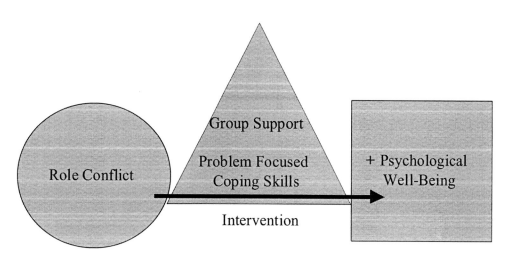

Figure 1. Figure of the Moderating Effects of the Lifestyle Modification Intervention

DISCUSSION

The results of this study support the efficacy of this six-session psychoeducational intervention in a community based setting. Treatment group participants had higher self-esteem and lower depression and role conflict scores when compared with control group scores. Both control and treatment groups had a significant reduction in life events over time. There were no significant differences in satisfaction with life scores, Male or Female scores (instrumentality).

The psychoeducational program was a viable intervention that reduced multiple stresses through an increase in support networks and awareness of personal and political issues contributing to role conflict that was both culture- and gender-appropriate. (Napholz, 1999, 2001, 2002). The intervention supported change in patterns of coping through increased awareness of behaviors, change symptoms associated with those behaviors and decrease maladaptive response strategies. Additionally, this study has advanced knowledge on stressors that African American working women experience and identified stress-reduction strategies that enhanced psychological well-being in regards to increasing self-esteem scores and decreasing depression and role conflict scores. These findings are important in that, despite the increasing levels of emotional distress reported by African American women, there are few reports of clinical interventions designed to address this issue among at-risk segments of employed African American women who carry out multiple roles. The stress from the multiple roles that African American women in the labor force experience was evident in the control group. The group without an intervention significantly increased their level of depression and increased their role conflict while decreasing their self-esteem. In contrast, the treatment group significantly decreased their level of depression, decreased their role conflict, while increasing their self-esteem.

Further refinement and testing of the intervention is needed to develop areas related to life satisfaction and instrumentality (Male and Female scores). Perhaps changing life satisfaction among this group may take much longer especially since the intervention cannot change the occurrence of life events. Additionally, life satisfaction may be a more embedded construct that evolves over time and is dependent on other circumstances held stable. Possibly, as self-esteem and depression improve and stabilize, one develops a more positive outlook on life which is eventually reflected in a feeling of satisfaction with life. There was no change in instrumentality possibly due to the length of the intervention and that this construct, like life satisfaction, evolves over time.

There is a need for the development of the needed knowledge to support an expanded perspective of women's roles and work. Knowledge of the coping styles and life-styles of African American women is necessary to design interventions that build on the strengths of African American women. Psychoeducational support groups may be a viable alternative to facilitate the problem solving and support once afforded by informal support networks. The scope of mental health threats can be more adequately defined and appropriate interventions more effectively focused by building on the existing research on role conflict and psychological well-being among African American working women.

Participants were able to make social comparisons of work environments and differentiate the possible personal and structural contributions to work and nonwork stressors. Sharing of adaptive ways to cope with role conflict provided an opportunity for others with maladaptive coping strategies to judge the effectiveness of individual actions.

The participants discussed significant changes in important informal support systems. These women identified that they had been socialized to be strong, to take care of their kin, and to handle their own problems within the kinship network (Green, 1994). Informal network changes are the result of increases in mobility with resultant decreases in available family support networks (Barnett & Hyde, 2001). Loss of informal family support systems once afforded these participants resulted in a perceived greater role strain when role conflicts occurred. Psychoeducational support groups may be a viable alternative to facilitate the problem solving and support once afforded by these informal networks. A second important issue was a fear that that their cultural behaviors and beliefs would be viewed as pathological rather than as legitimate and valuable learned survival skills. From this, it was thought important to focus on strengths and shared problem solving rather than on maladaptive coping strategies.

The intervention highlights multiple sources of stress for African American women and supports the development of culture- and gender-appropriate community interventions as viable methods for stress reduction. These stressors provide impetus for developing community-based partnership education programs designed to self-empower African American women. There is a need to establish more community support groups – through church groups, community centers, and work sites. Currently, one of the research sites found the intervention so helpful, it has funded a continuation of the intervention and support group.

It was found that the participants had multiple demands on their off-work time. Future recommendations to encourage recruitment and retention include: providing intervention sites that are convenient, childcare, transportation costs, a light meal, pre-session phone call reminders and certificates of completion (Napholz, 1998).

A summation of the foundational and summative research for the psychoeducational intervention has been presented and an overview of its intervention components. It is hoped that the results will foster the further development of culturally sensitive theories and research, as well as other programs to help reduce stress among low-income African American working women.

In summary, it was challenging and exciting to learn how to better tailor (McClowry, 2000) the interventions for this diverse group of women, rather than depend on standardized protocols that many African American women would not find welcoming or personally relevant. Culturally sensitive intervention strategies incorporating gender, racial, cultural and societal realities are first steps toward facilitating African American women's growth toward an optimal level of psychological well-being. The diversity of African Americans must be considered in program development, program implementation, and policy making (C. Tucker, 2002). We need to empower African American women to choose actions benefiting self and family to successfully promote the knowledge necessary for more accurate and comprehensive perspectives on the roles and work of African American women.

REFERENCES

Austin, R. (1992). Despair, distrust and dissatisfaction among Blacks and women. *The Sociolog Quart, 33*, 579-598.

Barnett, R. & Hyde, J. (2001). Women, men, work, and family. *American Psychologist, 56*(10), 781-796.

Blau, F., & Ferber, M. (1986). *The economics of men, women and work*. Englewood Cliffs, NJ: Prentice Hall.

Bowman, P. (1991). Work life. In Jackson J (Ed.) *Life in Black America*. Newbury Park, CA: Sage.

Bullock, S. & Houston, E. (1987). Perceptions of racism by Black medical students attending White medical schools. *J of the National Med Ass* 79: 601-608,

Burchfield, S. (1985). Stress: An integrative framework. In S. Burchfield (Ed.) *Stress psychological and physiological interactions* (pp. 381-394). New York: Hemisphere.

Clark, R. & Anderson, N. Clark, V. et al (1999). Racism as a stressor for African Americans. *Amer Psych 54*(10), 805-816.

Cox, T. & Nkomo, S. (1990). Invisible men and women: A status report on race as a variable in organization behavior research: Special issue: The career and life experiences of Black professionals. *J. of Organizational Beh., 11*, 419-431.

Feagin, J. (1991). The continuing significance of race: Antiblack discrimination in public places. *Amer socio Review, 56*, 101-116.

Feagin, J., & Sikes, M. (1994). *Living with racism: The Black middle class experience*. Boston: Beacon Press.

Fernando, S. (1984). Racism as a cause of depression. *International J of Soc Psych, 30*, 41-49.

Greene, B. (1994). African American women. In L. Comas-Diaz (Ed.): *Women and therapy* (pp 10-29). New York: Guilford.

Conchran, S. & Mays, V. (1994). Levels of depression in homosexually active African-American men and women. *Amer J of Psych, 151*, 524-529.

Harris, O. (1989). Black working women: Introduction to a life span perspective. In R. Jones (Ed.) *Black adult development and aging*. Berkeley, CA: Cobbs & Henry.

Hatchett, S., Cochran, D. & Jackson, J. (1991). Family life. In J. Jackson (Ed.) *Life in Black America*. Newbury Park, CA: Sage.

Holahan, C. & Moos, R. (1987). Personal and contextual determinants of coping strategies. *Journal of Personality and Social Psychology, 52*, 946-955.

Holt, R. (1982). Occupational stress. In L. Goldberger & S. Breznitz (Ed.) *The handbook of stress* (pp 419-444). New York: Guilford.

Hughes, D., & Dodge, M. (1997). African American women in the workplace: Relationships between job conditions, racial bias at work, and perceived job quality. *Amer. J. of Community Psychology 25*(5).

James, K., Lovato, E. & Khoo, G. (1994). Social identity correlates of minority workers' health. *Academy of Management J, 37*, 383-396.

Johnson, N. (2001). Changing outcomes in women's health. *Monitor on Psychology 32*(9), 5.

Jones, J.(1997). *Prejudice and racism*. New York: McGraw-Hill.

King, D. (1988). Multiple jeopardy, multiple consciousness: The context of a Black feminist ideology. *Signs, 14*, 42-72.

Lazarus, R. & Folkman, S. (1984). Stress, appraisal, and coping. New York: Springer.

Marsh, C. (1993). Sexual assault and domestic violence in the African American community. *Western Journal of Black studies, 17*,149-155.

Mays, V. (1995). Black women, work, stress, and perceived discrimination: The focused support group model as an intervention for stress reduction. *Cultural Diversity and Mental Health, 1*(1), 53-65.

McClowry, S., Tommasini, N., Giangrande, S. et al (2000). Daily Hassles of married women with children: An empirical foundation for a preventive program. *J of Amer Psych Ns Ass 6*(4),107-111.

McNeilly, M., Anderson, N., Robinson, E., et al (1996). The convergent, discriminant, and concurrent criterion validity of the perceived racism scale: A multidimensional assessment of White racism among African Americans. In R. Jones (Ed.) *Handbook of tests and measurements for Black populations* (pp 359-374). Hampton, VA: Cobb.

Mortimer, J. & Sorenson, G. (1984). Men, women, work, and family. In K. M. Borman, D. Quarm , S. Gideonse (Eds) *Women in the workplace: Effects on families* (pp. 139-168). Norwood, NJ, Ablex.

Napholz, L. (1994). Sex role orientation and psychological well-being among working Black women. *The Journal of Black Psychology, 20*(4), 469-481.

Napholz, L. (1998). Enhancing research participation and retention for three ethnically diverse groups. *Journal of Cultural Diversity, 5*, 117-119.

Napholz, L. (1999).   A preliminary analysis of the effects of a stress reduction psychoeducational intervention on African American working women. *J of Gender, Culture, and Health, 4*(2), 153-168.

Napholz, L. (2001). An effectiveness trial to increase psychological well-being and reduce role conflict among African American blue-collar working women. In programs and Abstracts (pp. 42-50) of the *15th APNA Conference on Integrated Knowledge Development for Psychiatric-Mental Health Nursing*, Reno.

Napholz, L. (2002). Stress-reduction psychoeducational interventions for Black working women. *Nurs Clin N. Am* 37, 263-272.

Peterson, C., Maier, S. & Seligman, M. (1993). *Learned helplessness: A theory for the age of personal control.* New York: Oxford University Press.

Sanchez-Hucles, J. (1997). Jeopardy not bonus status for African American women in the work force: Why does the myth of advantage persist? *Amer J of Com Psych 25*(5), 565-580.

Selye, H (1976). *The stress of life.* New York: McGraw-Hill.

Tucker, C. & Herman, K. (2002). Using culturally sensitive theories and research to meet the academic needs of low-income African American children. *American Psychologist, 57*(10), 762-773.

Urban, W. (2001). Lifestyle psychotherapy. *California Psychologist, 34*(10),12-13.

Williams, D., Yu, Y., Jackson, J. et al (1997). Racial differences in physical and mental health: Socioeconomic status, stress, and discrimination. *Journal of Health Psych, 2*:335-352.

In: Psychology of Stress
Editor: Kimberly V. Oxington, pp. 35-52

ISBN 1-59454-246-5
©2005 Nova Science Publishers, Inc.

Chapter III

STRESS MANAGEMENT INTERVENTIONS FOR MEDICAL POPULATIONS

Wendy G. Lichtenthal, Norah S. Simpson and Dean G. Cruess
Department of Psychology
University of Pennsylvania

ABSTRACT

In this chapter, we will review the empirical support for stress management (SM) interventions developed for various medical patient populations, focusing on those applied to patients with human immunodeficiency virus (HIV) infection/acquired immune deficiency syndrome (AIDS) and cancer. SM interventions for other patient populations will also be briefly discussed. The emphasis throughout this chapter will be on those interventions for which randomized controlled clinical trials have been conducted. We will also summarize the various stress management strategies that have been implemented in these interventions, as well as the range of psychological and physiological health outcomes that have resulted from these studies. Reducing or managing responses to stress has different health implications for each disease, and we will consider the benefits of SM interventions in this context. Additionally, we will briefly discuss the implications of these findings and suggest directions for future research.

Why is it important to investigate the efficacy of stress management (SM) interventions for medical populations? The psychological implications of reducing levels of stress are straightforward, as most individuals have experienced the negative impact of stress on their mood, attitudes, and overall psychological state. Medical illnesses, acute and chronic, are often accompanied by a number of disease-related *stressors*, or events that produce stress. These stressors include, but are not limited to: physical pain, loss of control, financial strain, role changes, death anxiety, social stigma, and general life uncertainty (Andersen, 2002; Antoni, Cruess, D. G., et al., 2000). There is therefore little debate that reducing the psychological burden of medical conditions and related stressors is a worthwhile venture for improving at least some aspects of psychosocial functioning.

In the last two decades, however, it has become clear that the benefits of stress reduction are not limited to the psychological realm. It appears that there are also positive physiological effects of lowering stress levels, such as decreasing physical symptoms, altering neuroendocrine and immune functioning, delaying disease progression, and perhaps even increasing the probability of survival. Because these outcomes may have particular value for medical populations, we will focus our discussion on reviewing the literature on effective SM interventions designed for specific medical patient groups.

WHAT ARE STRESS MANAGEMENT INTERVENTIONS AND HOW DO THEY WORK?

SM interventions often incorporate a variety of techniques to help individuals manage and reduce stress in their lives. We present descriptions of some frequently utilized techniques in Table 1.

Table 1. Frequently Used Stress Management Techniques

Technique	Description
Cognitive restructuring	Identify distorted or dysfunctional cognitions and shape them into more accurate and adaptive thoughts
Problem-solving training	Consider realistic solutions to problems by choosing options, trying them out, and repeating until resolution is achieved
Coping skills training	Learn about and appropriately apply problem-focused and emotion-focused coping strategies
Social support training	Learn and practice social and communication skills and focus on developing a social network
Guided imagery	Visualize described scenes in an effort to relax and refocus the mind
Self-disclosure	Write or speak about a specified topic repeatedly over a given period of time
Progressive muscle relaxation	Systematically tense and relax specific muscle groups throughout the body
Biofeedback	Utilize electronic devices which receive and transmit signals from the body to learn to recognize and voluntarily induce a state of relaxation
Deep breathing	Focus on inhalation and exhalation, filling the lungs with air to their capacity
Mindfulness meditation	Enhance non-judgmental awareness and acceptance through focusing on breathing

Additional intervention components include support groups, exercise, and hypnosis. This is not an exhaustive list of SM strategies, and interventions may use only one or a combination of these techniques. In addition, many SM interventions also employ some psycho-education of the human stress response in order to help individuals understand how stress affects cognitive, affective, behavioral, physical and social aspects of functioning. Typically, SM techniques are taught to study participants by a skilled professional or graduate student who has undergone specific training for this purpose. Because stress may promote engagement in unhealthy behaviors that can lead to additional negative psychological and physical health effects, many interventions also contain behavioral components that target aspects of health other than direct stress reduction, such as diet, exercise, and smoking. Some interventions are specifically formulated as SM, whereas others use components that are widely-believed to be stress reducing or which result in decreased stress levels as a by-product of targeting other areas of functioning. Therefore, it is useful to characterize many, if not all, psychosocial and behavioral interventions as SM.

Through the application of an assortment of techniques, SM interventions can help mitigate the response to stressful life events such as medical illness. They can also improve psychosocial functioning in a variety of domains, including reducing distress, anxiety, and depression; and increasing the identification of positive consequences of the illness experience and overall quality of life (Andersen, 2002; Antoni, Cruess, D. G., et al., 2000; Antoni et al., 2001; Fawzy, Fawzy, Arndt, & Pasnau, 1995). Improvements in adaptive coping may also be observed. Folkman (1999) pointed out that unlike personality characteristics, coping strategies are presumed to be modifiable and thus are appropriate targets for intervention. Positive changes in active coping can lead patients to acquire necessary information for treatment and can help them to find alternatives to engaging in negative health behaviors when distressed (Folkman, 1999). Some SM interventions teach participants how to modify lifestyle behaviors that exacerbate medical conditions. There are thus at least two routes by which successful SM interventions can produce physical health benefits. The first is by directly reducing stress and its harmful physiological effects, and the second is by increasing healthy lifestyle behaviors.

PHYSIOLOGICAL EFFECTS OF STRESS

Kemeny (2003) recently reviewed the numerous physiological responses to stressors. These include activation of both the sympathetic adrenomedullary (SAM) system and the hypothalamic-pituitary-adrenal (HPA) axis, which are two components of the endocrine system that are associated with the physiological stress response. Stress can also enhance the inflammatory response of the immune system. In the short term, this may be beneficial; however, chronic inflammation can adversely affect health and exacerbate several illnesses. It has also been found that exposure to stressors can decrease immune system functioning. Thus, chronic stressors, such as medical conditions, can negatively impact health outcomes because of their deleterious effects on both the endocrine and immune systems (Kemeny, 2003).

This chapter will discuss some of the major research initiatives that have examined SM interventions, focusing on those applied to patients with human immunodeficiency virus (HIV) infection/acquired immune deficiency syndrome (AIDS) and cancer. SM for other patient groups will also be briefly discussed. We will review interventions that have been specifically designated as SM and also those that can be construed as SM because of their presumed impact on psychosocial and/or physiological functioning. Reducing or managing responses to stress has different health implications for each disease, and we will consider the benefits of SM interventions in this context. We will argue that although the evidence of positive effects on significant disease-related health parameters (i.e., disease progression, survival) among some patient groups is inconclusive, the significant psychological benefits and measurable effects in numerous health-related physical parameters provide evidence that these interventions are useful to medical patient populations.

There are a number of studies of SM interventions in the research literature that have not used randomization and control comparison groups. However, the focus of this chapter will be on more scientifically rigorous investigations, and thus we will concentrate on discussing results only from randomized controlled trials.

HIV/AIDS

HIV and AIDS are chronic illnesses that require lifelong treatment and are often accompanied by financial, social, and psychological burdens. Individuals with HIV and AIDS are subject to a number of stressors that, while not unique to these diseases, often combine to present a formidable challenge with which to cope. Given the potentially harmful effects of stress and maladaptive coping techniques, clinical researchers have become interested in stress reduction interventions as a tool for improving psychological and physical health states among individuals living with HIV infection (Leserman, 2003). Distress, denial (a coping strategy that is often maladaptive), and low adherence to behavioral health interventions have been found to predict faster disease progression in gay men infected with HIV (Ironson et al., 1994). Early studies suggested the benefits of SM interventions on immunological and health-related indices among HIV-infected individuals and more recent studies have further demonstrated the significant beneficial effects of SM interventions in this population. (Robinson, Mathews, & Witek-Janusek, 2000).

Initial research on SM interventions for HIV-positive patients tested their effects on changes in affective and immune functioning changes following notification of HIV serostatus (a frequently stress-producing event) among groups at high risk for contracting HIV. One study tested the effects of an exercise program (LaPerriere et al., 1990), and another examined the effects of a short cognitive-behavioral stress management (CBSM) intervention on a population of HIV-positive gay men prior to serostatus notification (Antoni et al., 1991). The CBSM intervention was developed by researchers at the University of Miami and has been utilized in numerous behavioral medicine studies (see Antoni, Cruess, D. G., et al., 2000; and Antoni et al., 2001; among others). CBSM involves teaching various coping strategies, conflict resolution techniques, and assertion training; encourages emotional expression; and uses cognitive restructuring, progressive muscle relaxation, and relaxing imagery (Antoni et al., 1991; Antoni, Cruess, D. G., et al., 2000; Antoni et al., 2001). Both the exercise and the CBSM intervention studies found a significant buffering effect on increases in depressed mood among seropositive intervention participants compared to seropositive controls after notification about their HIV-positive status (LaPerriere et al., 1990; Antoni et al., 1991). The exercise intervention also prevented HIV-infected intervention participants from exhibiting the decrease in natural killer cell levels and increase in anxiety levels observed among HIV-infected control participants (LaPerriere et al., 1990). Seropositive CBSM intervention participants demonstrated an increase in several beneficial immune markers, including CD4+ and natural killer cell counts (Antoni et al., 1991). This research documents both positive psychological and immune changes resulting from SM interventions in an HIV-positive population. These findings suggested that interventions employing a variety of SM techniques could buffer the distress response and immunological changes following notification of HIV positive serostatus (Antoni et al., 1991).

Other early studies also found psychological and physiological benefits of SM in HIV-positive populations. An investigation of the effects of a specialized stress reduction intervention that incorporated training in biofeedback, guided imagery, and hypnosis found significant decreases in stress symptoms and increases in vigor and hardiness among HIV-positive symptomatic men assigned to the intervention group when compared to control participants (Auerbach, Oleson, & Solomon, 1992). In a later study, Eller (1995) tested the effects of guided imagery compared to progressive muscle relaxation among a group of HIV-positive men at various disease stages. The author found significant increases in CD4+ cell counts in the progressive muscle relaxation group and significant decreases in fatigue in the guided imagery group (Eller, 1995). Both treatment groups also reported reductions in depression levels compared to a control group (Eller, 1995). Beneficial effects on mood and immune function have also been demonstrated in other studies of different SM techniques, including massage (Ironson et al., 1996), relaxation and education (Nicholas & Webster, 1996), and a combination of progressive muscle relaxation and electromyograph biofeedback-assisted relaxation training, meditation, and hypnosis (Taylor, 1995) among HIV-positive individuals.

A more recent research initiative on the effects of SM in HIV investigated the effects of a 10-week CBSM intervention among HIV-positive gay men (Antoni, Cruess, D. G., et al., 2000; Antoni, Cruess, S., et al., 2000). As described earlier, the CBSM intervention involved multiple SM components. Participation in this intervention resulted in a number of psychological and physiological changes. Improvements in relaxation skills, cognitive coping strategies, and social support were demonstrated among CBSM participants, and were subsequently found to mediate resulting changes in mood. These mood changes were also associated with alterations in adrenal hormone regulation (Antoni, Cruess, S., et al., 2000).

Additional endocrine changes were observed, including decreases in urinary cortisol levels and increases in serum dehydroepiandrosterone sulfate (DHEA-S) and testosterone levels that were related to reductions in depressed mood (Cruess, Antoni, Schneiderman, et al., 2000). Reductions in norepinephrine levels were associated with decreases in anxiety (Antoni, Cruess, D. G., et al., 2000). The CBSM intervention also appeared to buffer decreases in DHEA-S and increases in the cortisol/DHEA-S ratio. The latter shift in endocrine levels was associated with reductions in mood disturbance and perceived stress among HIV-seropositive men (Cruess et al., 1999). Cruess, Antoni, Kumar, and Schneiderman (2000) specifically examined the relaxation training component of CBSM and found that levels of salivary cortisol assessed prior to in-session relaxation training decreased over the course of the intervention. These reductions were associated with decreases in levels of stress during home relaxation training, overall mood disturbance, and anxiety (Cruess, Antoni, Kumar, et al., 2000). In addition, those participants who practiced the prescribed home relaxation more frequently demonstrated greater decreases in their cortisol levels in the first three CBSM sessions.

These hormonal changes were also found to be associated with immune changes. Increased DHEA-S/cortisol ratios were partially related to short-term changes in IgG antibody titers to herpes simplex virus-2 (HSV-2; Cruess S. et al., 2000). In a separate study of CBSM, individual decreases in dysphoria significantly predicted lower HSV-2 herpes simplex antibody titers by the end of the intervention, although no changes in HSV-Type 1 antibody titers or in lymphocyte subpopulations (CD4+ or CD8+ cell numbers) were observed (Lutgendorf et al., 1997). Longer-term changes in lymphocyte subpopulations in association with shifts in hormone levels were also observed, including changes CD8+ suppressor cytotoxic cells that were related to reductions in norepinephrine output (Antoni, Cruess, D. G., et al., 2000) and increases in transitional naïve CD4+ cells that were associated with reductions in urinary cortisol output (Antoni et al., 2002). Antoni (2003) provides a more thorough review of this collection of studies.

Additional studies have focused on the psychosocial impact of SM in HIV-positive populations. Chesney et al. (2003) examined HIV-seropositive gay men randomized into a coping-effectiveness training, informational control, or wait-list control group. After 10 90-minute group sessions that took place over three months, the coping-effectiveness group demonstrated significantly greater decreases in perceived stress and burnout compared to the informational control group. Participants were re-evaluated at 6 and 12 months, and although the differences in perceived stress and burnout between the groups were not maintained, optimism levels in the coping-effectiveness and informational control groups continued to rise (Chesney et al., 2003).

Another recent study examined the effects of a supportive-expressive group intervention on long-term psychosocial adjustment in HIV-positive gay men (Weiss et al., 2003). At each of four assessments conducted over 15 months, there were no differences between the treatment and control groups on measures of distress, coping, or social support; however, it was noted that distress levels in both groups decreased over time (Weiss et al., 2003). The authors offered explanations of the null results, including the fact that study participants were well-adjusted at the baseline assessment and that they participated during a time when HIV treatments were rapidly improving. Thus, these events may have minimized the effects of this SM intervention (Weiss et al., 2003).

SM interventions have also been developed to assist HIV-infected patients with medication adherence, which is often perceived by patients as a stressful burden. Jones et al. (2003) examined the impact of a CBSM intervention on medication adherence among women with AIDS. They found that women who demonstrated low adherence to their medication regimens improved their level of adherence, although not significantly. Intervention participants also demonstrated significant decreases in denial-based coping (Jones et al.,

2003). As adherence to medical regimen is a critical component of health maintenance in HIV-infected populations, further investigations of medication adherence are of particular importance.

The effects of expressive writing have also been examined among HIV-positive individuals (O'Cleirigh et al., 2003; Petrie, Fontanilla, Thomas, Booth, & Pennebaker, 2004). In a recent study, 37 HIV-positive participants were randomly assigned to write about either an emotional or neutral control topic for 30 minutes on four consecutive days (Petrie et al, 2004). Compared to the control participants, the emotional writing participants demonstrated a significant increase in CD4+ lymphocyte counts. These changes in lymphocyte levels were also associated with a drop in HIV viral load (Petrie et al., 2004). The results from this study demonstrate how writing interventions can significantly impact physiological parameters among patients with HIV.

Overall, SM interventions for HIV-infected populations appear to significantly improve both psychological and physical health. Additional benefits may include increases in positive health behaviors, such as medication adherence. With recent improvements in medical treatments, HIV has become a chronic disease. Consequently, SM interventions may become an important supplement to standard treatment regimens for this medical population. Future research will reveal whether SM interventions can actually reduce morbidity and mortality in this population.

CANCER

Although the effectiveness of medical treatments for various forms of cancer has improved throughout the years, a cancer diagnosis can still cause patients a great deal of distress. In addition, patients often feel anxiety about treatment and its side effects, fear of recurrence, and feelings of isolation (Antoni et al., 2001). Because patients commonly experience distress, several types of SM interventions have been developed targeting disease-related psychosocial issues. Fawzy et al. (1995) suggested that psychosocial interventions for cancer patients might be particularly helpful soon after diagnosis or in the beginning stages of treatment. There are also a variety of long-term stressors that can be targeted by SM, such as sexual dysfunction, interpersonal relationships, employment, and finances (Andersen, 2002).

One of the largest research initiatives of SM among cancer patients has involved the investigation of the efficacy of a 10-week CBSM intervention for individuals with early-stage breast cancer (Antoni et al., 2001; Cruess, Antoni, McGregor, et al., 2000; Cruess et al., 2001; McGregor et al., 2004). Antoni et al. (2001) examined 100 women who were randomized into either CBSM approximately six to eight weeks after their surgical treatment or a one-day seminar of information from the CBSM intervention approximately 16-18 weeks post-surgery. The women were assessed at four time points. Results showed that CBSM participants demonstrated decreased prevalence of at least moderate or more severe depression at all follow-up assessments and reported significantly more benefit-finding (i.e., finding positive consequences of their cancer experience) immediately following the intervention (Antoni et al., 2001). In addition, there was an interaction between benefit-finding and optimism that indicated that less optimistic women in the CBSM condition, who reported lower baseline levels of benefit-finding, increased their levels of benefit-finding to those of the more optimistic women. This suggested that the intervention was most helpful to those with the greatest need (Antoni et al., 2001). This increase was sustained until the nine-month assessment, but the increase in benefit-finding observed among more optimistic women was not. Optimism levels also increased among those women in the active intervention (Antoni et al., 2001).

Cruess, Antoni, McGregor, et al. (2000) also found that an increase in benefit-finding was related to a reduction in cortisol levels that occurred among breast cancer patients who participated in CBSM. Participants in the CBSM intervention had significantly lower serum cortisol levels immediately following the intervention than those of subjects in the control group. This reduction in cortisol levels was not related to changes in distress, but rather to increases in benefit-finding that appeared to be a result of the CBSM intervention. Furthermore, Cruess, Antoni, McGregor, et al. (2000) demonstrated that benefit-finding mediated the relationship between group assignment and post-intervention cortisol levels, thus partially explaining the decrease in cortisol levels observed among CBSM participants. Cruess et al. (2001) found a similar reduction in serum testosterone levels among CBSM participants when compared to a wait-list control group. In this investigation, CBSM participants demonstrated levels of testosterone comparable to levels of healthy women following the intervention. These reductions were likewise inversely associated with the observed increases in benefit-finding following the intervention (Cruess et al., 2001).

While the changes in hormone levels resulting from CBSM interventions were not directly related to health outcomes in these studies, alterations in hormone levels do have significant immunosuppressive effects. McGregor et al. (2004) explored whether or not the increases in benefit-finding exhibited among participants of the CBSM intervention were related to enhanced immune functioning. They examined in vitro lymphocyte proliferation in response to specific activation of the T cell receptor, CD3+, because prior studies demonstrated that lymphocyte proliferation in response to non-specific mitogen (reflecting how well lymphocytes function and respond) was predictive of better prognoses among breast cancer patients. Both this measure of immune functioning and benefit-finding were assessed prior to the CBSM intervention among 29 breast cancer patients (McGregor et al., 2004). Benefit-finding was then assessed again at the conclusion of the 10-week intervention (Time 2), while immune functioning was measured for a second time three months after the completion of the intervention (Time 3) so that the effects of adjuvant therapy (e.g., chemotherapy, hormonal therapy, and radiotherapy) on immune functioning would not confound the results. The authors found that lymphocyte proliferation significantly increased among CBSM participants by Time 3, whereas it marginally decreased in the comparison group; however, these changes were not related to levels of distress (McGregor et al., 2004). In fact, the change in proliferation over time was associated with the change of benefit-finding observed. The correlation between these changes was stronger in the intervention group than in the comparison group (McGregor et al., 2004).

The efficacy of CBSM has also been examined in other cancer patient populations. Penedo et al. (2004) tested the effects of a modified version of CBSM for prostate cancer patients who had undergone treatment. They found that participants in the experimental group reported greater quality of life following the intervention when compared to the control group. This effect was mediated by increases in perceived SM skills, suggesting that the acquisition (and presumably implementation) of SM strategies can positively impact quality of life.

Other cognitive-behavioral interventions designed to reduce distress among cancer patients have also been studied. Improvements in quality of life, in addition to reductions in anxiety, were observed among malignant melanoma patients who participated in a cognitive-behavioral intervention targeting distress (Trask, Paterson, Griffith, Riba, & Schwartz, 2003). Although there was no treatment effect on distress two or six months post-intervention when a conservative intent-to-treat analysis was employed, reductions in distress at two months were observed using an effect-of-intervention analysis (Trask et al., 2003). It is worth noting that the effect-of-intervention results may be a closer approximation of the efficacy of this intervention because nearly half those randomized to the treatment condition did not participate in the intervention, frequently because of traveling inconveniences (Trask et al., 2003).

It is therefore encouraging to note that Allen and colleagues (2002) found that a problem-solving and education intervention delivered largely over the telephone was efficacious in improving emotional health and practical needs being met at a four-month follow-up among breast cancer patients under the age of 50. Interestingly, although women in the intervention group whose baseline social problem-solving skills were moderate or good showed decreased difficulties related to their cancer eight months post-treatment, those with either poor or excellent problem-solving abilities fared worse. There were too few participants with excellent problem-solving skills to speculate on the cause of this surprising treatment effect. The authors posited that those with poor problem-solving skills might have been overwhelmed by the additional burden of participation and noted that targeting interventions to the appropriate population is an important issue to consider (Allen et al., 2002).

Researchers have also examined the application of self-disclosure techniques among cancer patients in randomized clinical trials. Walker, Nail, and Croyle (1999) examined written emotional expression among a small sample of breast cancer patients, but did not find that the intervention improved psychological adjustment to their disease. However, Stanton et al. (2002) found that written exercises focusing on emotional expression or benefit-finding resulted in a reduction in physical symptoms and medical appointments among breast cancer patients. The authors posited that these exercises helped to buffer patients' reactions to their physical symptoms, in addition to having a potential impact on immune functioning. At the three month follow-up, they found physical symptoms were significaantly reduced in the emotional expression group, and participants in both the emotional expression and benefit-finding groups had significantly fewer medical appointments than the control group. It appears that emotional expression and more directive writing exercises may impact physical health among cancer patients, although further investigation with other types of cancer patients should be conducted.

Many researchers have examined the impact of mindfulness meditation interventions for SM among cancer patients; however, few have been randomized controlled trials. Speca, Carlson, Goodey, and Angun (2000) found that cancer patients who were randomized to a seven-week mindfulness-based stress reduction program that involved group meetings and at-home practice experienced numerous psychological and physical symptom benefits following participation when compared to a wait-list control group. The treatment group reported reductions in global mood disturbance, including decreases in depression, anxiety, anger, and confusion; as well as in overall stress levels, including cognitive, emotional, and physical symptoms of stress. Increases in vigor were also observed. This study was also unique in its investigation of both men and women with a diverse range of cancer types (Speca et al., 2000). These studies provide important preliminary evidence that mindfulness meditation may be an effective SM intervention, which warrants further investigation using randomized controlled study designs.

A relatively small number of studies have examined the impact of psychosocial interventions on cancer survival in cancer populations. Spiegel, Kraemer, Bloom, and Gottheil (1989) tested the efficacy of supportive-expressive group psychotherapy among breast cancer patients and found that women randomized to the treatment condition survived approximately 18 months longer than those in the control group. However, Fox (1998) argued that the initial finding of increased survival might have been due to the particularly low survival rate of the control group rather than a true effect of the psychosocial intervention.

Fawzy et al. (1990) investigated a psychiatric intervention for malignant melanoma patients that consisted of 10 sessions of coping skills training, progressive relaxation, and group support. Those randomized to the intervention demonstrated enhanced coping skills and natural killer cell activity, an immune measure that has been shown to be particularly relevant for cancer, when compared to patients in the control group. More patients in the treatment condition survived six years later (Fawzy et al., 1993), but this effect did not persist at the 10-year follow-up except when controlling for sex and tumor thickness (Fawzy, Canada, & Fawzy, 2003).

A number of trials examining the impact of psychosocial/SM interventions on survival outcomes have demonstrated null results. Cunningham et al. (1998) randomized metastatic breast cancer patients into either 35 weeks of a cognitive behavioral therapy (CBT) and support group (based on that of Spiegel et al., 1989) or a control condition. However, their inability to detect effects of the intervention may have been due to the small sample size, as well as the use of relaxation (stress-reduction) tapes in the control group. In a separate study, Edelman, Lemon, Bell, and Kidman (1999) likewise did not find increased survival among metastatic breast cancer patients randomized into a CBT group when compared to a standard care control group. In reconciling the differences in findings between their study and Spiegel et al.'s (1989), the authors posited that the absence of a survival advantage in the treatment group of their study may have been due to the short-lived nature of the psychological benefits observed (which were not present by a three-month follow-up assessment) or because their eight-week intervention was not long enough to produce effects (Edelman et al., 1999). In an attempt to replicate the Spiegel et al. (1989) study, Goodwin et al. (2001) found psychological benefits and reductions in pain (especially among women reporting higher distress) among intervention participants, but not increased survival.

In summary, the literature on the impact of SM interventions on survival is inconclusive, but there is evidence that SM interventions can positively affect psychosocial functioning. Furthermore, these interventions appear to induce physiological changes, including altering stress hormone levels and enhancing immune functioning. After reviewing investigations of the application of educational, behavioral training, individual psychotherapy, and group psychosocial interventions among cancer patients, Fawzy et al. (1995) concluded that patients are able to experience mental and physical health benefits from interventions employing a diverse range of techniques. In an extensive review of the literature on psychological interventions for cancer patients, Andersen (2002) used a biobehavioral model to organize the literature, highlighting how changes in stress levels, treatment compliance, and physiological parameters can affect health outcomes like disease progression and survival. This perspective is useful way to synthesize the vast direct and indirect effects SM interventions can have on mental and physical health functioning.

OTHER MEDICAL ILLNESSES

Cardiovascular Disease

As discussed earlier in the chapter, perceived stress may lead to increased sympathetic nervous system arousal. Such activation may then contribute to adverse cardiovascular effects such as myocardial ischemia (insufficient blood flow to heart) or cardiac arrhythmias (Claar & Blumenthal, 2003). Several large-scale studies have been conducted studying the effects of SM interventions on cardiovascular disease (CVD); however, these studies have produced mixed results. A meta-analysis of early studies examining the efficacy of SM interventions in CVD populations demonstrated that supplementing standard care with SM interventions was related to increased quality of life and reduced mortality (Linden, Stossel, & Maurice, 1996); however, a more recent review has cast doubts on the ability of SM interventions to significantly reduce cardiac related morbidity and mortality (Claar & Blumenthal, 2003).

Although SM interventions among populations with or at-risk-for CVD may not reliably decrease disease-related morbidity and mortality, a number of studies have demonstrated that SM interventions can lower risk-markers for CVD, and thus should be considered as a useful adjunct therapy along with standard medical care (Sundin et al, 2003; Blumenthal et al, 1997). Conclusions from these studies suggest that behavioral interventions offer additional benefit over and above usual medical care in patients with CVD. It has been noted that the assessment of behavioral medicine interventions (such as SM) is more difficult when focused on health outcomes with low incidence rates, such as CVD, with its relatively sporadic markers of disease progression (Rutledge & Loh, 2004). As the majority of SM interventions in this population have shown positive, if weak effects, further investigations are warranted to better assess the impact of these interventions on cardiovascular health.

Rheumatoid Arthritis and Asthma

Emotional disclosure has also been studied as an intervention targeting psychological and physiological stress responses in both asthma and rheumatoid arthritis populations. An early study conducted by Kelley and colleagues (1997) found that patients with rheumatoid arthritis who were assigned to participate in verbal emotional disclosure sessions on four consecutive days showed less affective disturbance and better physical functioning in daily activities than the control group three months later. A more recent study focused on the effect of written emotional disclosure among individuals with asthma or rheumatoid arthritis (Smyth, Stone, Hurewitz, & Kaell, 1999). In this study, 112 patients were randomly assigned to write about either the most stressful event of their lives or an emotionally neutral topic for 20 minutes on three consecutive days. Four months after treatment, asthma patients in the experimental group showed improvements in lung function compared to control participants, and rheumatoid arthritis patients in the experimental group showed improvements in overall disease activity compared to control participants. Combining all completing patients, nearly half of the experimental patients had clinically relevant improvement compared to only approximately a quarter of the control group (Smyth et al, 1999).

Results from these expressive writing and emotional disclosure studies, along with the others mentioned earlier in the chapter (O'Cleirigh et al., 2003; Petrie et al., 2004; Stanton et al., 2002, Walker et al., 1999), suggest that expressive wtiting is a viable SM technique that can be utilized in isolation or as part of multi-component SM interventions. Expressive writing reliably produces significant changes in health and physiology in both healthy and medical populations. Further research should be done to learn how to better (more frequently) implement this powerful, low-cost intervention that is easy to implement in medical settings.

Headache

A recent study also applied SM to medical treatment of chronic tension type headaches, reporting an increased rate of treatment success when both treatments are used together (Holroyd et al., 2001). This study compared the effects of a tricyclic antidepressant, placebo, SM plus antidepressant, and SM plus placebo on reductions in headache symptoms. The SM intervention utilized in this study combined relaxation and cognitive coping techniques. The authors stated that while both therapies (antidepressant and SM) resulted in improvements in treatment groups, the combined therapy was more likely to produce significant reductions in headache symptoms. To date, few studies have investigated the efficacy of SM treatment of chronic headaches using randomized controlled designs; however, results from the study by Holroyd and colleagues (2001) indicate that this application of SM intervention to headache populations warrants future study.

ISSUES OF CONSIDERATION AND FUTURE DIRECTIONS

In addition to research on HIV/AIDS, cancer, CVD, rheumatoid arthritis, asthma, and headache, SM interventions have also been examined among patients with hypertension (Schneider et al., 1995); epilepsy (Deepak, Manchanda, & Maheshwari 1994); Crohn's disease (Garcia-Vega & Fernandez-Rodriguez, 2004); and a number of other medical illnesses. Future studies will likely explore the numerous applications of SM interventions to additional medical populations.

Among the most intriguing findings from these studies is that of the potential for prolonged survival for participants in psychosocial SM interventions with life-threatening illnesses such as HIV/AIDS, cancer and CVD. However, because of the inconsistency of the results in the literature, it has been argued that it is important not to overstate such findings until they have been replicated so that patients (and their healthcare practitioners) are not misled (Palmer & Coyne, 2004). An important question remains, however; if randomized controlled trials consistently demonstrated that SM does *not* prolong survival, would SM interventions still be valuable? We argue, as have others (Spiegel & Giese-Davis, 2004), that they are valuable insofar as they provide patients with tools to cope with disease-related stressors and can lead to enhanced psychosocial functioning and quality of life.

Another major issue is how researchers determine whether or not their findings are clinically significant or meaningful. Some outcomes, such as prolonged survival, are fairly straightforward to interpret. The implications of others, such as changes in specific neuroendocrine or immune parameters, are less clear. Researchers from different fields (e.g., health psychologists versus immunologists) may have distinct interpretations of what qualifies as clinically significant. Some psychosocial outcomes are ambiguous as well. One way that investigators can get a better sense of the utility of SM interventions is by assessing consumer satisfaction. SM interventions that are rated as helpful or valuable by participants, but that do not demonstrate treatment effects, may still be beneficial in ways that were not measured.

Still, there are numerous remaining questions that should be addressed in future studies. For example, what are the active ingredients of effective SM interventions? The use of multiple techniques makes it difficult to determine which ones are producing the observed effects (Claar & Blumenthal, 2003). It is also not clear whether SM interventions are more effectively administered in individual or group formats. Future studies should attempt to answer these questions, and should additionally explore individual differences in patient responses to appropriately tailor the interventions for maximum effectiveness as well as realistic and practical application (Allen et al., 2002). Additionally, it is critical to more clearly establish the clinical significance of specific findings. Researchers should continue to explore whether or not the psychological benefits produced by these interventions translate into physiological benefits and attempt to better understand how interventions that do not appear to be reducing distress are affecting biological outcomes. The results of investigations of SM interventions thus far are promising, and through replication and effectiveness trials, SM has the potential to become an integral part of medical patients' treatment regimens.

REFERENCES

Allen, S. M., Shah, A. C., Nezu, A. M., Nezu, C. M., Ciambrone, D., Hogan, J., & Mor, V. (2002). A problem-solving approach to stress reduction among younger women with breast carcinoma. *Cancer, 94,* 3089-3100.

Andersen, B. L. (2002). Biobehavioral outcomes following psychological interventions for cancer patients. *Journal of Consulting and Clinical Psychology, 70,* 590–610.

Antoni, M. H. (2003). Stress management effects on psychological, endocrinological, and immune functioning in men with HIV infection: Empirical support for a psychoneuroimmunological model. *Stress, 6,* 173-188.

Antoni, M. H., Baggett, L., Ironson, G., LaPerriere, A., August, S., Klimas, N., Schneiderman, N., & Fletcher, M. A. (1991). Cognitive-behavioral stress management intervention buffers distress responses and immunologic changes following notification of HIV-1 seropositivity. *Journal of Consulting & Clinical Psychology, 59,* 906-15.

Antoni, M. H., Cruess, D. G., Cruess, S., Lutgendorf, S., Kumar, M., Ironson, G., Klimas, N., Fletcher, M. A., & Schneiderman, N. (2000). Cognitive-behavioral stress management intervention effects on anxiety, 24-hr urinary norepinephrine output, and T-cytotoxic/suppressor cells over time among symptomatic HIV-infected gay men. *Journal of Consulting & Clinical Psychology, 68,* 31-45.

Antoni, M. H., Cruess, D. G., Klimas, N., Maher, K., Cruess, S., Kumar, M., Lutgendorf, S., Ironson, G., Schneiderman, N., & Fletcher, M. A. (2002). Stress management and immune system reconstitution in symptomatic HIV-infected gay men over time: Effects on transitional naive T cells (CD4$^+$CD45RA$^+$CD29$^+$). *American Journal of Psychiatry, 159,* 143-145.

Antoni, M. H., Cruess, S., Cruess, D. G., Kumar, M., Lutgendorf, S., Ironson, G., Dettmer, E., Williams, J., Klimas, N., Fletcher, M. A., & Schneiderman, N. (2000). Cognitive-behavioral stress management reduces distress and 24-hour urinary free cortisol output among symptomatic HIV-infected gay men. *Annals of Behavioral Medicine, 22,* 29-37.

Antoni, M. H., Lehman, J. M., Kilbourn, K. M., Boyers, A. E., Culver, J. L., Alferi, S. M., Yount, S. E., McGregor, B. A., Arena, P. L., Harris, S. D., Price, A. A., & Carver, C. S. (2001). Cognitive-behavioral stress management intervention decreases the prevalence of depression and enhances benefit finding among women under treatment for early-stage breast cancer. *Health Psychology, 20,* 20-32.

Auerbach, J. E., Oleson, T. D., & Solmon, G. F. (1992). A behavioral medicine intervention as an adjunctive treatment for HIV-related illness. *Psychology and Health, 6,* 325-334.

Blumenthal, J. A., Jiang, W., Babyak, M., Krantz, D. S., Frid, D. J., Coleman, R. E., Waugh, R., Hanson, M., Applebaum, M., O'Connor, C., & Morris, J. J. (1997). Stress management and exercise training in cardiac patients with myocardial ischemia: Effects on prognosis and evaluation of mechanisms. *Archives of Internal Medicine, 157,* 2213–2223.

Chesney, M. A., Chambers, D. B., Taylor, J. M., Johnson, L. M., & Folkman, S. (2003). Coping effectiveness training for men living with HIV: Results from a randomized clinical trial testing a group-based intervention. *Psychosomatic Medicine, 65,* 1038-46.

Claar, R. J., & Blumenthal, J. A. (2003). The value of stress-management interventions in life-threatening medical conditions. *Current Directions in Psychological Science, 12,* 133-137.

Cruess, D. G., Antoni, M. H., Kumar, M., Ironson, G., McCabe, P., Fernandez, J. B., Fletcher, M., & Schneiderman, N. (1999). Cognitive-behavioral stress management buffers decreases in dehydroepiandrosterone sulfate (DHEA-S) and increases in the cortisol/DHEA-S ratio and reduces mood disturbance and perceived stress among HIV-seropositive men. *Psychoneuroendocrinology, 24,* 537-49.

Cruess, D. G., Antoni, M. H., Kumar, M., McGregor, B., Alferi, S., Boyers, A. E., Carver, C. S., & Kilbourn, K. (2001). Effects of stress management on testosterone levels in women with early-stage breast cancer. *International Journal of Behavioral Medicine, 8,* 194-207.

Cruess, D. G., Antoni, M. H., Kumar, M., & Schneiderman, N. (2000). Reductions in salivary cortisol are associated with mood improvement during relaxation training among HIV-seropositive men. *Journal of Behavioral Medicine, 23,* 107-122.

Cruess, D. G., Antoni, M. H., McGregor, B. A., Kilbourn, K. M., Boyers, A. E., Alferi, S. M., Carver, C. S., & Kumar, M. (2000). Cognitive-behavioral stress management reduces serum cortisol by enhancing benefit among women being treated for early stage breast cancer. *Psychosomatic Medicine, 62,* 304–308.

Cruess, D. G., Antoni, M. H., Schneiderman, N., Ironson, G., McCabe, P., Fernandez, J. B., Cruess, S. E., Klimas, N., & Kumar, M. (2000). Cognitive-behavioral stress management increases free testosterone and decreases psychological distress in HIV-seropositive men. *Health Psychology, 19,* 12-20.

Cruess, S., Antoni, M., Cruess, D., Fletcher, M. A., Ironson, G., Kumar, M., Lutgendorf, S., Hayes, A., Klimas, N., & Schneiderman, N. (2000). Reductions in herpes simplex virus type 2 antibody titers after cognitive behavioral stress management and relationships with neuroendocrine function, relaxation skills, and social support in HIV-positive men. *Psychosomatic Medicine, 62,* 828-37.

Cunningham, A. J., Edmonds, C. V. I., Jenkins, G. P., Pollack, H., Lockwood, G. A., & Warr, D. (1998). A randomized controlled trial of the effects of group psychological therapy on survival in women with metastatic breast cancer. *Psycho-Oncology, 7,* 508–517.

Deepak, K. K., Manchanda, S. K., & Maheshwari, M. C. (1994). Meditation improves clinicoelectroencephalographic measures in drug-resistant epileptics. *Biofeedback Self Regulation, 19,* 25–40.

Edelman, S., Lemon, J., Bell, D. R., & Kidman, A. D. (1999). Effects of group CBT on the survival time of patient with metastatic breast cancer. *Psycho-Oncology, 8,* 474–481.

Eller, L. S. (1995). Effects of two cognitive-behavioral interventions on immunity and symptoms in persons with HIV. *Annals of Behavioral Medicine, 171,* 339-348.

Fawzy, F. I., Canada, A. L., & Fawzy, N. W. (2003). Malignant melanoma: Effects of a brief, structured psychiatric intervention on survival and recurrence at 10-year follow-up. *Archives of General Psychiatry, 60,* 100-103.

Fawzy, F. I., Cousins, N., Fawzy, N. W., Kemeny, M. E., Elashoff, R., & Morton, D. (1990). A structured psychiatric intervention for cancer patients: I. Changes over time in methods of coping and affective disturbance. *Archives of General Psychiatry, 47,* 720–725.

Fawzy, F. I., Fawzy, N. W., Arndt, L. A., & Pasnau, R. O. (1995). Critical review of psychosocial interventions in cancer care. *Archives of General Psychiatry, 52,* 100-113.

Fawzy, F. I., Fawzy, N. W., Hyun, C. S., Elashoff, R., Guthrie, D., Fahey, J. L., & Morton, D. L. (1993). Malignant melanoma: Effects of a structured psychiatric intervention, coping, and affective state on recurrence and survival six years later. *Archives of General Psychiatry, 50,* 681–689.

Folkman, S. (1999). Thoughts about psychological factors, PNI, and cancer. *Advances in Mind-Body Medicine, 15,* 236-281.

Fox, B. H. (1998). A hypothesis about Spiegel et al.'s (1989) paper on psychosocial intervention and breast cancer survival. *Psycho-Oncology, 7,* 361–370.

Garcia-Vega, E., & Fernandez-Rodriguez, C. (2004). A stress management programme for Crohn's disease. *Behaviour Research & Therapy, 42,* 367-383.

Goodwin, P. J., Leszcz, M., Ennis, M., Koopmans, J., Vincent, L., Guther, H., Drysdale, E., Hundleby, M., Chochinov, H. M., Navarro, M., Speca, M., & Hunter, J. (2001). The effect of group psychosocial support on survival in metastatic breast cancer. *New England Journal of Medicine, 345,* 1719-1726.

Holroyd, K. A., O'Donnell, F. J., Stensland, M., Lipchik, G. L., Cordingley, G. E., & Carlson, B. W. (2001). Management of chronic tension-type headache with tricyclic antidepressant medication, stress management therapy, and their combination: A randomized controlled trial. *Journal of the American Medical Association, 285,* 2208-2215.

Ironson, G., Field, T., Scafidi, F., Hashimoto, M., Kumar, M., Kumar, A., Price, A., Goncalves, A., Burman I., Tetenman, C., Patarca, R., & Fletcher, M. A. (1996). Massage therapy is associated with enhancement of the immune system's cytotoxic capacity. *Neuroscience, 84,* 205-217.

Ironson, G., Friedman, A., Klimas, N., Antoni, M., Fletcher, M. A., LaPerriere, A., Simoneau, J., & Schneiderman, N. (1994). Distress, denial, and low adherence to behavioral interventions predict faster disease progression in gay men infected with human immunodeficiency virus. *International Journal of Behavioral Medicine, 1,* 90-105.

Jones, D. L., Ishii, M., LaPerriere, A., Stanley, H., Antoni, M., Ironson, G., Schneiderman, N., Van Splunteren, F., Cassells, A., Alexander, K., Gousse, Y. P., Vaughn, A., Brondolo, E., Tobin, J. N., & Weiss, S. M. (2003). Influencing medication adherence among women with AIDS. *AIDS Care, 15,* 463-474.

Kelley, J. E., Lumley, M. A., & Leisen, J. C. (1997). Health effects of emotional disclosure in rheumatoid arthritis patients. *Health Psychology, 16,* 331-340.

Kemeny, M. E. (2003). The psychobiology of stress. *Current Directions in Psychological Science, 12,* 124-129.

LaPerriere, A. R., Antoni, M. H., Schneiderman, N., Ironson, G., Klimas, N., Caralis, P., & Fletcher, M. A. (1990). Exercise intervention attenuates emotional distress and natural killer cell decrements following notification of positive serologic status for HIV-1. *Biofeedback and Self Regulation, 15,* 229-242.

Leserman, J. (2003). The effects of stressful life events, coping, and cortisol on HIV infection. *CNS Spectrum, 8,* 25-30.

Linden, W., Stossel, C., & Maurice, J. (1996). Psychosocial interventions for patients with coronary artery disease: A meta-analysis. *Archives of Internal Medicine, 156,* 745-752.

Lutgendorf, S. K., Antoni, M. H., Ironson, G., Klimas, N., Kumar, M., Starr, K., McCabe, P., Cleven, K., Fletcher, M. A., & Schneiderman, N. (1997). Cognitive-behavioral stress management decreases dysphoric mood and herpes simplex virus-type 2 antibody titers in symptomatic HIV-seropositive gay men. *Journal of Consulting & Clinical Psychology, 65,* 31-43.

McGregor, B. A., Antoni, M. H., Boyers, A., Alferi, S. M., Blomberg, B. B., & Carver, C. S. (2004). Cognitive-behavioral stress management increases benefit finding and immune function among women with early-stage breast cancer. *Journal of Psychosomatic Research, 56,* 1-8.

Nicholas, P. K., & Webster, A. (1996). A behavioral medicine intervention in persons with HIV. *Clinical Nursing Research, 5,* 391-406.

O'Cleirigh, C., Ironson, G., Antoni, M., Fletcher, M. A., McGuffey, L., Balbin, E., Schneiderman, N., & Solomon, G. (2003). Emotional expression and depth processing of trauma and their relation to long-term survival in patients with HIV/AIDS. *Journal of Psychosomatic Research, 54,* 225-235.

Palmer, S. C., & Coyne, J. C. (2004). Examining the evidence that psychotherapy improves the survival of cancer patients. *Biological Psychiatry, 56, 61-62.*

Penedo, F. J., Dahn, J. R., Molton, I., Gonzalez, J. S., Kinsinger, D., Roos, B. A., Carver, C. S., Schneiderman, N., & Antoni, M. H. (2004). Cognitive-behavioral stress management improves stress-management skills and quality of life in men recovering from treatment of prostate carcinoma. *Cancer, 100,* 192-200.

Petrie, K. J., Fontanilla, I., Thomas, M. G., Booth, R. J., & Pennebaker, J. W. (2004). Effect of written emotional expression on immune function in patients with human immunodeficiency virus infection: A randomized trial. *Psychosomatic Medicine, 66,* 272-275.

Robinson, F. P., Mathews, H. L., & Witek-Janusek, L. (2000). Stress reduction and HIV disease: A review of intervention studies using a psychoneuroimmunology framework. *Journal of Associated Nurses in AIDS Care, 11,* 87-96.

Rutledge, T., & Loh, C. (2004). Effect sizes and statistical testing in the determination of clinical significance in behavioral medicine research. *Annals of Behavioral Medicine, 27,* 138-145.

Schneider, R. H., Staggers, F., Alexander, C. N., Sheppard, W., Rainforth, M., Kondwani, K., Smith, S., & King, C. G. (1995). A randomised controlled trial of stress reduction for hypertension in older African Americans. *Hypertension, 26,* 820–827.

Smyth, J. M., Stone, A. A., Hurewitz, A., & Kaell, A. (1999). Effects of writing about stressful experiences on symptom reduction in patients with asthma or rheumatoid arthritis: A randomized trial. *Journal of the American Medical Association, 281,* 1304-1309.

Speca, M., & Carlson, L. E., Goodey, E., & Angen, M. A. (2000). A randomized, wait-list controlled clinical trial: The effect of a mindfulness meditation-based stress reduction program on mood and symptoms of stress in cancer outpatients. *Psychosomatic Medicine, 62,* 613-622.

Spiegel, D., & Giese-Davis, J. (in press). Examining the evidence that psychotherapy improves the survival of cancer patients: A reply. *Biological Psychiatry, 56,* 62-64.

Spiegel, D., Kraemer, H. C., Bloom, J. R , & Gottheil, E. (1989). Effect of psychosocial treatment on survival of patients with metastatic breast cancer. *Lancet, 334,* 888–891.

Stanton, A. L., Danoff-Burg, S., Sworowski, L. A., Collins, C. A., Branstetter, A. D., Rodriguez-Hanley, A., Kirk, S. B., & Austenfeld, J. L. (2002). Randomized, controlled trial of written emotional expression and benefit finding in breast cancer patients. *Journal of Clinical Oncology, 20,* 4160-4168.

Sundin, O., Lisspers, J., Hofman-Bang, C., Nygren, A., Ryden, L., & Ohman, A. (2003). Comparing multifactorial lifestyle interventions and stress management in coronary risk reduction. *International Journal of Behavioral Medicine, 10,* 191-204.

Taylor, D. N. (1995). Effects of a behavioral stress-management program on anxiety, mood, self-esteem, and T-cell count in HIV-positive men. *Psychological Report, 76,* 451-457.

Trask, P. C., Paterson, A. G., Griffith, K. A., Riba, M. B., & Schwartz, J. L. (2003). Cognitive-behavioral intervention for distress in patients with melanoma: comparison with standard medical care and impact on quality of life. *Cancer, 98,* 854-864.

Walker, B. L., Nail, L. M., & Croyle, R. T. (1999). Does emotional expression make a difference in reactions to breast cancer? *Oncology Nursing Forum, 26,* 1025-1032.

Weiss, J. L., Mulder, C. L., Antoni, M. H., de Vroome, E. M., Garssen, B., & Goodkin, K. (2003). Effects of a supportive-expressive group intervention on long-term psychosocial adjustment in HIV-infected gay men. *Psychotherapy and Psychosomatics, 72,* 132-140.

In: Psychology of Stress
Editor: Kimberly V. Oxington, pp. 53-82

Chapter IV

PHYSICAL HEALTH OUTCOMES OF PSYCHOLOGIC STRESS BY PARENTAL BEREAVEMENT: A NATIONAL PERSPECTIVE IN DENMARK

Jiong Li[1,2] and Jorn Olsen[2]

[1] Centre for Health Research and Psycho-oncology, NSW Cancer Council, University of Newcastle, Wallsend NSW 2287, Australia
[2]Danish Epidemiology Science Centre, Department of Epidemiology and Social Medicine, University of Aarhus, Denmark

ABSTRACT

Background

Bereavement represents a specific type of stressful life events. It could be detrimental to health both in the short-term and in the long run. The aim of the studies is to examine the possible health effects of parental bereavement. Only severe health consequences that may lead to death or hospitalization were studied.

Methods

The studies were based on a follow-up of cohorts from nationwide registers. We enrolled the 21,062 parents who lost a young child (below 18 years of age) in Denmark from 1980-96 into the exposed cohort, and 293,745 parents who did not lose a child to the unexposed cohort. Outcomes of interest were mortality, myocardial infarction (MI), stroke, cancer incidence, cancer survival, multiple sclerosis (MS) and inflammatory bowel diseases (IBD). Cox's proportional-hazards regression models were used to evaluate the relative risks.

Results

We observed a significantly increased mortality risk in bereaved mothers (HR 1.43, 95% CI 1.24-1.64), but not in bereaved fathers (HR 1.09, 0.95-1.23). The RRs for first MI event and MS were 1.28 (1.08-1.51) and 1.56 (1.05-2.31), respectively. A slightly increased cancer risk was observed (1.09, 0.99-1.20) in bereaved parents. The HR of dying from an incident of cancer in the bereaved was 1.23 (1.03-1.47). The risks of stroke and inflammatory bowel disease (IBD) in the bereaved parents were identical to that in non-bereaved.

Conclusions

We observed an increased mortality in bereaved mothers. The death of a child may lead to an increased risk of MI, MS, and a mildly increased risk of cancer as well as worse cancer survival in bereaved parents. The life event is not associated with the risk of stroke and IBD.

BACKGROUND

Definition of Stress

Systematic considerations of the possible effects of stress can be traced to the work of Cannon and Selye in the early 1930s. Cannon studied the effects of physical or emotional "stress" in his work on blood hormones, by which he meant stimuli that disrupted an individual's normal internal environment [1]. Selye's initial work used "stress" as a synonym for "stimulus", too. Later he proposed that the term referred, instead, to the non-specific response of an individual to such stimuli, which he called "stressors" [2,3]. With the fast development of stress research in the past several decades, researchers within the fields of psychology, physiology, social and behavioural sciences have produced a number of broad and narrow definitions of stress within the fields of psychology, physiology, social and behavioural sciences has been described by researchers. Lazarus and Foldman defined stress as a result of an imbalance between demands and resources[4]. Cox defined stress as "a perceptual phenomenon arsing from a comparison between the demand and coping ability" [5]. McGrath described the "overload" definition of stress as the result of environmental demands that are too heavy for the individual [6]. Levine suggested that stress is "anything that induces increased secretion of glucorticiods" [7]. A recent definition of stress by McEwen referred to "events, that are threatening to an individual, and which elicit physiological and behavioural responses" [8].

The choice of definition depends on either the psychosocial or psychobiological aspect of the stress in focus. The term encompasses both the stimulus (e.g., a biologic event like an infection and a social event like a change of residences, or merely a disturbing thought) and its effects, ranging from no effect, to a psychological response (anxiety, depression), physiological change, or even possibly disease activation, or any combination. Individuals may interpret a stressor as desirable or undesirable, for example, pain, sex, or threat of injury, for instance, usually elicits predictable responses. On the other hand, life events and other psychological processes have more varied effects, for example, a change of jobs may be of little concern to one person, yet lead to crisis in another person who views the event as a personal failure. Both a person's interpretation of an event as stressful or not and his/her response to it depend on one's personality, prior experience, attitudes, coping capacity, culture, general state of physical health, and genetic susceptibility [9]. Therefore, stress is often difficult to understand and even harder to study. However, over the last few decades, the innovation in strategies to refine concepts, measures, and research designs in the study of life experiences and health keeps improving the understanding of the association between stress and health [10-12].

Life Events Research on Health

Stressful experiences often include major life events, trauma, and, abuse, and they are sometimes related to the environment in the workplace, neighbourhood, or home. Sudden traumas are at the most discrete end. This class of stressor includes single, unanticipated, and overwhelming experience and they are discrete because the onset and offset of the stressor are often short-term by nature, e.g., natural disasters or severe accidents. Life change events are normally represented as slightly less discrete on average than sudden traumas, e.g., divorce and serious illnesses, although some of the classic life events are more like traumas in terms of discreteness. Stress related to macro systems or the environment in the workplace, neighbourhood and home is often treated as chronic, together with non-events and other chronic stressors.

In their earlier works in the 1930s, Canon and Selye suggested that experimental stimuli produce adaptive physiological responses in animals [2,3]. The first human life experience of stress research involved the reactions of soldiers to battlefield traumas during World War II [13]. However due to the lack of good research models to measure life stress, the next two decades did not bring any major progresses. In the 1960s, the initial effort by Holmes and Rahe's Schedule of Recent Experiences (SRE) [14] broadened stress research to include catastrophic events arising in almost everyone's life. Their introduction of life events scales reactivated research on stress and disease and made it possible for investigators to examine the associations between events and a variety of disease outcomes. This checklist approach has been widely accepted across the world [11]. Numerous newer checklist instruments have also been developed in response to the concerns over the methodological flaws of the SRE, although most of them suffer from many of the shortcomings of their predecessors [11, 12]. Whereas Holmes and Rahe based their framework on a physiological understanding of the consequences of adaptation and change, Brown and colleagues used the Life Events and Difficulties Schedule (LEDS) [12] and concentrated on the psychological meaning of life events and the emotions they produce. This interview-based approach brought to light the importance of "expressed emotion", and it has contributed to the recent increasing interest in life events research. The LEDS possesses a number of methodological advances and it has been increasingly applied in the investigation of the relationship between stress and many health outcomes, e.g. psychiatric illness like depression, anxiety, schizophrenia, and physical illness like multiple sclerosis, myocardial infarction, appendectomy, abdominal pain, etc [12].

Studies on major life events can be, on one hand, divided into two groups, the aggregate life event studies (e.g. studies based on SRE [14] or LEDS [12]) and the studies focusing on single events (e.g. bereavement, job loss, retirement, divorce, etc). On the other hand, there are studies that focus on short-term effects on health and others that investigate long-term effects.

Earlier studies of life events on health have been concerned mainly with acute or short-term effects of life events (e.g. aggregate life event studies by SRE or LEDS, and some studies focusing on the short-term effect of specific life events, e.g., the consequences of unemployment, retirement, and especially widowhood). However, during the past two decades we have seen a new interest in the chronic or long-term effects of stress. This interest draws on a long-standing research tradition that has studied the health-damaging effects of chronic work stress, chronic strains, on-going difficulties, stress in organizations, war-related trauma, and long-term stress in daily life.

Biological Mechanisms Underlying the Association Between Stress and Health

Controversy has always been a part of stress research because of the complexity of concepts, measures and research designs. In the late 1980s, Heston stated that there was no compelling evidence to support a causal association between stressful life circumstances and illness. He also urged for a reorientation of the stress research into redistribution of "human and material resources to hard ball biology" [15]. With the rapid progress in biological science in the last two decades, an explosion of research has been published on the underlying mechanisms of relationships between stress and health outcomes.

The biological response to stress is the set of neural and endocrine adaptations that restore the body systems through changes. The immediate and acute stress response is the activation of the autonomic nervous system (fight or flight response). This 5 to 10 minute long process releases hormones such as norepinephrine and epinephrine, which maintain a readiness state for between 1 to 2 hours [9, 16]. The long-term stress response involves a series of systems, including the central and peripheral neural system, the hypothalamic-pituitary-adrenal (HPA) axis, the sympathetic adrenomedullary systems, and immune systems, which interact to mediate the stress response. [9,16] The main proposed mechanisms involve:

- HPA axis and neuroendocrine-immune changes
- Homeostasis and allostasis

HPA Axis and Neuroendocrine-Immune Pathways

The main axes of neuroendocrine response are the HPA axis, and the sympathetic adrenomedullary system. The HPA axis is led by the hippocampus, a region of the brain that exerts an inhibitory effect on the secretion of corticotrophin releasing hormone (CRH). The hypothalamus releases CRH, which stimulates corticotrophins-cells in the pituitary secreting adrenocorticotrophic hormone (ACTH). ACTH induces the adrenal cortex to secrete cortisol, which acts on the hypothalamus and the hippocampus in a negative feedback loop (by binding to glucocorticoid receptors) to decrease CRH release. The sympathetic adrenomedullary system is located in the medulla (center) of the adrenal gland, which secretes catecholamines-norepinephrine (NE) and epinephrine (E), with NE additionally found in neurons secreting neuropeptide Y (NPY). The metabolism of these hormones interacts with the HPA axis. Psychological stress could affect the function of the central nervous system and its hormonal and cellular inflammatory / immune connections in a variety of body systems. Acute stress could activate the HPA and end a negative feedback loop to the brain. The body then shuts off the hormonal stress response and restores a steady state. With chronic stressors, this negative feedback mechanism is comprised by a larger hypothalamic production of CRH and a reduction of the number of cortisol receptors. This leads to hippocampal neuronal damage, loss of inhibitory cortisol feedback, and perpetually increased serum cortisol levels, which are related to many deleterious effects on body systems [9,16,17].

Homeostasis and Allostasis / Allostatic Load

The term "homeostasis" refers to the feedback mechanisms that maintain constant internal conditions in the face of environmental change [9,16,18]. Homeostatic systems such as blood oxygen, blood PH, and body temperature are often maintained within narrow ranges. The concept of allostasis, the ability to achieve physiological stability through change, extends the idea of homeostasis to include broader processes leading to disease [9]. The long-term effect of the physiological response to stress has been referred to as allostatic load. It is the price that the body pays for the adjustments. A stressful life event like bereavement may challenge the neuroendocrine systems to an extent that a cascade of secretion of hormonal changes is activated. That may cause short- and long-term interruptions in the hormonal balance, leading to an allostatic load that results from the chronic over-activity or under-activity of body systems. Emotional and behavioural changes following an exposure to stress could also influence the balance of hormones, and on the other hand, the imbalance of this internal environment may further affect the emotions and behaviour in men [9,16,18]. These interactions could have adverse effects on various systems and lead to diseases in the long run.

Epidemiological Studies on the Association Between Psychological Stress and Clinical Health Outcomes, and Possible Biological Pathways

Much research has been conducted on the association between stress and the onset and course of many diseases like cardiovascular diseases, autoimmune diseases, infectious diseases, malignant diseases, etc. Some have also studied the specific mechanisms of these associations.

Myocardial Infarction (MI) and Stroke

The most extensive literature has been based on the association between stress and coronary heart disease (CHD) [9,12,18]. Two recent reviews by Rozanski et al [19] and Hemingway and Marmot [20] connect various psychosocial factors, e.g., depression and anxiety, personality factors, social isolation, work characteristics, and chronic life stress with CHD.

Short-term stress could act as a trigger of MI in already predisposed individuals [21]. However, the long-term effect has become a major concern for the understanding of the aetiological role of stress in the development of CHD [19,20]. The application of longitudinal design in life events research provided valuable insight into this association. Recent work has developed operational and theoretical models, e.g., the job-control-demands-support model, effort-reward imbalance, to explore the effects of stress on CHD [19,20]. In addition, researchers have shown that stress could lead to various pathophysiological effects, such as myocardial ischemia, arrhythmogenesis, platelet and endothelial dysfunction, accelerated development of coronary artery atherosclerosis, and even necrosis [19,20]. The body of evidence for the association has increased continuously for the past two decades.

On the other hand, Macleod recently argued that psychological stress is an important determinant of coronary heart disease may be spurious [22]. His study, which was based on the use of a superficial subjective scale for exposure (Reeder stress inventory) and self-reported angina (Rose questionnaire), has provoked substantial debate [23]. The discussion echoes Heston's [15] criticism of life events research once more, raising the concern that previous studies have been suffering from methodological limitations [24].

In contrast to the large body of evidence on the association between stress and CHD, few have examined the effect of stress on stroke, and the existing evidence remains inconclusive. Depressive symptoms and self-reported stress were reported to be associated with an increased risk of stroke [25,26]. However, one study by Abel et al reported lack of an association between social readjustment and stroke [27].

Cancer Incidence and Survival

The belief that psychological stress causes cancer has a long history [28], however, so far the scientific evidence for such an association remains contradictory [29]. Some case-control studies have shown that stress has a strong effect on the incidence of cancer [30], while others reported negative findings [31]. Most cohort studies have shown no evidence of an association [32,33], but two recent studies showed an increased risk of breast cancer [34,35].

Some have pointed out the underlying biological mechanisms of the association, e.g., stress could influence tumour growth and metastasis by increasing the level of corticosterone, prolactin, oestrogen, or by decreasing the number and activity of lymphocytes and natural killer (NK) cells [36].

Multiple Sclerosis

Psychological stress has been suggested to be associated with MS since the 19th century [37]. Warren and Grant reported that more stressful life events have been reported in MS patients than in controls [38], and that an increased occurrence of life events was found to precede disease exacerbations in several other studies [38]. However, Nisipeanu and Korczyn documented that stress caused by the threat of missile attacks during the Gulf War of 1991 did not produce increased numbers of relapses [39]. The discrepancies in findings may be explained by methodological variations and limitations in these studies. There is a need for well-designed follow-up studies using a more rigorous definition of stress exposure [38].

Some have observed that stress disrupts the blood-brain-barrier [40], others have observed the stress-induced alterations of the cytokine production and T cell activation against CNS protein in MS patients [41]. Down-regulation of the immune system like higher CD4+ cell numbers and percentage [42], and increased activity of hypothalamic corticotropin-releasing hormone neurons have been found in MS patients [43].

Other Autoimmune Diseases

Inflammatory bowel disease (IBD) has been related to stress for decades [44]. In some case-series studies, higher proportions of psychological symptoms have been reported, and psychosocial stress is suggested to lead to the onset or exacerbation of IBD [44]. Two case-control studies reported more symptoms of depression, anxiety, or psychopathological diagnoses in IBD patients, yet another two case-control studies found no differences in terms of stress [44]. *Psoriasis* has also been related to stress. Studies evaluating the effects of stress on the course of psoriasis support the role of stress as a modulator of disease and suggest that the severity of the stressor may be associated with the severity of the disease [45]. Other autoimmune diseases that have been proposed to be associated with psychological stress include *Rheumatoid arthritis (RA), Graves' thyroid disease*, and *insulin-dependent diabetes mellitus (IDDM)* [46-48]. However, the evidence supporting these associations is still weak due to the limitations in previous studies.

Infectious Diseases

Several studies have suggested that high levels of stress can increase an individual's susceptibility to infection, usually an upper respiratory viral infection like *the common cold* [49]. Stress-induced immune alterations may be associated with an increased susceptibility to activation of latent infection by the Epstein-Barr virus (EPV), and the human immunodeficiency virus (HIV) [50,51].

Conclusions Leading to the Present Study

Research into stress and health has always faced methodological challenges, such as: 1) Inconsistent definition and assessment of stress exposure. Different stress measures often yield conflicting results, making it difficult to compare or draw conclusions. 2) The intermixture of chronic stressors and acute stressors, which are often reported in life-event inventories. This makes the ascertainment of a clearly ordered temporal association between life events and health outcomes quite complicated because many physical and psychiatric diseases often take many years to develop. 3) Differential recall bias. Bias could hardly be disregarded in a case-control design or even in a longitudinal study where data are often obtained from self-reports or interviews. 4) Insufficient statistical power [11,15,22].

Parental bereavement is usually considered the most severe of all stressful life events [52-54]. Although most of the bereaved parents manage to come through this life event and find a path back to normal life, almost all have been affected deeply and permanently by the loss. The grief process incorporates diverse psychological and physical manifestations [52,55-58]. Consequently, the affected parents could be exposed to a higher disease and mortality risk. Furthermore, bereavement may lead to more adverse lifestyle behaviours that may result in various adverse health outcomes [60-62].

However, so far no study has systematically examined the effect of the death of a child on clinical health consequences in bereaved parents. Most published studies are small in size and often with limited follow-up. In addition, most studies have focused on short-term effects, mainly in terms of psychiatric, psychological, and somatic responses in affected parents [52,55].

Furthermore, very few clinical health outcomes, e.g., mortality, cancer, and some psychiatric disorders, have been investigated as primary endpoints in previous studies.

The death of a child is a single and objective event, and it has been ranked as one of the most severe and stressful life events [52,59]. This event may stress anybody regardless of coping capacities. By using this exposure, we expect to achieve a rather large stress exposure contrast. Several studies have examined the effect of miscarriage, the death of an infant, and the death of adult children, but the information on the effects of the loss of a young child is sparse.

In a country with a low infant and childhood mortality, a follow-up study needs a large study base and it may be difficult or even impossible to get this vulnerable group to follow a study protocol over long periods of time. Selection bias related to non-response to recruitment or compliance may easily invalidate internal inference, and long-term follow-up may be impossible in many countries. In the Nordic countries, register-based research could overcome these problems [63,64]. The price to pay for a register-based study is the limited options for confounder control, which, however, may be a smaller problem than selection bias, especially if the principles of deconfounding have been used.

We selected the endpoints of interest as both physical illness like cancer, vascular diseases, MS, and psychiatric illness, primarily according to the hypotheses based on the possible biological mechanisms [11,12,52]. We did not include some endpoints due to the limited number of cases or due to incomplete information in the registers.

AIM OF THE STUDIES

The overall aim of the study is to investigate and quantify the effect of the death of a child on physical health in bereaved parents.

The specific aims are to examine the effect of the death of a child in bereaved parents on the following health outcomes: overall and specific mortality, myocardial infarction (MI), stroke, cancer incidence, cancer survival, multiple sclerosis (MS), inflammatory bowel disease (IBD).

MATERIAL AND METHODS

Study Design and Participants

The study is based on the follow-up of cohorts identified from national registers in Denmark [65-71]. First we identified all children who died aged 17 or less from the Fertility

Database for each year from 1980 to 1996 [65-71]. A total of 12,512 deceased children were identified and linked to their first degree relatives by their CPR numbers. There were 440 children who had no links to any family, and the remaining 12,072 were linked to 12,037 families (35 children were from families with multiple cases), and 35,041 members from these families were included into the exposed cohort [65-71].

From the Fertility Database and for each exposed family, we randomly selected from the remaining population 15 families that did not have a deceased child below the age of 18 in the same calendar year. The matching was based on the family structure (family size, number of parents in the family, number of children in six age groups (less than 1 year, 1–2 years, 3–6 years, 7–9 years, 10–14 years, and 15–17 years) on January 1st of the year when the child died. In total, 184,413 families were found. The age matching criteria was relaxed for 1,981 families to keep the 1:15 ratio. Altogether 537,754 persons from these families were recruited to the unexposed cohort.

Information on the deceased children (age, sex, date of birth, date of death, cause of death) was obtained from the Fertility Database. Information on cohort members (date of birth, date of death, gender, school education, place of residence, cause of death, hospital records with date of admission, days in hospital, diagnosis at discharge, etc) was obtained from the Prevention Register, the Cancer Registry, and the Multiple Sclerosis Registry [65-71]. All register linkages were made by means of the CPR number. At the beginning, 19,361 parents were in the exposed cohort and 295,540 parents were in the unexposed cohort. During the follow-up, 1,701 unexposed parents lost a child and they were subsequently included into the exposed cohort. Due to incomplete information another 94 unexposed parents were further excluded. In the end we had 21,062 parents in the exposed cohort, and 293,745 parents in the unexposed cohort. The process of identification of cohorts and extraction of information are summarized in Figure 1.

Outcomes, Follow-Up and Statistical Analysis

Mortality

The main outcomes of interest in the mortality study were overall mortality (Danish version of ICD 8 codes 000-799, E800-E999 for the period 1980-1993, ICD 10 codes A00-R99, V01-Y98 for the period 1994-1997) and cause-specific mortality (natural deaths, ICD8 codes 000-799, ICD10 codes A00-R99, unnatural codes ICD8 codes E800-E999, ICD10 codes V01-Y98).

The follow-up started when the participants were recruited to the cohorts and ended when they died, emigrated, or at the end of 1997 when the follow-up ended, whichever came first. Survival analyses were performed using Cox proportional-hazards regression to estimate Hazards ratios (HRs) [67]. For parents who changed exposure status, a time-dependant variable for exposure was included in the models. Potential confounders (age, sex, school education, residence, number of children in the family, and number of parents in the family) were included in the models. We examined the differences in mortality between the exposed and the unexposed cohort members by gender of the parents (male, female), duration of follow-up (1-3 years, 4-8 years, 9-18 years), and also the three characteristics relating to the deceased child (age of the child [<1 month, 1-1 months, 1-2 years, 3-9 years, 10-17 years], cause of death [natural death, unnatural death as described above], type of death [unexpected death[1], other death]).

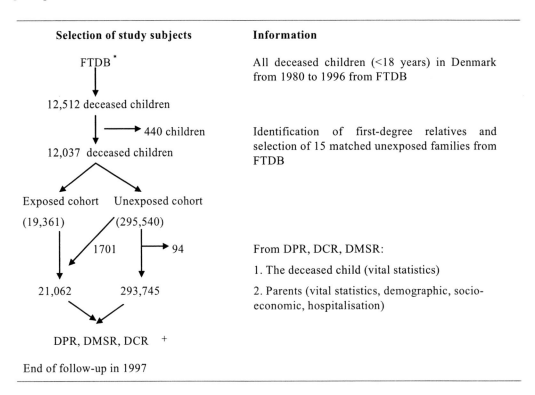

<table>
</table>

Selection of study subjects   **Information**

FTDB* — All deceased children (<18 years) in Denmark from 1980 to 1996 from FTDB

12,512 deceased children

440 children — Identification of first-degree relatives and selection of 15 matched unexposed families from FTDB

12,037 deceased children

Exposed cohort   Unexposed cohort
(19,361)   (295,540)

1701   94   —   From DPR, DCR, DMSR:
                          1. The deceased child (vital statistics)
21,062   293,745   2. Parents (vital statistics, demographic, socio-economic, hospitalisation)

DPR, DMSR, DCR +

End of follow-up in 1997

* FTDB = Fertility Database
+ DPR = Danish Prevention Register, DCR = Danish Cancer Registry, DMSR=Danish Multiple Sclerosis Registry

Figure 1 Identification of cohorts and extraction of information

Myocardial Infarction (MI)

The outcome of interest was MI as coded by the International Classification of Diseases (ICD), ICD 8 codes 4100 to 4109 for the period 1980-1993, and ICD 10 code I21 for the period 1994-1996. We recorded two MI events, namely, fatal MI and first MI. First MI during follow-up was either a hospitalisation due to MI or a MI death, whichever occurred first.

The follow-up started at study entry and ended at death, emigration, date of MI, or at the end of 1996, whichever came first. The relative risks (RRs) were obtained using the Cox proportional hazards regression model [65]. Several potential confounders (age, sex, school education, residence, number of children in the family, number of parents in the family, previous hospitalisation for hypertension, prior hospitalisation for diabetes) were included in

[1] unexpected death: sudden unexpected death, ICD 8 codes 795, ICD 10 codes R95-R97, motor vehicle accidents, ICD8 codes E810-E823, ICD10 codes V01-V89, suicide, ICD 8 codes E950-E959, ICD 10 codes X60-X84, and other accidents and violence, ICD8 codes E800-E807, E825-E949, E960-E999, ICD 10 codes V90-V99, W00-X59, X85-Y89.

the models. For parents who changed exposure status, a time-dependant variable for exposure was included in the models.

Stroke

All incident cases with discharge diagnoses of subarachnoid hemorrhage, intracerebral hemorrhage, ischemic stroke, and unspecified stroke were identified. All incident cases with discharge diagnoses of subarachnoid hemorrhage (ICD-8 code 430, ICD-10 code I60), intracerebral hemorrhage (ICD-8 code 431, ICD-10 code I61), ischemic stroke (ICD-8 codes 433, 434, ICD-10 code I63), and unspecified stroke (ICD-8 code 436, ICD-10 code I64) were identified from the register. We classified the stroke as fatal when stroke was listed as the primary or underlying cause of death.

The follow-up started when the participants were recruited to the cohorts, and ended on the date of stroke, death, emigration, or at the end of 1997, whichever came first. The RRs were calculated using the Cox proportional hazards regression models. Potential confounders were those in the MI study together with a variable for prior MI hospitalisation (yes, no) [69].

Cancer Incidence

The main outcomes of interest were: all incident cancers, breast cancer, smoking-related cancers (ICD 7 codes 140, 141, 143-149, 150, 157, 160-162, 180 and 181), alcohol-related cancers (ICD 7 codes 141, 143-146, 148-150, 155, 161), virus/immune-related cancers (ICD 7 codes 155, 171, 191, 200-202, 204), lymphatic/hematopoietic cancers (ICD 7 codes 200-205) and hormone related cancers (ICD 7 codes 170, 172, 175, 177).

The follow-up started when the participants were recruited to the cohorts and ended when they were diagnosed with cancer, died, emigrated, or at the end of 1997, whichever came first. The RRs were calculated using Cox proportional-hazards regression. The same potential confounders in the mortality study were included in the analyses [66].

Cancer Survival

The main outcomes of interest were overall cancer survival, survival for site-specific cancers, and five subgroups of cancers in which stress could play a role in the aetiology: smoking-related cancers (ICD7 codes 140, 141, 143-150, 157, 160-162, 180 and 181), alcohol-related cancers (ICD7 codes 141, 143-146, 148-150, 155 and 161), virus and immune-related cancers (ICD 7 codes 155, 171, 191, 200-202, 204), lymphatic/haematopoietic tissue cancers (ICD 7 codes 200-205) and hormone-related cancers (ICD 7 codes 170, 172, 175, 177).

Among all bereaved parents, 461 had a subsequent incident of cancer and they were selected to the exposed cohort. Among the parents who did not lose a child, 6,237 had an incident of cancer after the recruitment and they were included into the unexposed cohort. The follow-up started when the participants were diagnosed with cancer and ended at date of death, emigration, or 31 December 1997, whichever came first. The hazard ratio (HRs) of dying from cancer were estimated by Cox regression, and the same potential confounders as in the cancer incidence study were included in the analyses [68].

Multiple Sclerosis

The outcome of interest was diagnosed MS as recorded in the Danish Multiple Sclerosis Registry (DMSR). The follow-up started when the participants were recruited to the cohorts and ended when they died, emigrated, were diagnosed with MS, or at the end of 1997, whichever came first. The RRs were calculated using the Cox proportional hazards regression model. The same potential confounders as in the mortality study were included in the models. Time from exposure to onset of MS was treated as a time-dependent variable [70].

Inflammatory Bowel Disease (IBD)

The outcome of interest was the incidence of IBD, defined as the parents' first hospitalization due to IBD (Crohn's disease, ICD 8 codes 563.01, ICD 10 codes K50.0, K50.1, K50.9; ulcerative colitis ICD 8 codes 563.19, 569.04, ICD 10 codes K51.0, K51.1, K51.2, K51.3) in their life.

The follow-up started when the participants were recruited to the cohorts and ended when they died, emigrated, were diagnosed with IBD, or at the end of 1997, whichever came first. The RRs were calculated using the Cox proportional hazards regression model. The same potential confounders as in the mortality study were included in the models [71].

RESULTS

We observed an excess mortality rate of 40.04/100,000 in the bereaved parents, and an overall crude HR of 1.22 (95%CI 1.11-1.33) during the entire follow-up period. The main contributing factor was an excess death in bereaved mothers. Accidents, suicide, and myocardial infarction are the top three contributors to excess death events among all single causes (Table 1).

The average risk of any first hospitalisation was increased slightly by 4% (HR 1.04, 95% CI 1.01-1.06), yielding an excess rate of 131.28/100,000 person years (Table 1).

Mortality

The overall adjusted mortality was increased in bereaved mothers (HR 1.43, 95% CI 1.24-1.64), but not in bereaved fathers (HR 1.09, 95% CI 0.95-1.23). The mortality risks in bereaved mothers from natural and unnatural causes were increased by 26% and 145%, respectively.

Bereaved mothers experienced the highest HR of 3.84 (2.48-5.88) during the first three years. After that the rates decreased. For natural causes, an increased mortality (44%) was observed in mothers solely during the 10th–18th year of follow-up. For bereaved fathers, we observed an adjusted relative mortality rate of 1.57 (95% CI 1.06-2.32) from unnatural causes during the first three years. Mothers who had lost a child unexpectedly had a higher adjusted HR (1.67, 95% CI 1.37-2.03) than mothers who lost a child for other reasons (HR 1.14, 95%CI 1.04-1.24) (Table 2) [67].

Table 1 Mortality and morbidity in bereaved parents 1980-1997, Denmark

Cause / site	Deaths				Hospitalisation			
	E / U*	Excess cases†	Excess rate (1/100,000) ‡	Crude hazard ratio (95%CI)	E / U*	Excess cases†	Excess rate (1/100,000) ‡	Crude hazard ratio (95%CI)
Natural causes	384/4779	47.04	21.53	1.17 (1.03-1.30)	7050/98127	131.28	60.09	0.95 (0.88-1.07)
Infectious/ parasitic disease	12/57	7.98	3.65	2.99 (1.60-5.57)	36/535	-1.72	-0.79	0.96 (0.68-1.34)
Cancer	165 /2108	16.37	7.49	1.19 (0.95-1.31)	144/2247	-14.43	-6.6	0.90 (0.76-1.07)
Benign neoplasm	3/57	-1.02	-0.46	0.75 (0.23-2.39)	172/2795	-25.07	-11.48	0.87 (0.74-1.01)
Endocrine / metabolic disease	14/104	6.67	3.05	1.91 (1.09-3.43)	103/1421	2.80	1.29	1.02 (0.84-1.25)
Anaemias, other (blood organs)	0/0	-	-	1.37 (0.82-2.29)	16/164	4.44	2.03	1.91 (1.19-3.43)
Mental disorders	11/28	9.02	4.13	2.25 (1.19-4.25)	55/699	5.71	2.62	1.11 (0.84-1.46)
Disease of nervous system, eye, adnexa	10/83	4.14	1.90	1.72 (0.89-3.31)	213/3544	-36.88	-16.88	0.85 (0.74-0.98)
Multiple sclerosis	-	-	-	-		10.28	4.71	1.65 (1.06-2.72)
Disease of the circulatory system	116/1493	10.73	4.91	1.11 (0.92-1.34)	518/7573	15.95	-7.30	0.97 (0.89-1.06)
Myocardial infarction	43/521	6.27	2.87	1.30 (0.95-1.81)	168/2096	20.22	9.25	1.21 (1.02-1.76)
Stroke	11/228	-5.08	-2.32	0.72 (0.40-1.34)	117/1670	0.25	0.11	1.01 (0.84-1.27)
Disease of respiratory system	14/225	-1.86	-0.85	0.89 (0.52-1.53)	289/3684	29.25	13.39	1.11 (0.98-1.25)

Table 1 Mortality and morbidity in bereaved parents 1980-1997, Denmark (Continued)

Disease of digestive system	68/841	8.70	3.98	1.16 (0.91-1.49)	535/7898	-21.87	-10.01	0.95 (0.87-1.04)
Diseases of the genitourinary system	4/26	2.17	0.99	2.19 (0.76-6.28)	43/6239	-396.89	-181.69	0.97 (0.88-1.07)
Complications in pregnancy, childbirth and the puerperium		-	-	-	2524/33502	161.85	74.09	1.05 (1.01-1.09)
Disease of skin / connective tissue	0/27	-	-	-	605/8581	-0.02	-0.01	1.00 (0.92-1.09)
Congenital malformations, etc	8/172	-4.13	-1.89	0.67 (0.33-1.36)	86/1012	14.65	6.70	1.21 (0.97-1.51)
Perinatal conditions	12/129	2.90	1.32	1.31 (0.73-2.37)	274/3663	15.72	7.20	1.05 (0.93-1.19)
Symptoms, other ill-defined	19/286	-1.16	-0-53	0.95 (0.60-1.51)	365/4947	16.20	7.41	1.04 (0.94-1.16)
External causes	116/1072	40.41	18.50	1.54 (1.27-1.86)	647/7700	104.09	47.65	1.17 (1.08-1.26)
Accidents	48/423	18.18	8.32	1.61 (1.19-2.16)	558/6722	84.04	38.47	1.16 (1.07-1.27)
Suicide	55/541	16.85	7.71	1.44 (1.08-1.90)	3/58	-1.09	-0.50	0.73 (0.23-2.32)
Total	500/5851	87.46	40.04	1.22 (1.11-1.33)	7697/105827	235.38	107.74	1.04 (1.01-1.06)

E/U: exposed/unexposed; [†]Excess cases=Cases in the exposed-Person years in the exposed*(cases in the unexposed/person years in the unexposed). [‡]Excess rate= Cases in the exposed / person years in the exposed- cases in the unexposed / person years in the unexposed.

Myocardial Infarction (MI)

The excess rates for fatal MI and first MI hospitalisation were 2.87/100,000 and 9.25/100,000, respectively (Table 1). The average adjusted RRs for fatal MI and first MI were 1.36 (95%CI 0.98-1.88) and 1.28 (95%CI 1.08-1.51), respectively (Table 2).

The MI risk did not increase during the first six years of the follow-up, but from the 7th to the 17th year of the follow-up. Parents who lost a child from SIDS had higher relative risks than others [65].

Table 2 Adjusted HRs* in bereaved parents, Denmark 1980-1997

Outcomes	HR	95% CI
Mortality	1.22	1.12-1.35
MI	1.28	1.08-1.51
Stroke	1.00	0.83-1.20
Fatal stroke	0.69	0.37-1.26
Non-fatal stroke	1.03	0.85-1.24
Cancer incidence	1.15	1.02-1.30
Cancer Survival	1.23	1.03-1.47
MS	1.56	1.05-2.31
IBD		
Crohn's disease	0.97	0.62-1.53
Ulcerative colitis	1.01	0.76-1.34

*Adjusted for age, sex, school education, residence, number of children in the family, and number of parents in the family.

Stroke

The excess rate for first stroke hospitalisation was 0.11/100,000. The overall risk of stroke was the same for the exposed and non-exposed (RR, 1.00; 95%CI 0.83-1.20). The average RRs (95% CIs) for fatal and non-fatal stroke were 0.69 (0.37-1.26) and 1.03 (0.85-1.24), respectively. There were no differences in the risk of hemorrhage stroke or non-haemorrhage stroke between the exposed and unexposed either (Table 2) [69].

Cancer Incidence

The incidence rate for cancer was increased by a rate of 9.72/100,000 in the bereaved parents. That corresponded to a slightly increased risk (RR 1.15, 95%CI 1.02-1.30) in mothers. With regard to specific sites, we found no increased risk for breast cancer, but an increased risk for smoking-related cancers (RR 1.65, 95%CI 1.05-2.59) in mothers during the follow-up from the 7th to the 18th year (Table 2) [66].

Cancer Survival

The overall adjusted HR for dying from cancer in the exposed cohort was 1.23 (95%CI 1.03-1.47). The HRs for site-specific cancers and other groups of cancers in the exposed patients were almost identical to those in the unexposed (Table 2) [68].

Multiple Sclerosis (MS)

The excess rate for MS in the exposed was 4.71/100,000. Exposed parents had an adjusted RR of 1.56 (1.05-2.31) for all MS, and an adjusted RR of 1.42 (0.90-2.24) for definite/probable MS. Parents who lost a child unexpectedly had an adjusted HR of 2.13 (95% CI 1.13-4.03) for all MS, which is higher than that for other bereaved parents (Table 2) [70].

Inflammatory Bowel Diseases

There were 301 incident cases of Crohn's disease and 766 incident cases of ulcerative colitis in the unexposed, and the RRs of first hospitalization were 0.97 (0.62-1.53) and 1.01 (0.76-1.34), respectively (Table 2) [71].

DISCUSSIONS

Main Findings

Our studies were based on large population-based cohorts with a complete follow-up and an outcome registration that was carried out independently (and in most cases "blind") of the exposure. The studies show quite accurately how the incidence of various endpoints differed from parents who lost a child to parents who did not.

Mortality

Many studies have shown that spousal bereavement is associated with an increased risk of mortality [52,72]. The effects of child loss on mortality has not been studied very often. Unlike the small study by Rees in which mortality increased nearly five times, several large studies did not find an increase [32,73]. We observed a total of 87.46 excessive deaths in the bereaved, equal to an increase rate of 40.04 per 100,000 and a 30% increase on the relative scale. The contributions to the increase are mainly unnatural deaths like suicide and motor vehicle accidents, and that reflects a possible impact of the life event on the psychological and psychiatric well-being [52].The observed excess death from physical illnesses after the first several years of the follow-up may be explained by the allostatic load following the death of a child [9,18] and/or lifestyle changes induced by stress [16,56-58,60-62].

Myocardial Infarction and Stroke

Most empirical studies support a positive association between stress and coronary heart disease (CHD), but they present different risk estimates. The RRs for MI, for instance, range from 0.9 to 4.9 [19,20]. Even, Macleod et al. have suggested recently that the associations between psychosocial measures and CHD may be due to bias [22]. However, our study is in line with the studies that support a link between stress and MI, most of which were not based upon self-report or perceived stress, and also were based upon "hard" endpoints like fatal CHD, MI [19,20].

On the other hand, the link between stress and stroke is far more inconclusive [27,74]. Our finding of a 20 to 30% increased MI risk is consistent with the majority of the previous studies. However, our data indicate no association between the death of a child and the risk of stroke in young- and middle-aged parents. It could be that stress does not play a role in the development of cerebrovascular disease, or stress may only be a causal factor in an older population, or perhaps a longer induction is needed. To our knowledge, the present study is the first large follow-up study to examine the effects of parental bereavement on cerebrovascular diseases. Further investigation is needed to confirm our findings.

Cancer Incidence and Survival

The association between stress and the incidence of cancer is still controversial [29]. Most case-control studies tend to show a positive association, but recall bias is often a problem in these studies since exposure needs to be recalled far back in time. Longitudinal prospective studies revealed a slight but non-significant trend in favour of an increased risk of cancer in stressed people [75]. We found that the death of a child was associated with a slightly increased overall cancer incidence in bereaved mothers. In line with most of the previous studies, our study suggests that an increased overall risk of cancer attributed to stressful life events is small if it exists at all [29,32-34,75].

The observed weak associations to cancer survival may be due to adaptive lifestyle factors related to stress exposure, or poorer compliance to the medical treatment of the cancer diseases. Our study is small, and we had no information on co-morbidity, disease-related variables or treatment effects that may outweigh the influence of psychological stress on cancer survival. Furthermore, our ability to adjust for confounding by disease-related factors is limited. On the other hand, unless stress is strongly and causally related to cancer occurrence, we will expect severe confounding [68].

Multiple Sclerosis (MS)

Our observations are in line with the suggestions from some previous studies [40-44] that support an association between psychological stress and an increased risk of MS. The diagnosis of MS depends on symptoms, access to medical care, local medical expertise, availability of and accessibility to new diagnostic procedures, and the level of public awareness of the disease [77]. However, in Denmark all citizens have equal and easy access to neurological services of homogenous quality, and almost all MS patients are included in the MS registry that is based on standardized diagnostic criteria [70]. It is not likely that the difference in MS risk is due to stress induced symptoms suspected for MS, nor is it probable that more cases of MS were revealed from the exposed group as a result of focused medical attention. However, MS is a rare disease. Although the burden is severe for the diseased person and his/her family, the effect of parental bereavement may add little to the disease burden at the population level.

Inflammatory Bowel Disease (IBD)

Although studies in psychoimmunology have suggested that stress could influence the susceptibility of IBD by affecting the central nervous system and HPA axis, etc, the empirical evidence on the issue of stress and IBD is conflicting. Case-control studies in this area were often subject to recall bias because IBD could impact one's psychologic well-being. This study is the first large follow-up study to examine the etiologic role of stress on the development of IBD, and our study did not support the hypothesis of a strong association between psychologic stress and the risk of IBD in young- to middle-aged adults [71].

Short-Term Versus Long-Term Effect of Exposure

The most intense stress reactions are often seen shortly after the bereavement [52,59], which is in accordance with the observed short-term peak of mortality from unnatural death and the significantly increased relative risk of first psychiatric hospitalisation during the first year of bereavement in our study.

Studies on aggregate life events cannot properly observe the long-term effect of stress on health [12]. Most evidence on the chronic effects of stress focused on job strain or organizational stress. However, studies have shown that some single traumatic events, e.g. war and bereavement, could have long-term detrimental effects on the psychiatric well-being, e.g. PTSD, depression, and pathophysiological changes [78] although the onset and offset of the events are often short-term by nature. But few have studied the non-psychiatric diseases as outcomes. We found that the mortality rates from unnatural deaths and psychiatric admissions increased significantly throughout the entire follow-up period, indicating that this life event could have a long-term effect on the psychological well-being, especially for parents who lost a child from unexpected causes. We also observed a long-term increased risk of mortality from natural causes, e.g., increased incidence of MI, MS, indicating a long-term effect on physical health as well. These observations may contrast the observations from widowhood studies in which adverse clinical physical illness or mortality increased only shortly after the exposure. However, higher excess mortality from natural death shortly after the bereavement requires pre-existing severe diseases which are more prevalent in elders. Our cohort members are probably too young to have many chronic diseases at the time of exposure. For example, MI is often the end stage of a prolonged process in which abnormalities of arterial and myocardial structure and function precede the onset of a clinical event by many years [21]. We do not expect many cohort members to have advanced atherosclerotic diseases at the start of follow-up. The observed long-term increased risk of diseases support the hypotheses that dysfunction of the immune system and adverse health behaviours may be involved in the development of MS, and perhaps also in the development of some site-specific cancers.

The Nature of Bereavement

For long time, the loss of a child has been categorized as one of the most stressful life events [53,54], with a significant etiological role in the development of psychiatric disorders, particularly. Severe types of bereavement have been reported to cause more stress than other deaths [52,59,79]. Several recent studies have shown that bereavement by violent death could lead to more psychiatric disorders, especially depression and PTSD, than by other deaths [78]. The unexpected death of a child, e.g. from accidents, suicide, or SIDS, could be very traumatic for parents. The higher excess risk of mortality in parents who lost a child unexpectedly or from unnatural causes and the highest RR of MI and MS in parents whose children died unexpectedly, especially by SIDS, are consistent with the suggestions from previous studies.

Few studies have been big enough to examine the effect of the deceased child's age on health outcomes in parents [52,59,79]. We did not observe any obvious modifying effect of the deceased child's age on parents' mortality and other illnesses like cancer incidence, cancer survival, MS and IBD. The highest RR of MI in the second age group were mainly due to SIDS. Although the RRs for psychiatric admissions were different across age groups of the deceased child, the difference was not statistically significant. Similarly, we did not observe any significant effect in modifying the risk in other observed health outcomes. Our data suggested that the age of the deceased child does not play a large role in the age range we studied. But we have limited statistical power to study such an interaction.

Personal Characteristics of the Bereaved Parents

The form that grief takes, its outward expressions, and the length of the recovery process are all influenced by the personal, social and cultural context within which bereavement occurs. Individual differences in the ability to cope with stress are substantial [9,29,59,80,81]. Personal characteristics like age, gender, prior health, and socio-economic status may all play a role.

Most researchers suggested that mothers often suffer more health problems than fathers, which is in line with our results [52,56,59,80]. It could reflect differences in stress response, coping capacity, or the neuroendocrine or immune systems susceptibility between men and women.

The role of age in reaction to parental bereavement remains unclear [52,59]. Some have suggested that older parents have less coping capacity than younger parents [82]. We did not find higher RR of mortality in older parents. The risks of cancer incidence, cancer survival, MS, etc, were not modified by the age of the parents either. We observed lower RRs of MI in the oldest age group. This may be due to additional component causes that could attenuate the effect of the bereavement on the relative scale.

It has been suggested that socio-economic status modifies the stress effect on health outcomes [52,79,82]. Some have indicated that a higher education may reduce the effects of spousal bereavement on mortality [83]. Others have argued the opposite [84]. Our results suggested that a higher level of education does not modify the effects of bereavement substantially. There have been suggestions that people of low socio-economic status or people with limited social support may find it more difficult to cope with stress [81,85], and that may be the reason for the observed higher RRs for some outcomes in parents with limited education and in parents living in more remote areas, and in single parents.

Strengths and Weaknesses of the Study

The present study is based on the linkage between several national administrative registers. The CPR register provides good quality data on demographic information for all residents in Denmark for the study period. The CPR number, a unique personal identification number, is the key to the linkage of databases. The data from the registers are generally of high quality, too. Virtually all bereaved parents were enrolled into the exposed cohort and the cohort was established back in time to ensure a long follow-up. All data were extracted from the databases and collected independently of the research hypothesis. This minimises the risk of surveillance bias and differential misclassification of endpoints that could otherwise be a problem in follow-up studies. However, the problems of variations in the quality of diagnoses are known worldwide and mostly independent on the structure of the health system. Although the data quality of information systems varies from disease to disease, previous studies have shown that diagnoses such as cancer, MI, MS, stroke, etc, are reasonably reliable [86]. The fact that the collection and quality of data are not under the control of researchers may lead to potential problems in specific studies, but it has the advantage of being out of range for manipulation that could introduce bias.

Selection Problems

Selection bias may occur if the likelihood of participation in the study varies not only with respect to exposure but also with respect to risk of disease. If potential study participants are aware of the details of the hypotheses to be examined in the study, and they give their consent in the light of these hypotheses, selection bias is a risk. This was not the case in our studies. In the studies for physical illnesses and mortality, we included all exposed parents into the exposed cohort, and randomly selected 15 times as many unexposed families from the remaining population. In the study on psychiatric disorders, we included all parents who had a child under the age of 18 across the country, so we do not expect a selection bias here, either.

Another possibility for selection bias in the cohort study is loss during the follow-up. The complete follow-up through record linkage with nationwide population-based registers made this type of bias less likely. We could, of course, not follow those who emigrated to other countries, but it is not likely that emigration is correlated to the exposure-the death of a child.

Information Problems

Information bias may be present in exposure, outcomes, or confounders. One of the major advantages of this study is the usage of an objective exposure indicator: the death of a child. It is recorded accurately and thus free from misclassification and recall bias in general [86]. However, for specific causes, the grouping of ICD 8 and ICD 10 codes may lead to some misclassification. We do not believe this to be a big problem for deaths due to natural causes, unnatural causes, suicide, and motor vehicle accidents. On the other hand, although not all unexpected causes of death, like sudden death from heart failure, are included in the group of "unexpected death" in our study, we think that the majority of unexpected deaths in children have been included.

The uncertainty in endpoints will probably lead to bias towards no association and the bias is not present for studies using mortality as the endpoint because the registration of death cause is based on information in the death certificates [86]. The data on other outcomes of interest in our study are in most cases of reasonably high quality. Nearly complete registration of all hospital events in the entire population is one important advantage of using the Danish National Hospital Register [87]. A study by Madsen et al. reported that the predictive value of MI was more than 90%, and a combination of the national registers was found to be a valid and powerful tool for the monitoring of the population incidence of MI [88]. Johnsen et al. reported that the predictive value of a stroke discharge diagnosis has been reported to be as high as more than 80% [89]. Several other studies showed that the rates and trends in cancer incidence were fairly accurately calculated in the Danish Cancer Registry [66]. The Danish Multiple Sclerosis Registry has also been considered to have valid and complete data on MS incidence [70]. However, we cannot exclude the possibility of misclassification in any case among large datasets. But we believe that it would be non-differential and would not affect the estimates in relative scales.

The registers have complete records on variables like age, sex, education, and residence [65-71]. The possibility of misclassification of potential confounders would be small and non-differential, if it exists, in this study. Thus any major role of residual confounding due to misclassification seems unlikely.

Confounding

Confounders are factors that correlate with the exposure and are causes of the outcomes under study. Confounders will vary from endpoint to endpoint. They may be known or unknown. Most confounders will in fact be unknown and therefore it is impossible to control them even in a study with primary data. Since we have no access to the study subject for data protection policy reasons, the option for confounder control was limited to age, calendar time, sex, family structure, residence and social conditions. We believe that the adjustment for these factors will adjust for many life style factors by using the principal of de-confounding, namely, by means of controlling family characteristics in the study design and socio-demographic factors in the analyses. We hope the socio-economic characteristics correlate with strong determinants at baseline, such as dietary habits, physical activity, smoking, use of alcohol, coping style, and social support, which are very important risk factors for all the outcomes of interest in our study. But we have no guarantee that this is the case. Only a series of large randomized trials could provide some sort of quantitative guarantee against confounding as an explanation.

All results could in principal be explained in part by confounding but that would be unlikely. Some of the associations are strong, and strong confounding is needed to explain these associations. Even in situations where confounding can be disregarded, it is an entirely different question whether an association is due to stress exposure caused by the death of the child or something else. The latter question cannot be addressed empirically in this study. The only arguments for a stress explanation relates to other studies that have indicated that the death of a child is one of the most serious stressors that will cause stress in most situations, irrespectively of coping capacity, etc [52,53,59].

Chance-Statistical Precision

Our study population is quite young for some of the outcomes like MI, stroke, cancer, and MS. So, although the follow-up period is long and the population size is large, the number of outcomes was modest, particularly when we examined the subgroups of outcomes, or modifying effects related to characteristics of the parents, or differences in short-term or long-term effects. However, most of the findings were in line with previous studies or research hypotheses, and the directions of the findings in almost all analyses suggested that stress has a detrimental effect on health.

Although, the same data sets gave rise to different studies, no "data-fishing" took place in the sense that all possible endpoints were subject to screening and selective reporting. All studies are based on prior hypotheses and almost all studies have been published or are being published, irrespective of the outcome. Under this condition no adjustment for the "multiple comparison problem" is necessary, nor even known.

CONCLUSIONS

(1) We found an increased overall mortality in mothers who lost a child younger than 18 years of age. Mortality from natural causes in mothers increased significantly but only after more than nine years of the follow-up. Mortality from unnatural death in mothers increased throughout the entire follow-up period, but decreased with time. Mothers who lost a child unexpectedly or from unnatural causes had higher relative mortality rates than other mothers.

(2) We found an increased risk of MI in parents who lost a child, but only after six years of the follow-up. Parents who lost a child by SIDS had the highest relative risk of MI. However, we found no increased risk of stroke among parents who lost a child.

(3) We found that the death of a child was associated with a slightly increased overall cancer incidence in mothers. There was a slight excess risk for smoking-related cancers, but no excess risk of breast cancer, alcohol-related cancers, hormone-related cancers, or immune/virus-related cancers. Bereaved parents who lost a child had a slightly shorter cancer survival than the non-bereaved.

(4) The study indicates a higher MS risk in parents who lost a child than in parents who did not lose a child. Our data suggest that severe stress may play a role in the development of MS.

(5) The short-term effects of the life event are an increased risk of mortality from external causes. The long-term effects are mainly an increased risk of physical diseases like MI, MS.

(6) Unexpected deaths may cause more stress, and mothers are often affected more than fathers.

(7) Given the fact that the increases in absolute incidence risk for most of the endpoints were not substantial in the bereaved parents, we believe that almost all of them have been subject to severe stress but most managed to cope with the stress.

PERSPECTIVES FOR FUTURE RESEARCH

Implications for Future Studies in Bereaved Research

Our data suggest that parents exposed to the stress of a child loss have a higher mortality and morbidity for some diseases than unexposed parents. What has been seen may be an "iceberg phenomenon." We think that most bereaved parents will suffer from the loss without getting one of the serious diseases we studied. Parental bereavement is of a great concern in public health and of clinical relevance. As this is the first large-scale study examining the mortality and morbidity in bereaved parents, the findings need to be replicated in other studies, particularly from other regions of the world with a high infant mortality, or a different culture.

In addition, some aspects of bereavement for which we have no information need to be further explored:

- Characteristics associated with the deceased child. We only present the results for the age band of 0-18 years, whereas the loss of an adult child may be different. Apart from the type of the death of the deceased child, other aspects of a child's death would be worth investigating further.
- Coping strategy and personal susceptibility. Information on parents' baseline mental and physical health, personality factors, lifestyle and behavior factors, coping strategy, and genetic factors are important. How these factors interact with the exposure has not been well elucidated.
- Changes over time following the bereavement. Many diseases like heart disease, stroke, cancer, or psychiatric illness often need years or decades of incubation and latency time. Changes in life styles have been reported in bereaved populations and could be important mediators in the development of illnesses. Further studies need to include this information to estimate the relative importance of exposure in the disease's etiology
- Interaction with social context like social support and work environment. The social context is very important both for the coping strategy as well as the exposure itself.
- Possible positive aspects of bereavement, which is an emerging area that has been neglected in previous studies.

Implications for Future Studies in General Stress Research

Although we see continuous improvements in life event research, there is still considerable controversy on methodological limitations. It is an area of stress research where experimental studies in humans usually are not an option. Life events may span from minor events that would stress some but not all, to severe events that probably would stress all. Both types of studies are needed, and studies on major life events will often be easier to interpret, especially if the life events are extreme. Common genetic factors could lie behind familiar bereavement and health consequences. This source of error is eliminated if the exposure stems from the closing of factories or natural disasters. The following recommendations should apply to future research:

- Focus on a single severe event may be the most fruitful approach. Misclassification and recall bias for exposure could be avoided. The association between stress and health will be strengthened by evidence from studies on sudden traumas like natural disasters, accidents, war or terror attacks on people. From a follow-up design of reasonable sample size, we should expect to see both acute and long-term effects on various health outcomes, if they exist.
- Using valid "hard" endpoints could avoid recall bias or misclassification of outcome.
- Research on commonalities versus diversities between acute and chronic stressors could provide further understanding of the disease process.
- Biological stress mechanisms. Research on biological pathways would render concrete support on empirical evidence.
- The application of biological markers of stress. A subject's own description of the effect of stress may distort what is going on in his/her body, but a biological measurement could provide objective measurement of exposure and outcome, which could not be achieved by the traditional approach of self-reports.

ACKNOWLEDGEMENTS

The activities of Danish epidemiology Science Centre is financed by a grant from the National research Foundation. We thank Ms Gitte Nielson and Mrs Hanne Grand for their linguistic assistance.

REFERENCES

[1]   Cannon WB. Stresses and trains of homeostasis. *Amer.J.Med.Sci.* 1935;**189**:1-14.
[2]   Selye H. Syndrome produced by diverse nocuous agents. *Nature* 1936;**138**:32.
[3]   Selye H. *The stress of life.* New York: McGraw-Hill, 1956.
[4]   Lazarus RS, Folkman S. *Stress, appraisal and coping.* New York: Springer, 1984.
[5]   Cox T. *Stress.* London: Macmillan Education, 1980.
[6]   McGrath JE. *Social and psychological factors in stress.* New York: McGraw-Hill, 1970.
[7]   Levine S. Influence of psychological variables on the activity of the hypothalamic-pituitary-adrenal axis. *Eur.J.Pharmacol.* 2000;**405**:149-60.
[8]   McEwen BS,.Wingfield JC. The concept of allostasis in biology and biomedicine. *Horm.Behav.* 2003; **43**:2-15.
[9]   McEwen BS. Protective and damaging effects of stress mediators. *New Engl J Med* 1998;**338**:171-9.
[10] Stansfeld S, Marmot M. *Stress and the heart: psychosocial pathways to coronary heart disease.* **London**: BMJ Books, 2002.

[11] Avison WR, Gotlib IH. *Stress and mental health : contemporary issues and prospects for the future* . New York: Plenum, 1994.

[12] Brown GW, Harris TO. *Life events and illness* . New York : Guilford Press, 1989.

[13] Grinker R, Spiegel J. *Men under stress*. Philadelphia: Blakiston, 1945.

[14] Holmes TH, Rahe RH. The Social Readjustment Rating Scale. *J Psychosom Res* 1967;**11**:213-8.

[15] Heston L. What about environment? In Dunner D, Gershon E, Barrett J, eds. *Relatives at risk for mental disorder*, pp 205-13. New York: Raven, 1988.

[16] Goodkin K, Baldewicz TT, Blaney NT, et al. Physiological effects of bereavement and bereavement support group interventions. In Stroebe MS, Hansson RO, Stroebe W, Schut H, eds. *Handbook of bereavement research*, pp 671-704. Washington DC: American Psychological association, 2001.

[17] Sternberg EM, Chrousos GP, Wilder RL, Gold PW. The stress response and the regulation of inflammatory disease. *Ann.Intern.Med.* 1992;**117**:854-66.

[18] Brunner E. Stress mechanisms in coronary heart disease. In Stansfeld S, Marmot M, eds. *Stress and the Heart: Psychosocial Pathways to Coronary Heart Disease*, pp 181-99. London: BMJ Books, 2002.

[19] Rozanski A, Blumenthal JA, Kaplan J. Impact of psychological factors on the pathogenesis of cardiovascular disease and implications for therapy. *Circulation* 1999;**99** :2192-217.

[20] Hemingway H,.Marmot M. Evidence based cardiology: psychosocial factors in the aetiology and prognosis of coronary heart disease. Systematic review of prospective cohort studies. *BMJ* 1999;**318**:1460-7.

[21] Muller JE. Circadian variation and triggering of acute coronary events. *Am.Heart J.* 1999;**137**:S1-S8.

[22] Macleod J, Davey SG, Heslop P, Metcalfe C, Carroll D, Hart C. Psychological stress and cardiovascular disease: empirical demonstration of bias in a prospective observational study of Scottish men. *BMJ* 2002;**324**:1247-51.

[23] Rosch PJ. Psychological stress and cardiovascular disease. Paper doesn't clarify things. *BMJ* 2002;**325**:337.

[24] Monroe SM,.Roberts JE. Conceptualizing and measuring life stress: problems, principles, procedures, progress. *Stress Med.* 1990;**6**:209-16.

[25] Everson SA, Roberts RE, Goldberg DE, Kaplan GA. Depressive symptoms and increased risk of stroke mortality over a 29-year period. *Arch.Intern.Med.* 1998;**158**:1133-8.

[26] May M, McCarron P, Stansfeld S, Ben Shlomo Y, Gallacher J, Yarnell J *et al*. Does psychological distress predict the risk of ischemic stroke and transient ischemic attack? The Caerphilly Study. *Stroke* 2002;**33**:7-12.

[27] Abel GA, Chen X, Boden-Albala B, Sacco RL. Social readjustment and ischemic stroke: lack of an association in a multiethnic population. *Neuroepidemiology* 1999;**18**:22-31.

[28] Snow HL. *Cancer and Cancer process*. London: Churchill, 1893.

[29] McGee R. Does stress cause cancer? There's no good evidence of a relation between stressful events and cancer. *BMJ* 1999;**319**:1015-6.

[30]   Chen CC, David AS, Nunnerley H, Michell M, Dawson JL, Berry H *et al.* Adverse life events and breast cancer: case-control study. *BMJ* 1995;**311**:1527-30.

[31]   Protheroe D, Turvey K, Horgan K, Benson E, Bowers D, House A. Stressful life events and difficulties and onset of breast cancer: case-control study. *BMJ* 1999;**319**:1027-30.

[32]   Johansen C,.Olsen JH. Psychological stress, cancer incidence and mortality from non-malignant diseases. *Br.J.Cancer* 1997;**75**:144-8.

[33]   Levav I, Kohn R, Iscovich J, Abramson JH, Tsai WY, Vigdorovich D. Cancer incidence and survival following bereavement. *Am.J.Public Health* 2000;**90**:1601-7.

[34]   Jacobs JR,.Bovasso GB. Early and chronic stress and their relation to breast cancer. *Psychol.Med.* 2000;**30**:669-78.

[35]   Lillberg K, Verkasalo PK, Kaprio J, Teppo L, Helenius H, Koskenvuo M. Stressful life events and risk of breast cancer in 10,808 women: a cohort study. *Am.J.Epidemiol.* 2003;**157**:415-23.

[36]   Cohen S,.Rabin BS. Psychologic stress, immunity, and cancer. *J.Natl.Cancer Inst.* 1998;**90**:3-4.

[37]   Charcot JM. Lectures on the diseases of the nervous system. London: New Sydenham Society, 1897.

[38]   Goodin DS, Ebers GC, Johnson KP, Rodriguez M, Sibley WA, Wolinsky JS. The relationship of MS to physical trauma and psychological stress: report of the Therapeutics and Technology Assessment Subcommittee of the American Academy of Neurology. *Neurology* 1999;**52**:1737-45.

[39]   Nisipeanu P, Korczyn AD. Psychological stress as risk factor for exacerbations in multiple sclerosis. *Neurology* 1993;**43**:1311-2.

[40]   Esposito P, Chandler N, Kandere K, Basu S, Jacobson S, Connolly R *et al.* Corticotropin-releasing hormone and brain mast cells regulate blood-brain-barrier permeability induced by acute stress. *J.Pharmacol.Exp Ther.* 2002;**303**:1061-6.

[41]   van Noort JM, van Sechel AC, Bajramovic JJ, el Ouagmiri M, Polman CH, Lassmann H *et al.* The small heat-shock protein alpha B-crystallin as candidate autoantigen in multiple sclerosis. *Nature* 1995;**375**:798-801.

[42]   Foley FW, Traugott U, LaRocca NG, Smith CR, Perlman KR, Caruso LS *et al.* A prospective study of depression and immune dysregulation in multiple sclerosis. *Arch.Neurol.* 1992;**49**:238-44.

[43]   Erkut ZA, Hofman MA, Ravid R, Swaab DF. Increased activity of hypothalamic corticotropin-releasing hormone neurons in multiple sclerosis. *J.Neuroimmunol.* 1995;**62**:27-33.

[44]   Drossman DA. Psychosocial factors in ulcerative colitis and Crohn's disease. In Kirsner JB, ed. *Inflammatory bowel disesae*, pp 342-57. Philadelphia: W.B.Saunders, 2000.

[45]   Picardi A, Abeni D. Stressful life events and skin diseases: disentangling evidence from myth. *Psychother.Psychosom.* 2001;**70**:118-36.

[46]   Anderson KO, Bradley LA, Young LD, McDaniel LK, Wise CM. Rheumatoid arthritis: review of psychological factors related to etiology, effects, and treatment. *Psychol.Bull.* 1985; **98**:358-87.

[47]   Winsa B, Adami HO, Bergstrom R, Gamstedt A, Dahlberg PA, Adamson U *et al.* Stressful life events and Graves' disease. *Lancet* 1991;**338**:1475-9.

[48] Goldston DB, Kovacs M, Obrosky DS, Iyengar S. A longitudinal study of life events and metabolic control among youths with insulin-dependent diabetes mellitus. *Health Psychol.* 1995;**14**:409-14.

[49] Cohen S, Tyrrell DA, Smith AP. Psychological stress and susceptibility to the common cold. *N.Engl.J.Med.* 1991;**325**:606-12.

[50] Glaser R, Pearson GR, Jones JF, Hillhouse J, Kennedy S, Mao HY *et al.* Stress-related activation of Epstein-Barr virus. *Brain Behav.Immun.* 1991;**5**:219-32.

[51] Leserman J, Petitto JM, Perkins DO, Folds JD, Golden RN, Evans DL. Severe stress, depressive symptoms, and changes in lymphocyte subsets in human immunodeficiency virus-infected men. A 2-year follow-up study. *Arch.Gen.Psychiatry* 1997;**54**:279-85.

[52] Osterweis M, Solomon F, Green M. *Bereavement: Reactions, consequences, and Care.* Washington DC: National Academy Press, 1984.

[53] American Psychiatric Association. *Diagnostic and Statistical Manual of Mental Disorders.* Washington DC: National Academy Press, 1987.

[54] Skodol AE,.Shrout PE. Use of DSM-III axis IV in clinical practice: rating etiologically significant stressors. *Am.J.Psychiatry* 1989;**146**:61-6.

[55] Stroebe MS, Stroebe W, Hansson RO, Schut H. *Handbook of bereavement research: Consequences,coping, and care.* Washington DC: American Psychological Association, 2001.

[56] Vance JC, Najman JM, Boyle FM, Embelton G, Foster WJ, Thearle MJ. Alcohol and drug usage in parents soon after stillbirth, neonatal death or SIDS. *J.Paediatr.Child Health* 1994; **30**:269-72.

[57] Anda RF, Williamson DF, Escobedo LG, Mast EE, Giovino GA, Remington PL. Depression and the dynamics of smoking. A national perspective. *JAMA* 1990;**264**:1541-5.

[58] Camacho TC, Roberts RE, Lazarus NB, Kaplan GA, Cohen RD. Physical activity and depression: evidence from the Alameda County Study. *Am.J.Epidemiol.* 1991;**134**:220-31.

[59] Rubin SS, Malkinson R. Parental response to child loss across the life cycle: clinical and research perspecitves. In Stroebe MS, Hansson RO, Stroebe W, eds. *Handbook of Bereavement Research: Conequences,coping, and Care,* pp 219-39. Washington DC: American Psychological Association, 2001.

[60] Klatsky AL,.Armstrong MA. Alcohol use, other traits, and risk of unnatural death: a prospective study. *Alcohol Clin Exp Res* 1993;**17**:1156-62.

[61] Leistikow BN, Martin DC, Jacobs J, Rocke DM. Smoking as a risk factor for injury death: a meta-analysis of cohort studies. *Prev.Med.* 1998;**27**:871-8.

[62] Li G, Smith GS, Baker SP. Drinking behavior in relation to cause of death among US adults. *Am.J.Public Health* 1994;**84**:1402-6.

[63] Frank L. Epidemiology. When an entire country is a cohort. *Science* 2000;**287**:2398-9.

[64] Sorensen HT, Sabroe S, Olsen J. A framework for evaluation of secondary data sources for epidemiological research. *Int.J.Epidemiol.* 1996;**25**:435-42.

[65] Li J, Hansen D, Mortensen PB, Olsen J. Myocardial infarction in parents who lost a child: a nationwide prospective cohort study in Denmark. *Circulation* 2002;**106**:1634-9.

[66] Li J, Johansen C, Hansen D, Olsen J. Cancer incidence in parents who lost a child. *Cancer* 2002; **95**:2237-42.

[67] Li J, Precht DH, Mortensen PB, Olsen J. Mortality in parents after death of a child in Denmark: a nationwide follow-up study. *Lancet* 2003;**361**:363-7.

[68] Li J, Johansen C, Olsen J. Cancer survival in parents who lost a child: a nationwide study in Denmark. *Br.J.Cancer* 2003;**88**:1698-701.

[69] Li J, Johnsen SP, Olsen J. Stroke in parents who lost a child: a nationwide follow-up study in Denmark. *Neuroepidemiology* 2003;**22**:211-6.

[70] Li J, Johansen C, Bronnum-Hansen H, Stenager E, Koch-Henriksen N, Olsen J. The risk of multiple sclerosis in bereaved parents: a nationwide cohort study in Denmark. *Neurology* 2004; 62:726-9.

[71] Li J, Norgaard B, Precht DH, Olsen J. Psychological stress and inflammatory bowel disease: a follow-up study in parents who lost a child in Denmark. *Am. J. Gastroenterol.* 2004;99:1129-33.

[72] Schaefer C, Quesenberry CP, Jr., Wi S. Mortality following conjugal bereavement and the effects of a shared environment. *Am.J.Epidemiol.* 1995;**141**:1142-52.

[73] Levav I, Friedlander Y, Kark JD, Peritz E. An epidemiologic study of mortality among bereaved parents. *N.Engl.J.Med.* 1988;**319**:457-61.

[74] Macko RF, Ameriso SF, Barndt R, Clough W, Weiner JM, Fisher M. Precipitants of brain infarction. Roles of preceding infection/inflammation and recent psychological stress. *Stroke* 1996;**27**:1999-2004.

[75] Petticrew M. Cancer-stress link: the truth. *Nurs.Times* 1999;**95**:52-3.

[76] Tross S, Herndon J, Korzun A, Kornblith AB, Cella DF, Holland JF *et al.* Psychological symptoms and disease-free and overall survival in women with stage II breast cancer. Cancer and Leukemia Group B. *J.Natl.Cancer Inst.* 1996;**88**:661-7.

[77] Noseworthy JH, Lucchinetti C, Rodriguez M, Weinshenker BG. Multiple sclerosis. *N.Engl.J.Med.* 2000;**343**:938-52.

[78] Shalev AY, Freedman S, Peri T, Brandes D, Sahar T, Orr SP *et al.* Prospective study of posttraumatic stress disorder and depression following trauma. *Am.J.Psychiatry* 1998;**155**:630-7.

[79] Parkes CM. Bereavement in adult life. *BMJ* 1998;**316**:856-9.

[80] Vance JC, Boyle FM, Najman JM, Thearle MJ. Gender differences in parental psychological distress following perinatal death or sudden infant death syndrome. *Br.J.Psychiatry* 1995;**167**:806-11.

[81] Kaplan GA,.Keil JE. Socioeconomic factors and cardiovascular disease: a review of the literature. *Circulation* 1993;**88**:1973-98.

[82] Rubin SS. The death of a child is forever: the life course impact of child loss. In Stroebe MS, Stroebe W, Hansson RO, eds. *Handbook of bereavement*, pp 285-99. New York: Cambridge University Press, 1993.

[83] Martikainen P,.Valkonen T. Do education and income buffer the effects of death of spouse on mortality? *Epidemiology* 1998;**9**:530-4.

[84] Lusyne P, Page H, Lievens J. Mortality following conjugal bereavement, Belgium 1991-96: the unexpected effect of education. *Popul.Stud.(Camb.)* 2001;**55**:281-9.

[85] Mittleman MA, Maclure M, Nachnani M, Sherwood JB, Muller JE. Educational attainment, anger, and the risk of triggering myocardial infarction onset. The Determinants of Myocardial Infarction Onset Study Investigators. *Arch.Intern.Med.* 1997;**157**:769-75.

[86] Juel K,.Helweg-Larsen K. The Danish registers of causes of death. *Dan.Med.Bull.* 1999;**46**:354-7.

[87] Andersen TF, Madsen M, Jorgensen J, Mellemkjoer L, Olsen JH. The Danish National Hospital Register. A valuable source of data for modern health sciences. *Dan.Med.Bull.* 1999;**46**:263-8.

[88] Madsen M, Davidsen M, Rasmussen S, Abildstrom SZ, Osler M. The validity of the diagnosis of acute myocardial infarction in routine statistics: a comparison of mortality and hospital discharge data with the Danish MONICA registry. *J.Clin Epidemiol.* 2003;**56**:124-30.

[89] Johnsen SP, Overvad K, Sorensen HT, Tjonneland A, Husted SE. Predictive value of stroke and transient ischemic attack discharge diagnoses in The Danish National Registry of Patients. *J.Clin Epidemiol.* 2002;**55**:602-7.

APPENDIX: LIST OF ABBREVIATIONS USED IN THIS CHAPTER

CDH	coronary heart disease
CI	Confidence interval
CPR	the unique personal identification number for each individual in the Central Office of Civil Registration in Denmark
CRH	corticotrophin releasing hormone
DCR	Danish Cancer Register
DCPR	Danish Central Psychiatric Register
DFD	Danish Fertility Database
DPR	Danish Prevention Register
DSM-IV	Diagnostic and Statistical Manual of Mental Disorders - Fourth Edition
DMSR	Danish Multiple Sclerosis Registry
DSI	Depression Symptom Inventory
EPV	the Epstein-Barr virus
HIV	the human immunodeficiency virus
HPA	the hypothalamic-pituitary-adrenal axis
HR	Hazard ratio
IBD	Inflammatory bowel disease
IDDM	insulin-dependent diabetes mellitus
ICD	International Classification of Diseases
LEDS	Life Events and Difficulties Schedule
MI	Myocardial Infarction
MS	Multiple Sclerosis
NND	neonatal death
OR	Odds ratio

PTSD	Post-Traumatic Stress Disorder
RA	Rheumatoid arthritis
RR	Relative Risk
SB	Still birth
SIDS	Sudden Infant Death Syndrome
SRE	Schedule of Recent Experiences

In: Psychology of Stress
Editor: Kimberly V. Oxington, pp. 83-100

ISBN 1-59454-246-5
©2005 Nova Science Publishers, Inc.

Chapter V

STRESS AMONG STUDENTS IN DEVELOPING COUNTRIES- AN OVERVIEW

Shashidhar Acharya

ABSTRACT

Mankind since the dawn of history has been afflicted with various forms of diseases. Communicable diseases that took a heavy toll of human life in medieval and prehistoric times, have been replaced by non- communicable diseases and conditions in the recent times. Among the six factors which are responsible for the major share of these diseases, Stress occupies an important place (Rose, G.A. and Blackburn H. 1968). The Oxford English dictionary defines stress as pressure, tension or worry resulting from the problems in one's life. It is thus a condition of the mind, in which a person loses his calm tranquility and equanimity and experiences extreme discomfiture.

A BRIEF HISTORY

With advances in preventive medicine and the practice of public health, the pattern of disease began to change in the developed world; many of the acute illnesses were brought under control. However as old problems were solved, new health problems in the form of chronic non communicable diseases began to emerge, e.g., cancer, diabetes, cardiovascular diseases, alcoholism and drug addiction especially in the affluent societies. These diseases that required the understanding of their social and behavioral aspects led to a new phase of public health in the 1960's called the "Social Engineering Phase" (Anderson, C.L. et al, 1978). As our understanding of the dimensions of health grew, so did the list of dimensions. In addition to the physical dimension, other dimensions have gained importance. These dimensions have a direct or indirect effect on stress and stress induced illnesses. They are:

- **Mental Dimension**: Research has shown that psychological factors can induce conditions like hypertension, peptic ulcer and bronchial asthma. (WHO 1964).

- **Social Dimension**: It implies harmony and integration within the individual, between each individuals and the world in which they live (Cmich, D.E., 1984).
- **Spiritual Dimension**: Spiritual health refers to that part of the individual that reaches out and strives for meaning and purpose in life. It includes integrity , principals and ethics, the purposes in life ,commitment to some higher being and belief in concepts that are not subject to 'state of the art' explanation.(Eberst, R.M., 1984)
- **Emotional Dimension**: Historically the mental and emotional dimensions have been seen as one element or as two closely related elements. However new research has shown them to be distinct entities (Eberst, R.M., 1984).
- **Vocational Dimension**: It is a part of human existence. When work is fully adapted to human goals, capabilities and limitations, it often plays a role in promoting physical and mental health. Physical work is associated with improvement in physical capacity, while goal achievement and self-realization in work are a source of satisfaction and enhanced self-esteem (WHO, 1985).

STUDENTS AS A RISK GROUP

Among all groups in the population, students especially college students are a group who are particularly prone and susceptible to stress. As a college student, the life can be stressful. In moderate doses, stress challenges students to do their best and keeps them learning and growing. For example, finals are an especially stressful time. Since the final exam has a high percentage in the total score and the outcome is uncertain, there will be high level of stress. This stress can prompt students to study harder, longer, and learn more from the extra effort. So positive stress was defined as functional stress when it enhances our individual or group performance.

On the other hand, the body does not distinguish between negative and positive stress: both excitement and anxiety strain the body's resources and depress the immune system. Stress varies in intensity and duration. Stress that lasts a short period of time can rapidly motivate us. However, stressor that lasts too long, happens too often, or is too strong may bring us physical, behavioral, and psychological problems. Then it becomes the negative stress or dysfunctional stress.

Negative stress can affect a person physically. A person under stress may suffer reduced physical coordination and control, sleeplessness, reduction in the ability to concentrate, store information in memory. And it may be even worse. Research has revealed that at least 50% of all diseases, including peptic ulcer, colitis, hypertension, enuresis, migraine headache, insomnia, and other illnesses, can be attributed to constant stress-related origins. Stress also can affect the individual mentally such as reducing self-esteem, decreasing interpersonal and academic effectiveness and creating a cycle of self-blame and self-doubt. Without adequate coping skills, people often adopt irrational behaviors such as disruptive eating patterns, increased smoking or alcohol consumption, isolation, irritability, harsh treatment of others, compulsive shopping to escape from the over- stressed situation temporarily.

Being over-stressed can be harmful to students. Goldman has reported that being over-stressed can be harmful to students (Goldman et al, 1997). 167 college students participated the survey. The results were concluded from their Self-Perception Profiles, including intellectual ability, scholastic competence, job competence, appearance, social acceptance, close friendships, finding humor in one's life, and global self worth. From the survey data, the authors arrived the conclusion that stress did bring negative effects on college students' self-perception.

Many other authors expatiated that high pressure of college study, the conflicting role demands, and the fast-changing environment, all lead to the relative high level of stress in college students. Undoubtedly, a high level of stress is found to be harmful to the health of students both psychologically and physically.

This may be due to the transitional nature of college life (Towbes and Cohen, 1996).This transition creates a situation where regular contacts with traditional supports like old friends and family may be reduced.The ability of such social supports to mediate the effect of exposure to stress is wellknown (Ensel and Lin, 1991; Moss,1973; Schutt et al, 1994; Thoits, 1995).They must adjust to being away from home for the first time, maintain a high level of academic achievement and adjust to a new social environment. College students must learn to balance the competing demands of academics, developing new social contacts, and being responsible for their own daily needs. While these stressors do not cause anxiety or tension by themselves, they may do so by the interaction with the individual's perceptions and reaction to these stressors. (Romano, 1992) The amount of stress experienced may be influenced by the individual's ability to cope with stressful situations. If stress is not dealt with effectively, feelings of loneliness, sleeplessness, nervousness and excessive worrying may result. (Wright, 1967).

The dynamic relationship between the person and his environment in stress perception and reaction is especially magnified in college students. The problems and situations encountered by college students may differ from those faced by others.(Hirsh and Ellis, 1996).Unlike other vocations, the college student is continuously exposed to stressful situations like periodic tests , examinations, projects etc.(Wright, 1964).Earning high grades is not the only source of stress for college students. Other sources of stress include excessive homework, unclear assignments, uncomfortable class rooms (Kohn and Frazer, 1986), and relations with faculty members, time pressures (Sgan-Cohen and Lowental, 1988), relationships with family and friends, eating, sleeping habits, and loneliness (Wright, 1967).

College marks the period where new systems of support are being created. This process itself can cause stress. It has been shown that peer events and other social gatherings designed to reduce stress end up doing the opposite (Dill and Henley, 1998). Stress has been associated with a variety of negative fallouts like suicide ideation (Hirsch and Ellis, 1996), smoking, (Naquin and Gilbert, 1996) and drinking (Morgan, 1997; McCormack, 1996). It has been seen that females tend to perceive higher levels of stress than males (Megel et.al, 1994)

In short, it can be said that the reasons for student stress are: 1) Societal Pressure 2) Low self esteem 3) Exam stress 4) Educational System and 5) Pressure from parents and teachers.

STRESS AMONG STUDENTS IN THE HEALTH CARE PROFESSIONS

Students from health care professions like medicine, dentistry, nursing and other fields suffer from various degrees of stress like all the other students of various disciplines. However the challenges a medical or a dental student has to face are very much different than that of students of other disciplines. Since the health care profession is a healing profession, the students have to develop traits like empathy, patience, special communication skills, ethical values, an aptitude for social service in addition to didactic learning. It is for these traits that the society respects the health care profession and its practitioners and rates it so highly. In their quest to live up to the society's expectations medical students suffer tremendous stress. Stress in medical training has been the subject of numerous investigations (e.g. Special issue of Medical Education, Volume 28, 1994).

Medical school may be particularly stressful as students come into close contact with serious illness and death, in addition to meeting the demands of the curriculum. (http://www.gmc-uk.org/n_hance/med/student.htm). It could be argued that a certain amount of stress is necessary for students to perform well. An over relaxed attitude could lead to complacency and a failure to do sufficient work. Stress however leads to psychological ill health in medical students. Several studies have examined the relationship between the causes of stress and psychological morbidity. Depression and anxiety are associated with concerns about mastering knowledge, personal endurance and ability and lack of time for other activities (Vitaliano PP et al 1984; Stewart SM et al 1997). Anxiety is also associated with feelings of anonymity, peer competition, long hours and loss of social time (Vitaliano PP et al 1984; Stewart SM et al 1997). Studies that have tried to identify the sources of stress among medical students generally point to three main areas: academic pressures, social issues and financial problems. (Vitaliano PP et al 1984).

Academic Pressures

The majority of stressful incidents in traditional curricula are related to medical training rather than to personal problems (Coles C, 1994; Guthrie EA et al, 1995). Workload and feeling overwhelmed by the amount of information to be mastered are major sources of stress. Fears of failing or falling behind are particular preoccupations. Other significant academic sources of stress include disillusionment with medicine and the realities of medical school (Guthrie EA et al, 1995), perception of hurdle jumping (Coles C, 1994), relationship with teachers (Guthrie EA et al, 1995; Firth J, 1986) and dealing with death and suffering (Firth J, 1986).

During the undergraduate course, medical students are damagingly overloaded with content and the relevance of much of what they are taught often eludes them. Vast amounts of information are commited to memory for dubious reasons and doubtful benefit.In the clinical years students find themselves unable to apply in a professional setting what they know well enough for examinations. This situation is especially acute in non English speaking countries and those countries where English is not widely spoken. Since all the textbooks and literature are in English, many students who are not well versed with the language find it very difficult to understand the basic concepts.Even the examinations are sometimes not defensible educationally and to students appear as hurdles to be surmounted rather than opportunities for assessing progress. The situation is similar if not more pronounced in developing countries (Acharya S 2003, Rajab 2001). In studies done in India, academic factors were greater perceived than all other factors as a cause of stress (Supe 1998), however there was no differences among students at different levels of the medical course regarding academic factors. (Supe, 1998; Indrayan A et al 1985).

Generalized stressors which differentiate the basic science from the clinical years as well as stressors which are unique to each year have been identified (Keniston, 1967; Gaensbauer and Mizner, 1980; Coombs and St John 1981; Knight 1981; Bok 1984). A number of studies have been conducted on the perceived stressors, problems and concerns of medical students (Coburn and Joviasas 1975; Edwards and Zimet 1976; Bjorksten et al 1983; Lloyd and Gartrell 1983; Heins et al 1984; Levin and Franklin 1984; Linn and Zeppa 1984; Firth 1986; Rosenthal et al 1986; Carmel and Bernstein 1987; Wolf et al 1987, 1988). Common themes may be identified from these studies although they were conducted over a 15 year interval with students from different years, different schools and different cultures. Generally the academic demands were most problematic. Personal-interpersonal issues were also of concern perhaps stemming the magnitude of the academic demands. Regarding the academic demands, during the basic sciences the major themes dealt with the massive amount of material to be mastered in preparations for the stressful examinations, while in the clinical years , the major themes dealt with caring for the sick patients and dealing with medical personnel. Financial responsibilities were also a major concern to many students who graduate with loans to pay off. It is clear that many students forego their personal interests and interpersonal ties and experience feelings of emotional isolation and alienation (Gaensbauer and Mizner, 1980; Coombs and Fawzy, 1986) by tipping the balance in favour of academic superiority at the expense of personal growth and development.

Although the focus of much of the research has been on stress and its adverse effects on medical students, there are also some data about the positive aspects and uplifting experiences of medical students. In a retrospective study of graduating seniors, the most uplifting experiences were about recreation and relationships (Wolf et al 1988). The one exception was good examination performance which was rated as the second highest uplift. The fact that it was also rated as the most stressful item shows how the lives of medical students often revolve around examination schedules. With first year students, the most frequently endorsed uplifting items were related to hedonistic concerns (e.g. Having fun, laughing,). A common theme for the senior and first year students was the importance of maintaining contact with friends and family. The sense of belonging and social support are certainly preferable to possible feelings of social isolation and alieation that can arise from unmet psychologic needs.

Social issues that can cause stress include the effects of being a student on personal life, in particular managing leisure activities and social relationships. (Firth J, 1986; Stewart SM et al 1997,)The factors causing stress vary with the stage of the course. Concern about workload, performance, and personal competence seem particularly marked in first year.(Guthrie EA et al, 1995; Stewart SM et al 1997).In studies of medical students in later years factors inherent in medical training such as dealing with patients, disease and death, relationships with consultants and effects on personal life are important.(Firth J, 1986).

Attitudes Values and Personality Change During the Study Period

Medical training has traditionally been a long and arduous process. Despite this, admission into medical schools remains fiercely competitive. Silver described enthusiastic freshman medical students soon becoming cynical, depressed, dejected, frightened or frustrated (Silver H.K., 1982). Stress in medical students is common (Supe, 1994; Stewart S.M et al 1997), even in the early stages of training. There is evidence to suggest that there is a shift in personality, attitudes, and values during the course of medical education. It has been shown in both cross sectional and longitudinal studies that cynical attitudes increased and expressions of humanitarion feelings decreased as students progressed through medical school(Eron 1955,1958).Graduating medical students perceived that they became more cynical over the course of their medical education(Wolf et al 1989a). It has been shown that there is a shift to more hedonistic personality characteristics in two longitudinal studies (Burstein et al 1980; Whittmore et al 1985).In a longitudinal study on depressed mood in which assessments were conducted six times from first year to the last year, at least 12 % of the class showed depressive symptoms at any assessment during the first three years ,the highest being 25% during the end of the first year (Clark and Zeldov 1988). In a second longitudinal study with first and second year students, the incidence of major depression or probable major depression was 12 % (Zoccodillo et al 1986). The lifetime prevalence was 25 % or three times the rate in the general population.With first year medical students, the anxiety levels were one standard deviation above the mean relative to non-patient levels and the depression doubled over the course of the first year (Vitaliano et al 1989b).In another study ,self esteem and positive mood decreased while negative mood(Depression and hostility) increased over the course of the first year (Wolf et al 1991a). In a study of first and second year medical students, symptoms of anxiety were reported above the median of the population of psychiatric patients (Vitaliano et al 1984). In one study, 62 out of 172 first year students (36%) in the north of England had probable psychological disturbance according to a well recognized psychological questionnaire (Guthrie E.A et al, 1995). On entering medical school, students experience a rise in depression scores that persisted over time (Henning K et al , 1998). Trainees (students, interns, and residents) suffer high levels of stress, which lead to alcohol and drug abuse(Johnson N et al,1990) interpersonal relationship difficulties (Gallegos K et al ,1990) depression and anxiety(Pitts FN et al 1961;Salt P. et al 1984) and even suicide (Richings J.C 1986) Medical students have mean anxiety scores one standard deviation above those of non-patients, and their depression levels increase significantly throughout the first year of medical school(Vitaliano P et al 1989). Stress may also harm trainees' professional effectiveness: it decreases attention (Smith K, 1990) reduces concentration (Askenasy J, Lewin I,1996), impinges on decision-making skills(Lehner P et al,1997:Klein G et al, 1996) and reduces trainees' abilities to establish strong physician-patient relationships(Pastore FR et al, 1995). There are many causes for psychological distress in medical students. Training is long and hard, and character traits such as perfectionism have been associated with depression and anxiety both in medical students (Helmers K.F et al, 1997) and doctors

(Schreier AR, and Abramovitch H, 1997). Medical students with low A level grades, an anxious personality, and reliance on avoidance coping strategies are also at risk (Stewart S.M et al 1997). Students commonly worry about the curriculum, personal competence, endurance, and finding time to have a life outside medical school (Stewart S.M et al 1997). These results suggest that there is a shift to a more cynical and hedonistic orientation during medical school as well as significant elevations and increases in symptoms of depression and anxiety. These shifts may in part be attributable to coping with a stressful learning environment.

School Environment

Very considerable attention is now being given to medical school as a social environment. The interface between the teaching staff and the medical students has long been a focus of research. Three decades ago investigations at Cornell University found sufficient respect and courtesy on the part of the teaching staff and the institution to consider that students were explicitly considered as collegues (Merton et al 1957). In contrast, investigations from Chicago found that at Kansas, medical students were disparaged and isolated as a student body, distanced from their teachers(Becker et al 1961).A similar situation can still be seen in developing countries like India (Acharya S 2003). Some clinicians deploy a style of teaching by humiliation. The climate of medical education is often unsupportive and threatening where it should be collaborative. This situation is especially prevalent in countries like India where most of medical schools do not provide adequate support services for students and trainees to harmful effects of stress.In a study of 581 students at 10 medical schools across the United States, 96.5% of respondents reported at least one type of perceived mistreatment or harassment during their training (Baldwin W.C et al, 1991). The most frequently type reported was public humiliation. Someone else taking the credit for one's work or being threatened with unfair grades or physical harm was also reported. Sexual harassment was a common complaint (55%). Mistreatment was most frequently attributed to residents and attending physicians. Mistreatment has been found to be widespread and pervasive during medical education (Silver 1982; Rosenberg and Silver 1984;Wolf et al 1989b; Sheehan et al 1990; Baldwin et al 1991; Silver and Glicken 1990; Richman et al 1992). Percieved psychological mistreatment by interns / residents and clinical teachers were found to be most widespread and there was also evidence found for sexual harassment. Increased perceived mistreatment was found to be positively associated with a perceived increase in cynicism (Wolf et al 1991b). It is possible that psychological harm and injury can have a lasting effect on the students(Sheehan et al 1990;Silver and Glicken 1990; Richman et al 1992). For example in one study students who reported experiencing atleast one abusive experience were significantly more likely to experience depressive symptoms and drink for escape purposes(Richman et al 192). The harmful consequences of the assault and insults reflected in the term 'traumatic deidealisation ' refer to an undercutting of self esteem and lowering of ideals about teachers and the medical profession by medical students (Kay 1990). These assaults and insults make it particularly problematic for emotionally vulnerable medical students whose identities as doctors are largely established during medical school (Knight 1981; Sheehan et al 1990; Silver and Glicken 1990). This perceived mistreatment can be detrimental to the psychological development of the students and potentially interfere with developing a positive doctor – patient relationship.

Demographic Characteristics

It is also important to consider the demographic differences in the way students may respond to the stress of medical education. Regarding the sex differences during the first year, women students developed more psychiatric symptoms and tended to report less satisfaction with life by mid year and remained more symptomatic by the end of the year but to a lesser extent(Lloyd and Gartrell 1981).Women also reported more role conflict and described their families as less supportive of their career choice. In a second study women students reported more negative effect and physical symptoms during the first term of medical schools as well as reporting a greater decrease in positive emotions and perceived peer friendliness than men (Alagna and Morkoff 1986). In an Indian study on dental students ,it was found that males tended to have greater stress than females.(Acharya S,2003). Although minority students (Black and Hispanic) reported greater social supports, higher self esteem ,lower anxiety and more internal locus of control, upon entering medical school, after one year the black students manifested slightly lower self esteem and higher levels of hostility and external locus of control. The Hispanic students continued to report higher self esteem and greater social supports but showed increased external locus of control and higher alcohol consumption. In a second study , black students perceived more stressors than white medical students in the same environment during the first year (Strayhorn 1980). Regarding marital status , the stressors of medical school were more severe for the single students; moreover, stress levels of formerly single students declined after marriage (Coombs and Fawzy 1982). It is important to take these demographic variables into account in designing future studies and intervention programs. In an Indian study, no difference in stress was observed in perceived stress on the basis of sex, place of stay, Mother tongue or on the basis of place of school or junior college education(Supe et al 1998).

Coping in Medical School

The ways in which medical students cope with stress in medical education, rather than the stressors per se may be the primary determinant of their health (Lazaraus and Folkman 1984). Coping and perceived social support are important mediating variables between stress and health outcomes(Lazaraus and Folkman 1984).Three adaptive styles for coping with stressors seem prominent among medical students: 1) Vigorous efforts to master ,overcome or counteract them instead of trying to live with or escape them.2) Changing the environment rather than themselves. And 3) Translating their feelings into ideas , manipulating these ideas , and sometimes forgetting the original feelings (Keniston 1967). Problem focused coping directed at altering or managing the problem causing the distress and emotion – focused coping directed at regulating the emotional response to the problem are two strategies which have been identified for dealing with stress (Lazaraus and Folkman 1984). Problem focused coping was used most frequently in a 4 year retrospective study with graduating medical students (Wolf et al 1988). These students also reported using a diversity of coping strategies (Wolf et al 1988), which is common in dealing with stressful encounters (Lazaraus and Folkman 1984). In a longitudinal study with first year medical students , problem focused and seeking social support coping decreased while emotion focused strategies increased (Vitaliano et al 1989b). Satisfaction with social supports decreased over the course of the first year and did not exert a protective role against psychological distress (Vitaliano et al 1989b). In another study, social support and psychiatric symptomatology were positively associated by mid year for first year students (Foorman and Lloyd 1986).It is conceivable that in a medical school environment , social ties may place competing demands on the student's time and energy and have potentially detrimental effects on health.

Effect of Coping Styles on Stress

Research shows that students with active coping styles (those who can tackle problems in a positive and straightforward manner) have lower levels of psychological distress (Stewart S.M et al 1997). However in an Indian study , it was found that stress was more common in medical students who have a dominant strategy of coping as positive reappraisal ,accepting responsibility, and planful solving. Those with the dominant strategy of escaping and distancing from difficult situation reported less stress. (Supe 1998). Preliminary evidence suggests that teaching medical students more effective coping strategies reduces distress in the short term (Mosley TH, and Perrin SG, 1994), and provides long-term protective effects (Michie S and Sandhu S, 1994). Helping students develop better ways of dealing with stress at an early stage of their medical undergraduate training needs to be considered, as students who suffer from distress in the first year of the course are at the highest risk of developing symptoms of stress later on (Guthrie E and Black D, 1998) In view of the potential long term benefits of managing stress in a more effective way, it may be important for students to develop such skills early on in their medical career.

Stress, Coping and Health Outcome

There are considerable data supporting the relationship between stress and health outcome (Notman et al 1984; Vitaliano eta 1 1984; Carmel and Berbstein 1987; Strayhorn 1989;Wolf et al 1989b;1999a;Bramness et al 1991).In these studies ,stress was measured in diverse ways with different instruments and related to a variety of psychological and physical outcome measures , for example, 6 medical school pressures including intangible phenomena such as threat and anonymity and more practical problems such as limited personal time and long hours were related to anxiety(Vitaliano et al 1984),while in a second study the perceived stressfulness of patient contact and medical practice demands were correlated with trait anxiety (Cornell and Bernstein 1987). In a nine month longitudinal study ,with first year medical students , hassles (Wide range of personal and professional irritating and annoying experiences) predicted concurrent and subsequent mood(Wolf et al 1989b), while with another sample of first year students, hassles at the beginning of first year were related to psychological symptoms at the beginning and the end of the year(Wolf et al 1991a).

Percieved mistreatment has also been related to a variety of mental health status , outcome measures including depressive and anxiety symptoms, hostility problem and escapist drinking,alchohol consumption leves and gender role orientation(Richman et al 1992), with Norwegian students, stress was a good predictor of mental health and consistent with the findings of U.S schools(Bramness et al 1991).

Two studies merit highlighting because of the unique methodology employed of grouping stydents by perceived stress (Vitaliano et al 1989) and psychological symptoms(Miller and Surtees 1991). Four groups were identified in the first study: 1) Resistors – Stress scores began and ended low; 2) Persistors – Scores began and remained high 3) Adaptors – Scores decreased from high to low; and 4) Maladaptors - Scores increased from low to high. These four groups were distinguishable by a variety of psychosocial variables including type A personality, anger expression and coping (Vitaliano 1989a). For example, resistors and maladopters began the year with similar levels of suppressed anger, external locus of control and wishful thinking, while at the end of the year, the maladaptors had significant increases in these variables whereas the resistors did not. In the second study , a subgroup of students who were continuosly symptomatic were distinguished from other groups by the following factors: 1) They were slow to make friends 2) Had inappropriate support from relatives 3) Had a tendency to have rows 4) Had steady girl or boyfriends and 5) Had vulnerable personalities(Miller and Surtees 1991). Differentiating students on stress, psychological symptoms and relevant dimensions and relating these factors to psychosocial and health/disease variables is a valuable approach for gaining a better understanding of stress,coping and health during medical education.

In the Precursors Study , medical student reactions to stress as self reported on a checklist of habits of nervous tension reflected individual psychobiological differences that are linked with future health or disease(Thomas 1971,1976; Thomas and McCabe 1980). The differing behavioral and affective reactions to stress appear to precede the initial clinical manifestations of major disease states by upto 20 to 30 years (Thomas and McCabe 1980). In a recent report from the Precursors Study (Graves and Thomas 1991),two of the 25 items from the Habits of Nervous Tension Questionnaire which were the strongest predictors of suicide were irritability and urinary frequency. Both these irems suggest that the proposed psychological sensitivities may relate to physiologic reactivity(Graves and Thomas 1991).These findings certainly have important implications for a preventive approach to health for medical students.

Coping was related to psychological distress in a longitudinal study of medical students (Vitaliano 1989b).Problem-focused coping was negatively related to distress while emotion-focused coping was positively focused to distress. This finding is consistent with the previous study of 12 diverse samples (Vitaliano et al 1986), in which problem focused coping was significantly and negatively related with psychological distress in 11 of the 12 samples while wishful thinking was positively related to distress in 10 of the 12 samples (Vitaliano et al 1986). Therefore, how medical students cope with stress during medical education can relate to health outcome which has important implications for intervention programmes designed to enhance adaptive coping strategies.

Cultural and Social Factors in Developing Countries

A lot of research has gone into the factors affecting stress and the coping systems in western countries. The support systems in the developed countries are very advanced and refined with the latest in science to back them up. However the Asian situation is very different. Owing to the difference in culture, there are some differences when it comes to factors affecting stress and the support systems in Asian countries.

There are huge differences between the education systems of Asian countries and the west. The American system is very flexible in the sense that students can choose among a host of classes and courses in high school and college. This means that they can change their major midway through college. This usually means that students in U.S receive more exposure to a variety of subjects and hence are more aware of their career options and opportunities. The American education system is designed in such a way so as not to hurt or reduce the self esteem of a student and most of the students pass the high school level. Also the education system is geared towards satisfying the needs of the industry. Student expression is encouraged and the teacher plays more of a supportive role than that of an instructor.

The Indian education system is one of the toughest and most competitive in the world. This education system is very rigid in the sense that the students upon enrolling for a graduate course can under no circumstances change their majors midway. Numerous subjects are heaped on the students at the school level. This undue thrust ends up blunting the student's sensitivity. Secondly the stiff competition that is rampant nowadays at all levels of education is also responsible for the discomfiture. Competition is akin to gambling and there is resultant stress. The student is forced to go through the drudgery of carrying on with the course, which he or she doesn't like. This can affect their academic performance. The whole graduate program is exam oriented and does not focus on the all round development of the individual. The fear of examinations begins almost as early as the IIIrd grade and persists upto even postgraduate levels. A number of social and psychological factors such as parental pressure, lack of career opportunities, uncertain future and so forth may trigger them off.This fear of examination is very much evident in medical and dental students also(Acharya S ,2003).

The syllabus is strictly written. One has to know the textbooks very well and if possible understand the content or other wise just learn the answers with out understanding it. This is because there is a lot of stress on theory and not on practical work. Some of the textbooks are never updated. Students continue to study the textbooks that were written 10 years ago. In short, students lose interest in their studies, as it is very boring, monotonous and tedious. The purpose of the educational system is not specified. In spite of spending lots of money for a good education and finishing graduation, many students still don't get jobs. The high school education system is very tough and harsh on the students who are burdened with a huge curriculum which is sometimes equivalent to that of American majors programs. Many students find it difficult to cope with the stress and resort to suicide, drug abuse, delinquency etc. The' corporal' mentality of the teaching faculty, a legacy of the British rule is still rampant, resulting in the near dictatorial attitude of the faculty. The students are not encouraged to form their own opinions, and open discussions are clearly discouraged. Not agreeing with the faculty's orders may lead to punitive action ranging from being ridiculed publicly in front of other students to failure in the examinations. In spite of being officially banned, corporal punishment is still rampant in schools especially in the rural areas.. Because of the relative absence of support and counseling centers, the student has nowhere to turn to other than his family. In many cases, the family too is found wanting in giving support during this crucial period. It is the parents who constantly dump their own pent up or unfulfilled ambitions on their children. In the process the dreams and ambitions of the children get thwarted. Most parents want their off springs to be doctors or engineers, even if the children may not have inclinations or capabilities for the same. In fact, a child's academic record and performance becomes a prestige issue for the parents and even families.

Sometimes parents feel a big blow is given to their self-esteem if their child fails or gets very bad marks in the exams. So they emotionally torture their child, which, is also one of the reasons why the student is driven to extreme measures like suicides. This phenomenon is common to all the Asian families where emphasis on hard work, discipline and respect for authority is inherent. (Suzuki, 1980).

The families in their anxiety about their ward's future ride roughshod over any concerns that their child might have , and encourage them to just "Take it on the Chin". Children are many a time forced to join an educational graduate program by their parents against their wishes. Such students have been found to suffer from more stress than those who joined of their accord (Acharya, 2003). Students joining courses that do not guarantee gainful employment suffer from more stress than the others (Acharya, 2003). Sometimes students lose faith in themselves if they are constantly failing or because they only hear criticism from their teachers and parents. Due to this they feel that they are hopeless and cannot do anything in life. These factors lead to the student losing his or her self esteem and confidence. There are fights between friends or peers, on who is more intelligent than the other this also causes emotional stress and frustration on the student.

Medical students in developing countries like their counterparts in the west face a tremendous amount of stress during their period of education. But in addition to the common factors, students from developing countries have to face some special circumstances caused by the difference in socioeconomic and cultural factors. In the western countries the medical profession is always under public scrutiny and because of high awareness among the public, malpractice suits are common. This often leads to the doctor patient relationship deteriorating into a customer client relationship. Hence more emphasis is placed on collecting evidence from the patient like lab reports, special investigations, having witnesses etc, to prevent future career ruining lawsuits than on actual treatment. In their efforts to have an evidence-based practice, the basic ethos of the medical profession may get diluted. In developing countries, the amount of respect the doctors command in the society is phenomenal and sometimes intimidating. This is even more so in the rural areas where the concept of 'Vaidya Narayano Hari " the Sanskrit phrase meaning " Doctor is equivalent to God " still prevails. Any treatment given or suggested by the doctor is considered sacrosanct. This may be one of the reasons why the number of malpractice litigations is negligible and almost non-existent in the rural areas. Since any treatment the doctor advises is followed with no questions asked, the doctor is under tremendous moral pressure to deliver. Evidence based practice is very much limited to some select urban areas. It is virtually non-existent in rural and semi urban areas because of the lack of basic laboratory facilities. The facilities though available in the big cities, are not affordable to a majority of the population. This creates a difficult situation where a doctor has to rely solely on the clinical signs and symptoms and his clinical training and experience when prescribing treatment. The students may find it very stressful to fit into the society's image of the medical profession. The development of the 'Imposter Phenomenon' because of these factors cannot be ruled out.

Studies have shown that cultural factors can affect the symptom expression of stress. Reports have shown that depression and anxiety are expressed in somatic terms in non western cultures in comparison to western cultures(Gureje et al 1997;Simon et al 1996).Kleinmann noted that in non western cultures, feelings of sadness, worthlessness and guilt were less common while somatic complaints such as feeling tired ,stomach aches ,headaches were more common. These somatic complaints have also been reported to include dizziness , fatigue and abdominal pain(Cheung1985; Kleinmann1988; Youngmann et al 1999).

Dental Students

Dentistry has been widely acknowledged as being associated with high levels of stress.(Atkinson et al 1991; Gorter R.C 1999). Stressors associated with dentistry include time and scheduling pressures, managing uncooperative patients, commercial issues and the highly technical and intensive nature of work.(Atkinson et al 1991; Gorter R.C et al 1999). The origins of this stress may lie in the process of dental education (Westerman G.H et al 1993; Heath J.R., et al 1999;Lamis D.R, 2001). In recent years, the injurious effects of stress experienced by dental students have received much attention. Stress has been shown to manifest as fatigue, tension, dizziness, sleeplessness, tachycardia, gastro intestinal symptoms and also irritability, anxiety and cynicism(Martinez N.P 1977;Knudsen W,1978;Wexler M,1978; Grandy T.G et al 1988;Cecchini J.J et al 1987;Tedesco L.A, 1986) In addition to this, a negative association has been reported between stress and academic performance of dental students(Cecchini J.J et al 1987;Tedesco L.A, 1986).Studies on dental students have shown that they are not much different from medical students when it comes to sources of stress, and coping mechanisms.

Recommendations

Some recommendations evolving from this overview of stress , coping , and health among students of medicine and its allied branches are advanced for enhancing the well being of the students.

> It is advantageous to obtain a clear understanding and have realistic expectation about what it takes to become a doctor and road that has to be traveled prior even to entering medical school (Coombs et al 1990).

➤ It is important to place a greater emphasis on qualitative variables in the admission process(Walton 1987;World Federation for Medical Education 1988; McGaghie 1990;Coombs 1991)

➤ The undergraduate medical school curriculum should include a didactic grounding and clinical experience in health promotion and disease prevention(Newfeld and Barrows 1974; Coles 1985;Kaufman et al 1989; Tayloret al 1989; Altekruse et al 1991)

➤ Health promotion programs (e.g Dickstein and Elks 1986; Wolf et al 1990;Basmuke et al 1992) are helpful in developing and maintaining a balanced lifestyle and can enhance the personal well-being of medical students.

➤ Medical, psychiatric and academic counseling should be made available to all medical students.

➤ Additional research is needed regarding all aspects of medical education with an emphasis on longitudinal research designs tapping into the complex interplay of environmental, personality, coping, academic and health outcome variables.

➤ It would be desirable to foster an international collaboration on well being issues among medical schools to work on improving all aspects of medical education such as periodic conferences of World Federation for Medical Education

➤ Periodic interaction of the faculty with trained educational psychologists who can train the faculty in the latest educational methodologies to maximize student performance and minimize stress (Acharya S 2003).

➤ Parents should be counseled during their children's pre-university period about the ill effects of pressurizing them to join an educational program against their wishes. This can be done by drafting the help of the high school authorities in conducting workshops involving parents and teachers on a regular basis. Career fairs can also be used as a forum for parent counseling (Acharya S 2003).

➤ Since it has been shown that students from predominantly non western cultures most of which are in developing countries express symptoms of stress through somatisation rather than psychologically, more attention should be paid by the educators to identify these symptoms to effectively deal with student stress.

➤ Students should also be taught to identify these symptoms among themselves and their friends, so that they can seek help at the appropriate forum.

REFERENCES

Acharya S. Factors affecting stress among Indian dental students. *J Dent Educ.* 2003 Oct;67(10):1140-8.

Altekruse J.,Goldenberg K.,Rabin D.,Riegelman R.K., & Wiese W.H.Implementing the Association of Teachers of Preventive Medicine's recommendations into the undergraduate medical school curriculum.*Academic Medicine* 1991. ,6,312-316.

Anderson ,C.L. et al.*Community Health*, 1978. C.V.Mosby.

Askenasy J, Lewin I. The impact of missile warfare on self-reported sleep quality. *Sleep*.1996; 19:47 –51

Atkinson T.M., Millar K., Kay E.J., Blinkhorn A.S. Stress in dental practice. *Dent Update.* 1991; 18: 60-4.

Baldwin WC, Daugherty RS, Eckenfels EJ. Students perceptions of mistreatment and harassment during Medical School. A survey of ten United States Schools. *The Western Journal of Medicine* 1991;**155**(2):140-5.

Bramneess JG, Fixdal TC, Vaglun P. Effect of Medical School Stress on the Mental Health of Medical Students in early and later clinical curriculum. *Acta Psychiatrica Scandinavia* 1991;**84**(4):340-5.

Cecchini J.J., Friedman V. First year dental students: relationship between stress and performance. *Int J Psychosom.* 1987; 34: 17-19.

Cheung F.M. (1985). An overview of psychopathology in Hong Kong with special reference to somatic presentation. In W. Tseng and D.Wu (Eds).*Chinese culture and mental health.* (pp 287-304). Orlando: Academic Press Inc.

Cmich,D.E *Jr. School Health* 1984.54,(1)30-32

Coles C.Differences between conventional and problem – based curricula in their students' approaches to studying.*Medical Education* 1985.19,308-309.

Coles C.Medicine and Stress. *Med Educ* 1994;28: 3-4

Coombs R.H. Non cognitive components in the selection and training of medical students.*Med Educ* 1991.25,539-541.

Coombs RH, Perell K, Ruckh JM. Primary prevention of emotional impairment among medical trainees. *Academic Medicine* 1990;**65**(9):576-81.

Dickstein L.J. & Elkes J.,(1986).A health awareness workshop: Enhancing Coping skills in medical students.In:*Heal Thyself: The Health of health care professionals*(ed. by C.Scott & J. Hawk). Brunner/Mazel, New York.

Dill, Patricia L. and Tracey B. Henley. "Stressors of College: A Comparison of Traditional and Nontraditional Students." *Journal of Psychology* 1998. 132(1): 25-32.

Dismuke S.E., McCleary A.M., McCall J., & Runyan J.W.Integrating an educational program and health promotion ,disease prevention into a medical school: University of Tennessee. *American Journal of Health Promotion* 1992.6,363,372-379.

Eberst,R.M. *Jr.School Health* 1984.54(3)99-104

Ensel, Walter M., and Nan Lin. "The life stress paradigm and psychological distress." *Journal of Health and Social Behavior* 1991. 32: 321-341.

Firth J.Levels and sources of stress in medical students. *Br Med J* 1986; 292:1177-80

Firth-Cozens J. Predicting stress in general practitioners: 10 year follow up postal survey. *Br Med J* 1997;313:34-5.

Gallegos K, Bettinardi-Angres K, Talbott G. The effect of physician impairment on the family. *Maryland Med J.*1990; 39:1001 -7.

Gaughran F, Dineen S, Dineen M, Cole M, Daly RJ. Stress in medical students. *Ir Med J* 1997;90:184-5.

Goldrnan, Cristin S, and Wong, Eugene H. "Stress And The College Student." *Education*, Summer 97, Vol. 117 Issue 4, p604, 7p, 1 chart

Gorter R.C., Albrecht G., Hoogstraten J., Eijkman M.A.J. Professional burnout among Dutch dentists. *Community Dent Oral Epidemiol.* 1999; 27; 109-16.

Grandy T.G., Westerman G.H., Lupo J.V., Comb C.G. Stress symptoms among third year dental students. *J Dent Educ.* 1988; 52: 245-9.

Gurege. O, Simon.G, Ustus. T,Goldberg D.Somatization in a cross cultural perspective: A WHO study in primary care. *American Journal of Psychiatry* ,1997; 154(7); 989-995

Guthrie E, Black D, Bagalkote H, Shaw C, Campbell M, Creed F. Psychological stress and burnout in medical students: a five year prospective longitudinal study. *J R Soc Med* 1998;91:237-43.

Guthrie EA, Black D, Shaw CM, Hamilton J, Creed FH, Tomenson B. Embarking upon a medical career: psychological morbidity in first year medical students. *Med Educ* 1995;29:337-41.

Heath J.R., MacFarlane T.V., Umar M.S. Perceived sources of stress in dental students. *Dent Update.* 1999; 26: 94-100.

Helmers KF, Danoff D, Steinert Y, Leyton M, Young SN. Stress and depressed mood in medical students, law students, and graduate students at McGill University. *Acad Med* 1997;72:708-14.

Hirsch, J. K., & Ellis, J. B. Differences in life stress and reasons for living among college suicide ideators and non-Ideators. *College Student Journal* 1996. 30, 377-384.

Indrayan A, Rao S,Grover V,Agrawal K,Gupta A."Freshers perception of problems in medical education"*Indian J Med Educ* 1985;24:85-94

Johnson N, Michels P, Thomas J. Screening tests identify the prevalence of alcohol use among freshman medical students and among students' family of origin. *J South Carolina Med Assoc.*1990; 86:13 –4

Kaufmann A., Mennin S., Waterman R., Duban S., Hansbarger C., Silverblat H.,Obenshain S.C., Cantrowitz M.,Becker T.,Sammmet J., & Wiese W. The New Mexico Experiment: Education Innovation and Institutional Change.*Academic Medicine* 1989.64,285-294.

Klein G. The effect of acute stressors on decision making. In: Driskell J, Salas E (eds). *Stress and Human Performance.* Mahwah, NJ: Lawrence Erlbaum, 1996:48 -88.

Kleinmann A. *Rethinking Psychiatry: From Cultural Category to personal experience.* 1988; New York; Free Press

Kohn, J. P., & Frazer, G. H. An academic stress scale: Identification and rated importance of academic stressors. *Psychological Reports* 1986. 59, 415-426.

Lamis D.R. Perceived sources of stress among dental students at the University of Jordan. *J Dent Educ.* 2001; 65: 232-241.

Lehner P, Seyed-Solorforough M, O'Connor M, Sak S, Mullin T. Cognitive biases and time stress in team decision making. *Trans Systems, Man & Cybernetics.*1997; 27:698 -703.

Martinez N.P. Assessment of negative effects in dental students. *J Dent Educ.* 1977; 41: 31-36.

McCormack, Arlene Smith. Drinking in stressful situations: college men under pressure." *College Student Journal* 1996. 30 (1): 65-77.

McGaghie W.C. Qualitative variables in medical school admission. *Academic Medicine* 1990. 65,154-149.

Megel, Mary Erickson, Peggy Hawkins, Susie Sandstrom, Mary Ann Hoefler, and Kathleen Willrett "Health Promotion, Self-Esteem and Weight Among Female College Freshman." *Health Values*, 18 (4): 10- 19. 1994.

Michie S, Sandhu S. Stress management for clinical medical students. *Med Educ* 1994;28:528-33.

Miller P McC. The first year at medical school: some findings and student perceptions. *Med Educ* 1994;28:5-7.

Morgan, Sue. "Cheap drinks, heavy costs: students and alcohol." *Youth and Policy* 1997. 56: 42-54.

Mosley TH, Perrin SG, Neral SM, Dubbert PM, Grothues CA, Pinto BM. Stress, coping and well-being among third-year medical students. *Acad Med* 1994;69:765-7.

Moss, Gordon E. *Illness Immunity and Social Interaction.*1973. New York: John Wiley.

Naquin, M.R. and Glen G. Glibert. "College students' smoking behavior, perceived stress and coping styles." *Journal of Drug Education* 1996. 26 (4): 367-76.

Neufeld V.R, Barrows H.S, The 'McMaster Philosophy': An approach to medical education.*Joural of Medical Education* 1974.49,1040-50.

Pastore FR, Gambert SR, Plutchik A, Plutchik R. Empathy training for medical students. Unpublished manuscript, New York Medical College, 1995.

Pitts FN, Winokur G, Stewart MA. Psychiatric syndromes, anxiety symptoms and responses to stress in medical students. *Am J Psychiatry*. 1961;118:333 -40.

Richings JC, Khara GS, McDowell. Suicide in young doctors.*Br J Psychiatry*. 1986;149:475 –8

Richman JA, Flaherty JA, Rospenda KM, Christensen ML. Mental Health Consequences and correlates of reported medical student abuse. *JAMA* 1992; 267(5): 692-4.

Romano, J. L. (1992). Psychoeducational interventions for stress management and well-being. *Journal of Counseling and Development*, 71, 199-202.

Rose ,G.A.and Blackburn H.(1968)Cardiovascular Survey Methods, Geneva,WHO.

Salt P, Nadelson C, Notman M. Depression and anxiety among medical students. Paper presented at APA Annual Meeting, Los Angeles, CA, 1984.

Schreier AR, Abramovitch H. American medical students in Israel: stress and coping. *Br J Psych* 1997;171:519-23.

Schutt, Russell K., Tatjana Meschede and Jill Riordan. "Distress, suicidal thoughts and social support among homeless adults." *Journal of Health and Social Behavior,*1994. 35: 134-42

Sgan-Cohen, H. D., & Lowental, U. Sources of stress among Israeli dental students. *The Journal of the American College Health Association,*1988. 36, 317-321.

Sheehan KH, Sheehan DV, White K, Leibowitz A, Baldwin DC. A pilot study of medical student abuse and student perception of mistreatment and misconduct in Medical School. *JAMA* 1990;**263**:533-7.

Silver HK, Glicken AD, Medical Students abuse - incidence, severity and significance. *JAMA* 1990;**263**(4):527-32.

Silver HK. Medical Students and Medical School. *JAMA* 1982;**247**:309-310.

Simon.G, Gater.R, Kiseli.S,Piccinelli.M. Somatic symptoms of distress: An international primary care study. *Psychomatic Medicine* ,1996;58;481 – 488.

Smith A. Stress and information processing. In: Johnston M, Wallace L, et al (eds). *Stress and Medical Procedures*. Oxford Medical Publications. Oxford, England: Oxford University Press, 1990:184.

Stewart SM, Betson C, Lam TH, Marshall IB, Lee PW, Wong CM. Predicting stress in first year medical students: a longitudinal study. *Med Educ* 1997;31:163-8.

Suzuki, B. (1980). Education and the socialization of Asian Americans: A revisionist analysis of the "model minority" theses. In R. Endo, S. Sue, & N. Wagner (Eds.), *Asian-Americans: Social and psychological perspectives* (pp. 155-178). Palo Alto, CA: Science and Behavioral Books.

Taylor W.C.,Pels R.J.,& Lawrence R.S. A First year problem based curriculum in health promotion and disease prevention. *Academic Medicine*,1989.673-677.

Tedesco L.A. A psychosocial perspective on dental education experience and student performance. *J Dent Educ.* 1986; 50: 601-5.

Thoits, Peggy A. "Stress, coping and social support processes: Where are we? What Next?" *Journal of Health and Social Behavior*,1995. extra issue: 53-79.

Towbes, L. C., & Cohen, L. H. Chronic stress in the lives of college students: Scale development and prospective prediction of distress. *Journal of Youth and Adolescence*,1996. 25, 199-217.

Vitaliano P, Maiuro R, Russo J, Mitchell E. Medical student distress: a longitudinal study. *J Nerv Ment Dis.*1989; 177:70 –6

Vitaliano PP,Russo J,Carr JE,Heerwagen JH.Medical school pressures and their relationship to anxiety.*J Nervous Mental Dis* 1984;172:730-6.

Walton,H.J. Personality assessment of future doctors. *Journal of the Royal Society of Medicine.*1987.80,27-30.

Westerman G.H., Grandy T.G., Ocanto R.A., Eriksine C.G. Perceived sources of stress in the dental school environment. *J Dent Educ.* 1993; 57: 225-31.

Wexler M. Mental health and dental education. *J Dent Educ.* 1978; 42: 74-7.

WHO (1964).Techn.Rep.Ser.,275

WHO(1985)Techn Rep Ser., No.714

Wolf T.M., Randall H.,& Faucett J.A health promotion program for medical student: Louisiana State University Medical Center.American *Journal of Health Promotion.*1990 4,193-282.

Wolf TM, Randall HM, Von Almen K, Tynes LL. Perceived mistreatment and attitude change by graduating medical students: a retrospective study. *Medical Education* 1991;**25**:192-90.

World Federation for medical education. The Edinburgh Declaration. *Lancet*,1988. 8608,464.

Wright, J. J. Environmental stress evaluation in a student community. The *Journal of the American College Health Association.*1964, 12(5), 325-336.

Wright, J. J. Reported personal stress sources and adjustment of entering freshmen. *Journal of Counseling Psychology.*1967. 14(4), 371-373.

Youngmann.R, Minuchin-Itsigsolin.S, Miriam ,B. Manifestations of emotional distress among Ethiopian immigrants in Israel: Patent and Clinician Perspectives.*Transcultural Psychiatry.*1999;36(1), 45-63.

In: Psychology of Stress
Editor: Kimberly V. Oxington, pp. 101-112

ISBN 1-59454-246-5
©2005 Nova Science Publishers, Inc.

Chapter VI

CHRONIC VERSUS ACUTE STRESS SITUATIONS: A COMPARISON OF MODERATING FACTORS

Shifra Sagy[*]
Ben-Gurion University of the Negev

ABSTRACT

The research compared patterns of moderating factors explaining stress reactions during two kinds of states: chronic without acute versus chronic plus acute stress. We examined the hypothesis that during a prolonged stress state, personal dispositions would have more explanatory power to understand stress reactions than in an acute situation. The research was conducted with Israeli Jewish adolescents, living in West Bank settlements, in two different situations: during the prolonged state of the "*intifada*" (the chronic without acute state) period and in the chronic (plus acute) state, immediately after the assassination of Prime Minister Rabin. Five variables were examined as moderating factors: trait anxiety, sense of coherence, cognitive appraisal of the political situation, family sense of coherence, and sense of community. Two stress reactions were measured: state anxiety and psychological distress. Data were collected from 266 eighth grader pupils during the chronic stress state, and 448 pupils at the same grade level at the acute stress state. The overall magnitude of variance explanation was found to be different at each state: a relatively high explained variance of state anxiety and psychological distress was found in the chronic stress situation, but not in the acute state. These data support the value of developing a model that would recognize the different types of stress situations in the study of moderating effects of stress.

The importance of considering differential stress effects on individual reactions in the field of stress and anxiety has been highly evaluated by some researchers (e.g. Folkman & Lazarus, 1985; Magnusson, 1982). This approach claims to understand and explain individual reactions in terms of the patterns of cross-situational profile. Actually, only a few models or

---

[*] Prof. Shifra Sagy, Department of Education, Ben-Gurion University of the Negev, P.O.Box 653, Beer-Sheva 84105, Israel. Telfax: 972-7-6469148 E-mail address: shifra@bgumail.bgu.ac.il

theories on the effects of stress deal with the problem of differences in types of stress situations (Parkes, 1986). Moreover, only a few models differentiate between chronic strains the relatively enduring problems, conflicts, and threats that people face in their daily lives - and acute stressors (Timko, Moos & Michelson, 1993). Although prolonged or chronic stress may be perceived as one of the major types of stressful situations, which often have more pervasive and potentially detrimental effects (Pearlin, 1989), most theories of psychological stress have put greater emphasis on studying reactions to acute life events (Garbarino & Kostelmy, 1994; Moos, 1992). Moreover, there has been no systematic research regarding the comparative question of the differential determinants or factors explaining stress reactions in these two kinds of states: chronic versus acute stress situations (Moos, 1992; Pearlin, 1989).

Human condition, however, is stressful and stresses are ubiquitous (Antonovsky, 1987). Thus, the interesting question is not the comparison between chronic versus acute stress situations only. It is rather investigation of the prolonged or chronic stress situation in two different states: chronic without acute versus chronic plus acute stress.

This paper compares stress reactions of adolescents under these two divergent environmental circumstances. Specifically, our aim was to study some moderating factors that may serve a "buffering" role in attenuating the potential impact of stressor events (Billings & Moos, 1981). We compared patterns of these moderating effects during a chronic without specific acute stress situation with patterns of effects in a chronic plus acute state.

The prolonged "chronic" stress situation can be perceived as more similar to a "normal" situation, usually characterized by daily hassles (Elliot & Eisdrofer, 1982). Indeed, research from different parts of the world has tended to confirm that children exposed to political violence do not inevitably suffer serious psychological consequences (Cairns & Dawes, 1996). In fact, the majority exhibit what may be seen as "normal" anxiety (Dawes, 1994). Punamaki (1996) even referred to the possibility of habituation to the political violence and the threatening environment. If we assume the chronic without acute state as an habituated one, we would expect that the moderating factors would have a relatively low explanatory power of the stress reactions then in the chronic plus acute state, since moderating effects are interpreted as occurring at higher than at lower levels of stressfulness (Baron, & Kenny, 1986).

Our research, however, exploited a different theoretical framework. Crisis theorists (e.g. Caplan, 1964) argued that a powerful stressful acute event might minimize or even eliminate individual differences in psychological responses, since it initially overwhelms coping resources for all those affected. Following this theoretical approach, Gal and Israelshvily (1978) proposed an interaction model of reactions to stress, which emphasized the differential influence of situational versus personality factors as determinants of how an individual copes with stress in different states. According to their model, when a threat is perceived as acute, the characteristics of the situation will have greater influence on the person's behavior than his/her personal factors. As the perceived threat decreases, the contribution of personality factors will increase. Some empirical support for this model was found in a previous longitudinal study that was carried out on adolescents who were confronting a stressful acute situation before the evacuation of Sinai settlements in the framework of the peace treaty with Egypt (Sagy & Antonovsky, 1986). Two to three weeks before the evacuation, when the stress was acute, none of the moderating variables examined was found significant in explaining the emotional reactions of state anxiety. After the evacuation, when the acuteness of the stress decreased and became more similar to a "normal" or chronic stress situation (there were still components of stress in the new situation), the predictors for state anxiety showed a significant impact: the explained variance increased from 0% (acute state) to 38% (chronic situation).

According to Gal & Israelshvily (1978) model, we would expect that the moderating factors would have marked effects on the stress reactions in the chronic (without acute) stress situation. Conversely, in the chronic plus acute stress state, it can be hypothesized that the moderators would have a relatively low explanatory power.

Research Background

The research was conducted with Israeli Jewish adolescents living in West Bank settlements[1] in the context of two situations: the chronic prolonged stress of the Jewish settlers during the "*intifada*"[2] period, and the acute state immediately after the assassination of Prime Minister Rabin in November 1995.

What were the components of the prolonged or chronic stress situation? First, the settlers' population in the West Bank was exposed to political violence during the "*intifada*" period, which began in December 1987 and has continued in various forms even after the Oslo Accords between Israel and the Palestinians were signed in 1993. During this long period, the children of the settlers, for example, have been subjected to danger in their daily travels to and from schools. The dangers have included road blocks, stone throwing and gunfire aimed at vehicles.

Other elements of stress were introduced by the ambiguity and uncertainty regarding the future, as a result of the peace agreements between Israel and the Palestinians: an uncertainty about what would happen and what could be done about it. Shalit (1982) viewed ambiguity - "the inability to clarify what the environment is" (p. 7) - as possessing the highest threat potential in the hierarchy of situational variables.

The element of acuteness was introduced to the ongoing chronic stress state by the assassination of Prime Minister Rabin, which occurred just before the second sample of the study was examined (November, 1995). It was a collective traumatic experience for the whole Israeli society. However, public opinion in Israel was highly aroused against the Zionist religious sector, from which the assassin came, and especially since he said that the murder was performed in the name of its ideology.

---

[1] The area of the West Bank under Israel's control was populated by approximately 800,000 Palestinians and close to 130,000 Israelis, a large percent of whom belong to the Zionist religious sector. The Israeli settlements were scattered over a large expanse of territory. Most of the settlements are small, containing up to 1,500 inhabitants, and these were the source of our sample.

[2] "Intifada" is the Arabic word for uprising, and refers to the sudden outburst of Palestinian resistance to the Israeli military occupation, that was the outcome of the Six Days War in 1967.

Factors Explaining Stress Reactions

The present study focused on two emotional reactions that are commonly used in research as indicators of psychological stress (Lazarus, 1993): anxiety state reaction (Spielberger, 1972) and psychological distress as measured by psychosomatic symptoms (Ben-Sira, 1979). As mentioned above, our main comparative question related to the relative explanatory power of personal resources as moderating the negative effects of the stressor toward a lower level of stress reactions. These included three personal orientations or traits- trait anxiety, sense of coherence, cognitive appraisal of the situation-and the sociodemographic parameter of gender. Two environmental resources, as perceived by the adolescents, were introduced by the family sense of coherence and sense of community.

Current research on anxiety distinguishes between the individual's actual experiences of anxiety in a specific situation (i.e., state anxiety) and the individual predisposition to have anxious experiences or to engage in anxiety-provoking behaviors in a stressful situation. Trait anxiety is a relatively stable condition of the individual that represents, among other things, individual differences in the likelihood that, in certain situations, state anxiety will be experienced (Endler & Parker, 1990).

In his theoretical model, Antonovsky (1987) sought to explain the successful coping with stressors by what he calls sense of coherence (SOC). SOC is a global orientation, an enduring tendency to see the world as more or less comprehensible, manageable, and meaningful. The SOC, according to the model, has implications for the individual responses in various kinds of stress situations. The SOC model suggests that an individual with a strong SOC is less likely to perceive many stressful situations as threatening and would be more likely to appraise such situations as manageable. There is less likelihood, then, that a stressful situation would be perceived as anxiety-provoking by an individual who tends to be high on SOC than by one with a low SOC.

Lazarus (1966) introduced the concept of appraisal as the cognitive mediation of stress reactions, viewing it as a universal process in which people evaluate the significance of what is happening for their personal well-being. Phillips and Endler (1982) saw the implication of this assumption for research on anxiety: data on subjects' perceptions of a situation could provide valuable information regarding the degree to which cognitive appraisals moderate between situations and emotional response. It was hypothesized then, that the attitudes regarding the government functioning and the complex political situation after the peace agreements were signed, would influence the emotional responses.

The sociodemographic parameter of gender is considered as a structural context that can affect the ways in which stress outcomes are manifested (Pearlin, 1989). Based on research literature showing that teenage girls generally report higher level of anxiety than boys (e.g., Zeidner, Klingman & Itzkovitz, 1993), it was hypothesized that gender would be another personal factor that explain variability of stress reactions.

The environmental resources examined in this study were the family and the community as perceived by the adolescent. Regarding these kinds of variables, the research is still at a stage that does not enable a satisfactory operational translation of complex collective concepts (Walker, 1985). Sagy & Antonovsky (1992) discussed two dichotomous techniques reflecting theoretical approaches: the holistic approach, which is external and objective (e.g.,

Reiss's work with families, 1981) and, the internal and subjective reductionist approach (e.g., McCubbin & Patterson, 1983). In the present study, we adopted the second approach. This means that we did not inquire into the "objective" cognitive map of the collective group. Instead, we examined the cognitive representations of the individuals involved, as they were seen "in the eyes of the beholder."

The family's views and beliefs were found to be crucial resources for its members' adaptation to stressful events (Boss, 1987; Oliver & Reiss, 1984, Patterson & Garwick, 1994). On the assumption that the family is a salient socializing agent influencing patterns of behavior in adolescence (Coleman, 1980), including emotional responses to stress, the impact of the family sense of coherence on the adolescents' state emotions was examined. The coherence of the family represents the extent to which the respondent sees his or her family world view as coherent.

The two types of states investigated in this study were characterized as complex community stress situations, posing a threat to the entire gamut of communities of settlers in the West Bank. Community characteristics, then, may also contribute to the understanding of emotional reactions in stress situations. The community, in the eyes of the beholder, was investigated by the sense of community concept, that refers to a personal quality connoting a strong attachment between people and their communities (Davidson & Cotter, 1991). McMillan and Chavis (1986) defined this concept in terms of four elements: membership, influence, integration and fulfillment of needs, and shared emotional connections. Empirical research on the model suggests that these four elements are interrelated and comprise a relatively cohesive construct (Chavis, Hodge & McMillan, 1986; Davidson & Cotter, 1991; Pretty, 1990).

To sum up, the present study was formulated to extend our understanding of a variety of moderating factors in two different stress situations. The major hypothesis was that during the chronic without acute stress situation personal dispositions would contribute more to understanding stress reactions, whereas in the chronic plus acute state these factors would have less explanatory power.

METHOD

Participants

The research was carried out in two points of time: November-December 1994 (chronic without acute state) and November-December 1995 (chronic plus acute state). During the first situation data were collected in three schools in the West Bank settlements. The sample was composed of 266 eight-grade pupils (135 boys and 131 girls). On the basis of the pupils' reports, most of the pupils (86%) and their parents (57% of the fathers and 69% of the mothers) were born in Israel. Most of the parents (81% of the fathers and 86% of the mothers) had more than eleven years of education, and 34% of the pupils' fathers and 29% of the mothers had an academic degree.

In the second situation, after Rabin assassination, data were collected in four schools from 448 eight-grade students (213 boys and 235 girls). Pupils who were studying in grade eight in the first stage of the study had already left the school to study in high schools by the second data collection period. Therefore, the sample for the chronic plus acute state was actually a different group. There were no significant differences in the demographic characteristics between the two groups.

Procedure

Data were collected by self-completion questionnaires administered on classrooms during a normal class period. All the students in the grade were invited to participate. The questionnaires were administered by two M.A students, who provided a few general instructions and explanations relating to the anonymity of the data collected.

MEASURERS

The following inventories were used for collecting data in stress reactions:

State Anxiety was assessed using the Hebrew version of Spielberger, Gorsuch and Lushene's (1970) State-Trait Anxiety Inventory (STAI). The Hebrew STAI is a translation of the English STAI, which proved to be reliable, valid and equivalent to the English inventory (Teichman, 1978). State Anxiety scores were evaluated using the mean score of the relevant 20 - items (on a scale of 1-4) inventory of the STAI. In the chronic state of the study the Cronbach's alpha was .84 and .85 in the acute situation.

Scale of Psychological Distress (SPD) is a 6-item psychosomatic symptom scale, referring to frequency of occurrence of familiar psychological symptoms. The scale was developed in Hebrew (Ben-Sira, 1979) and has been used in a number of studies with satisfactory psychometric properties (Ben-Sira, 1988). Five of the items are culled from Langer's psychological-equilibrium index (Langer, 1962): pounding heart, fainting, insomnia, headache and sore hands. The scale was elaborated for use in a population of children (Sagy & Dotan, in press). Some of the symptoms were modified (for example, stomach ache instead of sore hands) and one item (nervous breakdown) was deleted. In this format, the questionnaire included five items and was scored on a scale of 1-4, low scores denoting a high level of psychological distress and high scores indication a low level of distress. In the present study the Cronbach's alpha was .66 in the chronic state group and .61 in the acute one.

The moderator variables were measured by the following inventories:

Trait Anxiety was assessed using the Hebrew version of the Trait Anxiety Inventory of Spielberger, Gorsuch and Lushen's (1970) (STAI). The Cronbach's alpha was .81 in the chronic state group and .78 in the acute one.

Sense of Coherence (SOC) was measured by a series of semantic differential items on a 7-point scale, with anchoring phrases at each end. High scores indicate a strong SOC. An account of the development of the SOC scale and its psychometric properties, showing it to be a reliable and reasonably valid scale, appears in Antonovsky (1987, 1993). In this study, the SOC was measured by a short form scale consisting of 13 items and was found to be highly correlated to the original long version (Antonovsky, 1993). In the present study, the Cronbach's alpha was .74 in the chronic state group and .73 in the acute one. The scale includes items such as: "Doing the things you do everyday is" - answers ranging from (1) "a source of pain and boredom" to (7) "a source of deep pleasure and satisfaction."

Cognitive Appraisal of the Political Situation was measured by a 5-item questionnaire scored on a 5-point Likert scale. It included questions on political attitudes, the chances of the peace process succeeding, the extent of confidence in the government and its ability to function. The Cronbach's alpha was .74 in both groups.

Sense of Family Coherence (SOFC) was measured by a scale consisting of 12 - items on a 7-point scale. This scale is an elaborated version on the family level of the SOC personal orientation scale (Sagy, 1998). The SOFC score is the mean score of all scale items, with high scores denote a strong sense of family coherence. The scale includes items such as: "When your family faces a difficult problem you usually feel that the choice of a solution is..." - answers ranging from (1) "always confusing and hard to find for the family" to (7) " How much does it seems to you that the family rules are clear to you?" answers ranging from (1) "the family rules are not clear al all" to (7) "the family rules are completely clear." Previous studies found Cronbach's alpha coefficients of .88 and .76 (Sagy, 1998, Sagy & Dotan, in press). In the present study the Cronbach's alpha of the scale was .74 in the chronic state group and .77 in the acute one.

Sense of Community was measured by a scale developed by Davidson and Cotter (1986) and was found to be reliable and valid (Davidson & Cotter, 1986, 1991). It consists of 17 questions, scored on a 4-point Likert scale. The scale was translated into Hebrew by Sagy, Stern and Krakover (1996). It includes items such as: "I feel like I belong here" (membership); "It is hard to make friends and meet people in this place" (influence); "It would take a lot for me to move away from this community" (shared emotional connection). In the present study the Cronbach's alpha was .82 in the chronic state group and .85 in the acute one.

RESULTS

Table 1 displays score means, standard deviations and t test results of the variables in the study, each state separately. The State Anxiety and the SPD scores were both at the high end of the scale. t-tests showed no significant differences in State Anxiety and SPD scores between the two states.

The results of stepwise multiple regression analyses, for each state separately, are presented in Tables 2 and 3. The predictor variables examined were: gender, Anxiety- Trait, Sense of Coherence, Sense of Family Coherence, Sense of Community and Cognitive Appraisal.

Table 1: Means, standard deviations and t-test results, for each state separately

Variable	chronic without acute state (n=266)		Chronic plus acute state (n=448)		t-test
	M	SD	M	SD	
State Anxiety	2.24	.57	2.21	.60	.68
Psychological Distress	2.18	.53	2.11	.50	1.67
Trait Anxiety	2.02	.45	1.97	.41	1.72
Sense of Coherence	4.32	.87	4.47	.77	-2.27*
Cognitive Appraisal	4.96	1.09	4.84	1.02	.71
Sense of Family Coherence	4.49	.84	4.76	.80	-4.17***
Sense of Community	2.90	.50	3.23	.49	-8.61***

*$p \leq .05$; **$p \leq .01$; ***$p \leq .001$

Table 2: Stepwise multiple regression results for State Anxiety for each state separately

Variable	chronic without acute state (n=266)		chronic plus acute state (n=448)	
	β	R^2 change	β	R^2 change
Anxiety Trait	.39	.24***	.34	.16***
Sense of Coherence	.00	____	- .05	.01*
Cognitive Appraisal	.11	.02*	-. 06	____
Family Coherence	- .10	.01*	- .01	____
Sense of Community	- .13	.02**	- .08	____
Gender	.09	.01*	.07	____
R^2		.30		.17

*$p \leq .05$; **$p \leq .01$; ***$p \leq .001$

Table 3: Stepwise multiple regression results for
Scale of Psychological Distress for each state separately

Variable	chronic without acute state (n=266)		chronic plus acute state (n=448)	
	β	R^2 change	β	R^2 change
Anxiety Trait	.23	.15***	.16	.07***
Sense of Coherence	- .14	.02*	- .10	.01
Cognitive Appraisal	.01	–	.07	–
Family Coherence	- .05	–	.02	–
Sense of Community	- .03	–	- .08	.01
Gender	.18	.04**	.03	–
R^2		.21		.09

*$p \leq .05$; **$p \leq .01$; ***$p \leq .001$

The main predictor in the two analyses was Anxiety Trait. This may be due to the intercorrelations among some of the moderators (Tabachnick & Fidell, 1983). In the chronic without acute state, however, other predictors (Cognitive appraisal, Sense of Family Coherence, Sense of Community, gender) contributed also to variance explanation, while in the chronic plus acute state no other variables entered the equation. The overall magnitude of variance explanation was also different at each state: in the chronic without acute state the predictor variables explained 30% of variance of State Anxiety, but only 17% in the chronic plus acute state. With regard to SPD, the variance accounted for 21% in the chronic without acute state but only for 9% in the chronic plus acute state.

DISCUSSION

The present study attempted to examine moderating factors related to stress reactions in two different situations: chronic without acute vs. chronic plus acute state. Some of the results indicate a strong similarity between the two chronic stress situations. First, the stress reactions in both situations were found to be similar in their intensity. Second, among the six different personal and environmental resources examined, the personality trait of anxiety was found as the main predictor of the emotional reactions in both situations. Although these findings may be explained in methodological terms, they still suggest that the same personality trait has a potential significance for moderating stress reactions in the two states.

The similar results between the two states can be explained on the background of the selective situations examined here. Since the normal situation was one of chronic stress (with the background of the *intifada*), it seems that the element of acuteness, introduced by the assassination of Rabin, had no additional effect. These results, however, reflect only one aspect of the comparison between the two states.

The more interesting findings of this study seem to reside in the different magnitude of variance explanation at each state: the moderators of stress were more significant in attenuating the reactions of the chronic without acute stress than of the chronic plus acute state. The relatively high explained variance of state anxiety and psychological distress, that was found in the chronic without acute situation, did not appear in the acute state. These findings give some support to our hypotheses regarding the explanatory power of moderating factors. As we suggested above, a possible criterion for buffering effect to occur may be the chronicity vs. the acuteness of the stress situation: the more acute the state the less is the explanatory power of the moderators. The results of this study, showing a significant decrease in the explained variance in the chronic with acute state, support this kind of distinction. A very similar, and even more dramatic tendency, was found in a longitudinal research, mentioned above, on adolescents who experienced an acute stress state before the evacuation of Sinai settlements (Sagy & Antonovsky, 1986). In that study, the explained variance increased from 0% in the acute state to 38% in the chronic situation.

To sum up, the findings of this study support, first and foremost, the value of developing a model that would recognize the different types of stress situations in the research of moderating factors explaining stress reactions. It hints for an important distinction such as chronic with or without acute state, that has received little attention in prior research.

Moreover, our findings support the hypothesis that in a chronic plus acute stress situation the variables of individual psychology have lower explanatory power than in the chronic without acute situation. These results may suggest that research of stress reactions should focus not only on the personal resources as moderators in a stressful acute state.

Despite these theoretically suggestive results, the generalizability of this study is obviously very limited, due to the relatively small samples and the selective and not strictly defined situations examined here. Moreover, this report, which is cross-sectional in nature, prevents causal interpretation. However, since much stress research still involves students and relatively non-stressed samples, research conducted in the field is, we believe, of special interest. "An investigator needs only go where the work is, look, listen and record," wrote Kurt Lewin some five decades ago (quoted in Marrow, 1969, p. 15). To a limited extent, we have attempted to answer this call. So, although the results of this study may reflect only the special, unique situations examined here, they raise theoretical issues that should be investigated in a wider spectrum of stress situations.

REFERENCES

Antonovsky, A. (1987). *Unraveling the mystery of health.* San Francisco: Jossey-Bass

Antonovsky, A. (1993). The structure and properties of the Sense of Coherence Scale. *Social Science & Medicine,* 36, 725-733.

Baron, R. M., & Kenny, D.A. (1986). The moderator-mediator variables distinction in social psychological research: Conceptual, strategic and statistical consideration. *Journal of Personality and Social Psychology,* 51, 1173-1182.

Ben-Sira, Z. (1979). A scale of psychological distress. Research Communications in Psychology, *Psychiatry and Behavior,* 4, 337-356.

Ben-Sira, Z. (1988). *Politics and primary medical care: Dehumanization and overutilization.* Aldershot: Avebury.

Billings, A.G. & Moos, R.H. (1981). The role of coping responses and social resources in attenuating the stress of life events. *Journal of Behavioral Medicine,* 4, 139-157.

Boss, P. (1987). Family stress. In M. Sussman & S. Steinmetz (Eds.) *Handbook of marriage and the family* (pp. 695-724), New York: Plenum Press.

Cairns, E. & Dawes, A. (1996). Children: Ethnic and political violence - a commentary. *Child Development,* 67, 129-139.

Caplan, G. (1964). *Principles of preventive psychiatry.* New York: Basic Books.

Chavis, D., Hodge, J. & McMillan, P. (1986). Sense of community through Brunswick's lens: A first look. *Journal of Community Psychology,* 14, 24-40.

Coleman, J.C. (1980). *The nature of adolescence.* London Methuen.

Davidson, W. B. & Cotter, P.R. (1986). The relationship between sense of community and subjective well-being: A first look. *Journal of Community Psychology,* 19, 246-253.

Davidson, W.B. & Cotter, P.R. (1991). Measurement of sense of community with the sphere of city. *Journal of Applied Social Psychology,* 16, 608-619.

Dawes, A. (1994). The emotional impact of political violence. In A. Dawes & D. Donald (Eds.), *Childhood and adversity: Psychological perspectives from South African research*. Capetown, David Philip.

Elliot, G.R. & Eisdorfer, C. (Eds.) (1982). *Stress and human health: Analysis and implications of research*. New York: Springer.

Endler, N.S. & Parker, J.D.A. (1990). Stress and anxiety: Conceptual and assessment issues. *Stress Medicine*, 6, 243-248.

Folkman, S. & Lazarus, R.S. (1985). If it changes it must be a process: Study of emotion and coping during three states of a college examination. *Journal of Personality and Social Psychology*, 48, 150-170.

Gal, R. & Israelshvily, M. (1978). *Personality traits vs. situational factors as determinants of an individual's coping with stress: A theoretical model*. Paper presented at the Second International Conference on Psychological Stress and Adjustment in Time of War and Peace. Tel-Aviv.

Garbarino, J. & Kostelmy, K. (1994). *The effects of political violence on Palestinian children: An accumulation of risk model*. Unpublished manuscript.

Langer, T.S. (1962). A twenty-two items screening score of psychiatric symptoms indication impairment. *Journal of Health and Human Behavior*. 3, 269-276.

Lazarus, R. S. (1966). *Psychological stress and the coping process*. New York: McGraw-Hill.

Lazarus, R. S. (1993). From psychological stress to the emotions: A history of changing outlooks. *Annual Review of Psychology*, 44, 1-21.

Magnusson, D. (1982). Situational determinants of stress: An international perspective. In: Goldberg, L. & Breznitz, S. (Eds.) *Handbook of stress: Theoretical and clinical aspects*, New York: The Free Press.

Marrow, A.J. (1969). *The practical theorist: The life and work of Kurt Lewin*. New York: Basic Books.

McCubbin, H.I. & Patterson, J.M. (1983). The family stress process: The double ABCX Model of adjustment and adaptation. In H. I. McCubbin, M.B. Sussman & J.M. Patterson (Eds.) *Social stress and the family: Advances and development in family stress theory and research* (pp. 7-37). New York: Haworth.

McMillan, D. & Chavis, D. (1986). Sense of community: A definition and theory. *Journal of Community Psychology*, 14, 6-23.

Moos, R. H. (1992). Understanding individuals' life contexts: Implications for stress reduction and prevention. In: M. Kessler, S.E. Goldstone & J. Joffe (Eds.) *The present and future of prevention research* (pp. 196-213). Newbury Park, CA: Sage.

Oliveri, M.E. & Reiss, D. (1984). Family concepts and their measurement: Things are seldom what they seem. *Family Process*, 23, 33-48.

Parkes, K.R. (1986). Coping in stressful episodes: The role of individual differences, environmental factors, and situational characteristics. *Journal of Personality and Social Psychology*, 51, 1277-1292.

Patterson, J.M. & Garwick, A. W. (1994). Theoretical linkages: Family meanings and sense of coherence: In H.I. McCubbin, E. A. Thompson & J.E. Fromer (Eds.) *Sense of*

Coherence and resiliency: Stress, coping and health. Madison WI: University of Wisconsin System, Center for Excellence in Family Studies.

Pearlin, L.I. (1989). The sociological study of stress. *Journal of Health and Social Behavior,* 30, 241-256.

Phillips, J.B. & Endler, N.S. (1982). Academic examination and anxiety: The interaction model empirically tested. *Journal of Research in Personality*, 16, 303-318.

Pretty, G. (1990). Relating Psychological Sense of Community to social climate characteristics. *Journal of Community Psychology*, 18, 60-65.

Reiss, D. (1981). *The family construction of reality.* Cambridge, MA: Harvard University Press.

Punamaki, R.L. (1996). Can ideological commitment protect children's psychosocial well-being in situations of political violence? *Child Development*, 67,55-69.

Sagy, S. (1998) Effects of personal, family and community characteristics on emotional reactions in a stress reaction: The Golan Heights negotiations. *Youth & Society*, 29, 311-329

Sagy, S. & Antonovsky, H.(1986). Adolescents' reactions to the evacuation of the Sinai settlements: A longitudinal study. *The Journal of Psychology*, 120, 6, 543-556.

Sagy, S. & Antonovsky, A. (1992). The family sense of coherence and the retirement transition. *Journal of Marriage and the Family*, 54, 983-993.

Sagy, S. & Dotan, N. (in press). Coping resources of maltreated children in the family: A salutogenic approach. *Child Abuse & Neglect: The International Journal*

Sagy, S., Stern, E. & Krakover, S. (1996). Macro and microlevel factors relating to Sense of Community: The case of temporary neighborhoods in Israel. *American Journal of Community Psychology,* 24, 657-676.

Shalit, B. (1982). Perceived perceptual organizations and coping with military demands. In C. D. Spielberger, I.G. Sarason, & N.A. Milgram (Eds.) *Stress and anxiety*, Vol. 8 (pp. 189-194), Washington, DC: Hemisphere.

Spielberger, C. D. (1972). Anxiety as an emotional state. In C.D. Spielberger (Ed.) *Anxiety: Current trends in theory and research.* New York: Academic Press.

Spielberger, C.D., Gorsuch, R.L. & Lushene, R.E. (1970). *Manual for the State-Trait Anxiety Inventory.* Palo-Alto, CA: Consulting Psychologists Press.

Tabachnick, B.G., & Fidell, L.S. (1983). *Using multivarient statistics.* New York: Harper and Row.

Timko, C., Moos, R.H. & Michelson, D.J. (1993). The context of adolescents' chronic life stress. *American Journal of Community Psychology*, 21, 397-420.

Teichman, Y. (1978). *Manual for the Hebrew State-Trait Anxiety Inventory.* Tel-Aviv: Tel-Aviv University Press.

Walker, A.J. (1985). Reconceptualizing family stress. *Journal of Marriage and the Family,* 47, 827-837.

Zeidner, M., Klingman, A. & Itzkovitz, R. (1993). Anxiety, control, social support and coping under threat of missile attack: A semi-projective assessment. *Journal of Personality Assessment,* 60, 435-457.

In: Psychology of Stress
Editor: Kimberly V. Oxington, pp. 113-127

ISBN 1-59454-246-5
©2005 Nova Science Publishers, Inc.

Chapter VII

A COMPARISON BETWEEN THE EFFORT-REWARD IMBALANCE AND DEMAND CONTROL MODELS

Aleck S. Ostry[1,], Shona Kelly[1], Paul A. Demers[1],*
Cameron Mustard[2] and Clyde Hertzman[1]
[1] Department of Health Care and Epidemiology, UBC
[2] Institute of Work and Health, Toronto

ABSTRACT

Background

To compare the predictive validity of the demand/control and reward/imbalance models, alone and in combination with each other, for self-reported health status and the self-reported presence of any chronic disease condition.

Methods

Self-reports for psychosocial work conditions were obtained in a sample of sawmill workers using the demand/control and effort/reward imbalance models. The relative predictive validity of task-level control was compared with effort/reward imbalance. As well, the predictive validity of a model developed by combining task-level control with effort/reward imbalance was determined. Logistic regression was utilized for all models.

---

[*] Aleck Ostry Dept. of Health Care and Epidemiology 5804 Fairview Avenue, Vancouver BC V6T 1Z3 Phone:604-822-5872 Fax: 604-822-4994 e-mail: ostry@interchange.ubc.ca

Results

The demand/control and effort/reward imbalance models independently predicted poor self-reported health status. The effort-reward imbalance model predicted the presence of a chronic disease while the demand/control model did not. A model combining effort-reward imbalance and task-level control was a better predictor of self-reported health status and any chronic condition than either model alone. Effort reward imbalance modeled with intrinsic effort had marginally better predictive validity than when modeled with extrinsic effort only.

Conclusions

Future work should explore the combined effects of these two models of psychosocial stress at work on health more thoroughly.

BACKGROUND

A strong body of evidence indicates that exposure to adverse psychosocial work conditions is a major hazard for the health of workers in modern economies. Much of this evidence, accumulated over the past two decades, is based on the demand/control model [1] in which task-level work conditions characterized by low control and high demand have been shown to predict high rates of cardiovascular disease as well as high rates of sickness absence [2,3].

One of the criticisms of this model is its reliance on "objective" measures of the work environment only [4]. According to many critics, workers will respond differently to the same constellation of control and demand conditions leading to varied biological outcomes so that a measure of individual worker differences, specifically in coping style, must therefore be included in any job strain model.

In the early 1990s, the effort-reward imbalance model was developed [5]. This model postulates that jobs characterized by a perceived imbalance between high effort and low rewards are stressful and will lead to negative health outcomes, particularly in persons with limited coping abilities. This model is meant to tap the attribute of an individual's "need for control"; a personality characteristic related to flexibility in coping. According to the model, a person with high need for control will respond in an inflexible way to work situations of high effort and low reward; and will therefore be more stressed and disease prone than a person in the same situation who has less need for control.

Using well designed epidemiological studies both models have succesfully predicted "hard" disease outcomes (particularly CHD) [6,7]. In the first comparative study with both models, Bosma has demonstrated independent predictive effects for new coronary heart disease of a component of the demand/control model (low control) as well as effort/reward imbalance [1], in a cohort of English white-collar workers [8].

---

[1] In this study effort and reward variables were constructed from questionnaire items which were similar to but were not the same as items used by Johannes Siegrist in his effort/reward imbalance instrument.

The models overlap to some extent as "extrinsic demands" in the effort/reward imbalance model is similar to "psychological and physical demands" in the demand/control model. However, the models also differ. The effort/reward imbalance model includes a measure of coping ability (need for control) which has no counterpart in the demand/control model. On the other hand, effort/reward imbalance excludes any measurement of task-level control. This is important, for as Bosma notes, "recent publications increasingly underscore the special importance of low job control for a range of health outcomes, including cardiovascular disease and sickness absence" [8, p68].

The purpose of this investigation is to compare the predictive validity of the demand/control and effort reward/imbalance models for self-reported health status and the self-reported presence of any chronic disease condition in a sample of former and current sawmill manufacturing workers. As well, because task-level control is the only element which is absent from the effort/reward imbalance model, and because this variable has been consistently predictive of a range of health outcomes for the past 2 decades, the predictive validity of the effort/reward imbalance model in combination with task-level control is also tested.

METHODS

This investigation is based on a sample of 3,000 male sawmill workers drawn randomly from a cohort that was originally gathered to study the impact of chlorophenol anti-sapstain chemicals on British Columbia (BC) sawmill workers [9,10].

Selection of Sawmills and Workers for the Original Study

Fourteen medium to large sized sawmills, located mainly in Southwest BC, participated in the original cohort study. Study sawmills were selected on the basis of a long-term history of chlorophenol use and availability of intact personnel records. A total of 26,221 workers were enrolled in the cohort, representing approximately 20 percent of all BC sawmill workers. (This increased to approximately 29,000 as workers hired in study mills between 1986 and 1996 were added to the cohort.) To be eligible, a worker had to be employed at a study mill for at least one year between January 1, 1950 and December 31, 1996.

The investigation of this sample of 3,000 workers was originally designed to study the impact of a recession and major restructuring of sawmills which began in 1980. Accordingly, the year 1979 was chosen as the pre-recession/restructuring "baseline" year. All workers enrolled in the cohort during 1979 were included in this baseline sub-cohort. A sample of 3,000 workers was randomly selected from the 9,806 workers working in a study sawmill in 1979.

Locating Interviewees

In order to locate interviewees the 1979 sub-cohort was linked to the British Columbia Linked Health Database (BCLHDB). This database includes provincial health ministry files on physician services, hospital discharges, drug prescriptions for the elderly, long term care services, deaths, and births for the years 1985 through to 1996. These data are useful for finding individuals because they include patient postal codes at time of contact with a physician. Ethical approval limited our access to the first 3-digits of the 6-digit postal codes. This allowed us to identify the community where cohort members lived, so that we could then find them through public information sources.

The 9,806 workers employed at a study mill in 1979 were linked probabilistically to the BCLHDB. Linkage efficiency was 94.7% so that 3-digit postal codes were obtained for 9,282 workers; including 2,920 (97.3%) of the 3000 randomly sampled workers. Searches of union pension plans, electronic telephone databases, and telephone books (by hand) were undertaken to obtain full addresses for the 3,000 workers. For the unlinked workers in the sample, address searches were undertaken using names only.

Administering the Interviews

Face-to-face interviews were conducted between November 1997 and March 1999. Subjects living in remote regions of the province were interviewed by telephone. A short version of the questionnaire (requiring about 20 minutes compared to one hour) was administered by telephone when a respondent was only willing to conduct a brief interview or when proxy interviews were conducted for deceased or incapacitated interviewees. However, because work-related variables were incompletely determined with the short version of the questionnaire, only the long version of the questionnaire was used in this investigation.

The Instrument

The instrument was developed after a thorough review of the literature on technological change, restructuring, unemployment, and health and work. Two focus groups were conducted with experienced sawmill workers to finalize the questionnaire; it was then pilot tested on 29 retired sawmill workers.

Socio-demographic information and health behaviours (smoking and alcohol consumption) were measured. Income was measured for the year preceding interview as was the number of dependants supported by each subject. Income per dependant over the year prior to interview was categorized into quartiles. Education status was categorized as completed elementary, secondary, apprentice training, community college, and university.

Because of downsizing/restructuring over the follow-up period, many workers moved out of the sawmill sector and in and out of employment. Variables measuring non-psychosocial work conditions, which may confound associations between current psychosocial work conditions and self-reported health outcomes, such as history of unemployment, sector of employment and occupational category at time of interview were developed as follows. Data on current work sector was obtained and dichotomized (currently employed in the sawmill sector vs currently employed outside the sawmill sector). Data on unemployment history was also obtained and categorized as follows: no unemployment, 1 episode less than 1 year in duration, 1 episode greater than 1 year in duration, 2 episodes or more less than 1 year in duration, 2 episodes of more greater than 1 year in length.

All job titles obtained in the interviews were re-coded using the Canadian Standard Occupational Classification [12] and then translated into the Pineo16 Occupational Status Scale [13]. This 16 category scale was collapsed into 4 basic categories; professional/managerial, trades, semi-skilled, and unskilled to measure current occupational category.

Task-level work characteristics were measured using a shortened version [10] of Karasek's demand/control instrument [14,15]. Scores for control and psychological demand were divided into high and low categories at the median. Jobs which were high in psychological demand and low in control were categorized as high strain.

Esteem reward, status control, extrinsic effort, and need for control were measured in the "full" effort/reward imbalance model [5]. The two effort scales were constructed by summing across questions and dichotomizing the scale score with zero for the two bottom tertiles and one for the highest tertile representing high extrinsic effort and high need for control. Two reward scales were constructed by summing across questions and dichotomizing the scale score with zero for the two top tertiles and one for the bottom tertile representing low esteem reward and low status control. This "full" model was thus based on four variables, intrinsic demand, extrinsic demand, esteem reward, and status control. These four dichotomous variables were used to create the effort/reward imbalance indicators consisting of three categories: 1=neither high effort nor low reward; 2=either high effort or low reward; and 3=both high effort and low reward used in the "full" effort/reward imbalance model[5,8, 16].

A "partial" effort/reward imbalance model was also developed by eliminating one of the four components, intrinsic effort, from the full model. This "partial" model was thus based on three variables of the variables (extrinsic demand, esteem reward, and status control) utilized in the full model. Because the demand/control model contains no information on the personal characteristics of the worker, using a partial effort/reward imbalance model, i.e., with the psychological measure (intrinsic demand) removed, allows for a comparison of the "objective" elements of both models.

The combined effect of task-level control and the effort-reward imbalance models (full and partial) was tested by categorizing effort/reward imbalance into three categories (none, medium, and high) and task-level control into the two categories high and low. In this way workers were categorized into, at one extreme, a reference category of no effort/reward imbalance and high task-level control and, at the other extreme, a category of high effort/reward imbalance and low task-level control with 4 categories representing the possible combinations of effort/reward imbalance and task-level control between the two extremes.

Two outcome variables were used in this investigation; self-reported health status, and the presence of one self-reported chronic condition. Self-reported health was reported on a 5 point scale for current job and dichotomized into "good" (good or excellent) and "poor" (fair, poor, bad) health status for use in logistic regression analysis. Self-reported health is dichotomized, with a cut point between good and fair in most studies of work stress of this type [17]. And, any worker who reported one or more of the following conditions at time of interview was considered to have a chronic disease: asthma, back problems (excluding arthritis), chronic bronchitis or emphysema, diabetes, CHD, hearing loss; or any other non-specified chronic condition.

Analyses

Logistic regression was used to determine the association between self-reported health status or self-reported chronic disease status and with various exposure variables. In the first model, the association between both outcome variables and sociodemographic variables was examined (Table 3). In the second model, sociodemographic variables and current smoking status were included as adjustment variables in a model examining the association between the outcome variables and three non-psychosocial work variables, current sector, current occupational category, and unemployment history (Table 4).

In the third model, after controlling for socio-demographic variables, smoking, and non-psychosocial work conditions, associations with demand/control and effort/reward imbalance (full and partial) were tested (Table 5). In the fourth model associations were tested after combining effort/reward imbalance (full and partial) with task-level control (Table 6, 7).

RESULTS

Table 1 shows that the overall response rate was 72 percent, the refusal rate was 4.2 percent, and 19% of respondents were not located. The proportion of workers not located was highest in isolated "mill towns" with a younger more transient workforce than at other sawmills in the cohort. Refusal rates did not vary by age category but the "not found" rate was higher in younger age groups and workers with lowest duration of work in a study sawmill.

Some respondents did not speak English well enough for the interview. Cantonese and Punjabi speaking translators were hired to administer interviews to subjects who spoke these languages. Eight people, with other languages required translators but due to expense and logistics these interviews were not conducted.

Table 1: Interview status of 3,000 randomly sampled workers

Interview Status	Number	Percent
Long questionnaire	1885	62.9
Short questionnaire	270	9.1
Questionnaire Respondents sub-total	2155	72.0
Refusals	126	4.2
Deceased	18	0.6
Needs translator	8	0.3
Not located	693	22.8
Total	3000	100.0

Table 2 shows that 1,421 (75.4%) of the 1,885 long questionnaire respondents were aged 64 or less. Of these, 1170 (82.3%) were employed at time of interview, 131 (9.2%) were retired, 69 (4.9%) were unemployed, 40 (2.8%) were disabled, and 11 (0.8%) were in at home looking after children, performing voluntary work, or attending educational institutions at time of interview. Of the 1170 workers employed at time of interview, 600 (51.3%) were employed in a sawmill and 570 (48.7%) were employed outside the sawmill sector. The analyses described in this paper were based on the 1170 respondents who answered the long questionnaire and who were aged 64 or under and employed at time of interview.

Table 2: Age and labour force status of long questionnaire respondents at time of interview

Current Status	Number	Percent
Age Status		
65 Years or Over	464	24.6
64 Years or Less	1421	75.4
Total	1885	100.0
Labour force Status		
Sawmill Sector	600	42.3
Non-Sawmill Sector	570	40.1
Early Retired	131	9.2
Unemployed	69	4.8
Disabled	40	2.8
Other	11	0.8
Total	1885	100

Table 3 presents age-adjusted associations between self-reported health status and chronic conditions and sociodemographic variables, smoking, and self-reported health status in 1979. The presence of a chronic condition was associated in a step-wise gradient with increasing age. For the remaining variables, no statistically significant associations were observed with either outcome variable.

Self-reported health status declined step-wise with increasing age. Increasing education was positively associated, in gradient fashion, with increasing self-reported health status. This was statistically significant for university education (OR=0.60). Current smoking was associated with worse self-reported health status (OR=1.55).

Table 4 shows that, after adjustment, none of the non-psychosocial work variables demonstrated a statistically significant relationship with the presence of a chronic condition. In the case of self-reported health status, current employment in the sawmill sector was associated with greater odds (statistically significant) for reporting poor health (OR=1.57) and decreasing occupational status was associated with a (non-significant) gradient for worse self-reported health.

Table 3: Age adjusted associations of socio-demographic and smoking factors with poor self-reported health status (SRHS) and self-reported chronic condition (Chronic)

Variable	Chronic	SRHS
Age		
35-39	1.00	1.00
40-44	0.99	1.69*
45-49	1.37	1.77*
50-54	1.88**	1.72*
55-59	2.32**	2.06**
60-64	4.25**	2.50**
Birthplace		
Canada	1.00	1.00
Outside Canada	0.66**	1.32
Education		
Elementary	1.00	1.00
Secondary	0.99	0.75
Apprentice	1.34	0.76
Community College	1.05	0.75
University	0.71	0.60*
Marital status		
Married	1.00	1.00
Unmarried	1.08	1.05
Income/dependant		
<$12,999	1.00	1.00
$13,000-18,749	1.31	0.87
$18,750-28,229	1.34	0.75
>$28,00	1.20	0.65*
Current Smoking status		
No	1.00	1.00
Yes	1.11	1.55**

*p=0.05-0.01; **p=<0.01

Table 5 shows that low control (OR=1.60; CI=1.12-2.28) and high psychological demand (OR=1.65; CI= 1.21-2.26) predicted poor self-reported health. Effort/reward imbalance and job strain both predicted poor health status. The risk of reporting poor health status for subjects with high job strain was approximately twice as high as those with low strain (OR=2.07; CI= 1.18-3.66). And, for both the full and partial effort/reward imbalance models the risk of reporting poor health status for subjects with both high effort and low reward was approximately 3 times higher than those with low effort and high reward (full model; OR=3.35; CI= 2.10-5.51) and (partial model; OR=3.13; CI= 1.96-4.85).

**Table 4: Socio-demographic and smoking adjusted
associations of non-psychosocial work condition variables
with poor self-reported health status and self-reported chronic condition**

Variable	Chronic	SRHS
Sector		
Non-Sawmill	1.00	1.00
Sawmill	1.09	1.57**
Current Occupational Category		
Manager	1.00	1.00
Trades	1.30	1.08
Unskilled	0.89	1.26
Unemployment History		
1 episode< 1 year	1.00	1.00
1 episode > 1 year	1.19	1.12
2 episodes or more <1 year	1.01	0.88
2 episodes or more >1 year	1.21	1.22

*p=0.05-0.01; **p=<0.01

**Table 5: Associations between the demand/control and effort/reward imbalance models
(full andpartial) and poor self-reported health status and any chronic condition**

	Self-reported HealthStatus	Any Chronic condition
Control		
High	1.00	1.00
Low	1.60** (1.12-2.28)	1.09 (0.81-1.45)
Psychological demand		
Low	1.00	1.00
High	1.65** (1.21-2.26)	1.13 (0.86-1.48)
Physical demand		
Low	1.00	1.00
High	1.01 (0.68-1.50)	1.25 (0.86-1.81)
Job Strain		
Low	1.00	1.00
High	2.07* (1.18-3.66)	1.31 (0.77-2.22)
Partial Effort/reward Imbalance Model		
None	1.00**	1.00*
Medium	1.60* (1.06-2.45)	1.12 (0.0.84-1.44)
High	3.13** (1.96-4.85)	1.59** (1.12-2.24)
Full Effort/reward Imbalance Model		
None	1.00**	1.00**
Medium	1.87** (1.26-3.34)	1.22 (0.91-1.85)
High	3.35** (2.10-5.61)	1.70** (1.17-2.37)

Numbers in parentheses are 95% confidence intervals*p=0.05-0.01;**p=0.01-0.0001

Effort/reward imbalance (full and partial models) was the only variable which predicted the presence of a chronic condition. The risk of reporting a chronic condition for subjects with both high effort and low reward was 59 percent greater than those with low effort and high reward in the case of the partial model and 70 percent greater with the full model. The risk of reporting a chronic condition for subjects with high job strain was approximately 30% greater than those with low strain jobs.

For self-reported health status, combining effort/reward imbalance with task-level control produced odds ratios which increased in a regular gradient moving from the reference category (no effort/reward imbalance with high task-level control) to the "worst" category (effort/reward imbalance with low task-level control) (Table 6). For the full effort/reward imbalance model, the odds ratio for this latter category was 3.50 (CI=2.04-6.08). For the partial model the odds ratio for this latter category was 3.23 (CI= 2.01-5.18). In the case of chronic conditions, for the full effort/reward imbalance model, the odds ratio for the worst" category (effort/reward imbalance with low task-level control) was 1.98 (CI= 1.23-3.18) and for the partial model the odds ratio was 1.80 (CI= 1.14-1.80) (Table 7).

Table 6: Associations between effort/reward imbalance (full and partial) model combined with task-level control and poor self-reported health status

	Full Model	Partial Model
NO Imbalance with HIGH control	1**	1**
NO Imbalance with LOW control	0.75 (0.37-1.48)	0.71 (0.41-1.25)
MEDIUM Imbalance with HIGH control	40 (0.77-2.69)	1.16 (0.66-2.02)
MEDIUM Imbalance with LOW control	1.74 (0.97-3.10	1.54 (1.07-2.55)
HIGH Imbalance with HIGH control	2.20** (1.25-3.99)	2.09** (1.25-3.50)
HIGH Imbalance with LOW control	3.50** (2.04-6.080)	3.23** (2.01-5.18)

Numbers in parentheses are 95% confidence intervals*p=0.05-0.01;**p<0.01

Table 7: Associations between effort/reward imbalance (full and partial) model combined with task-level control and poor self-report of any chronic condition

	Full Model	Partial Model
NO Imbalance with HIGH control	1*	1
NO Imbalance with LOW control	1.04 *(0.63-1.72)	0.97 (0.67-1.58)
MEDIUM Imbalance with HIGH control	13 (0.70-1.83)	1.0 (0.65-1.56)
MEDIUM Imbalance with LOW control	38 (0.83-2.27)	38 (0.83-2.27)
HIGH Imbalance with HIGH control	1.57 (0.95-2.49)	1.38 (0.86-2.20)
HIGH Imbalance with LOW control	1.57 (0.95-2.49)	1.38 (0.86-2.20)

Numbers in parentheses are 95% confidence intervals*p=0.05-0.01;**p<0.01

Finally, in the case of self-reported health status, the Model Chi Square for the full effort/reward imbalance model combined with task-level control was 71.95 compared to 65.1 for effort/reward imbalance alone. Results were similar in size and trend for the partial effort/reward imbalance model combined with task-level control. In the case of "any chronic condition" the Model Chi Square for the full effort/reward imbalance model combined with task-level control was 46.67 compared to 44.97 for effort/reward imbalance alone. Results were similar in size and trend for the partial effort/reward imbalance model combined with task-level control

Discussion

In this investigation, effort/reward imbalance and job strain independently predicted self-reported health status and both the full and partial effort/reward imbalance models predicted the presence of a chronic condition. As well, both the full and partial effort/reward imbalance models in conjunction with task-level control predicted self-reported health status and the presence of a chronic condition.

The odds ratio for self-reported health status with the combination high effort/reward imbalance (full model) and low task-level control was 3.50 and the odds ratio in the case of the partial effort/reward imbalance model in combination with low task-level control was 3.23. These odds ratios were slightly higher than those obtained using the effort/reward imbalance model alone and approximately 50 percent greater than odds rations obtained using the demand control model (i.e., the job strain variable) alone. Similarl results were obtained for the outcome "any chronic condition".

Is the combined model (effort/reward imbalance with task-level control) a better predictor of the two outcome variables than effort/reward imbalance or task-level control alone? As noted, odds ratios were slightly higher for the combined models compared to effort/reward imbalance and task-level control on their own. The full effort/reward imbalance task-level control model explained 11.7% and 41.1% more variance in self-reported health status than the effort/reward imbalance model and task-level control alone. Results for the partial effort/reward imbalance task-level control model were similar. And, similar, but less pronounced trends were observed for the outcome "any chronic condition". These results both confirm those obtained from the Whitehall study [8,18] and extends it.

The predictive ability of the full compared to the partial (i.e., without intrinsic effort) effort/reward imbalance model was only marginally greater for both health outcomes. While intrinsic effort is a major theoretical component of the effort/reward imbalance model, its did not, in this study, contribute markedly to enhanced predictive ability for the model. The use of the partial effort/reward imbalance model should be further explored with other data, with "hard" outcomes, to determine empirically whether or not intrinsic effort adds substantially to the predictive ability of the model.

Major strengths of this study are that 1) both effort/reward imbalance and demand/control measures were obtained for each individual, 2) the sample was large (1,170 workers), 3) the workers, were at the time of the survey, employed across many sectors including manufacturing and the service, transportation, and construction sectors, and 4) the occupational status of workers ranged from unskilled to skilled professionals. Thus, in spite of the original sampling frame (which meant that all those sampled had been employed in the sawmill industry approximately 20 years prior to the survey), the sample represented a fairly heterogeneous group of middle-aged, male, former resource manufacturing workers.

The most serious, limitation of this study arises because both explanatory and outcome variables are based on self-reports at time of interview. It is possible that "soft" dependent variables such as self-reported health status may derive from the same conception of self as explanatory variables like psychosocial work conditions. In this case, there is a problem of common methods' variance in which the independent and dependent variables are hardly distinguishable [19] resulting in the possibility of contamination between measures [20].

Bias arising from common methods' variance may be a greater problem for the full effort/reward imbalance model relative to both the partial effort/reward balance model and the demand/control model. The intrinsic effort measure included in the full effort-reward imbalance model is essentially a measure of coping ability which because of its subjective nature may be more vulnerable to common methods' variance than the other variables in the effort/reward and demand/control models. Use of the partial effort/reward imbalance model may mitigate any common method's variance related to the intrinsic effort variable.

As well, some researchers have argued that any associations observed between self-reports of psychosocial work conditions and health outcomes may be confounded by the subjective "state" or personality of the worker [21,22,23]. According to this perspective, the major factor responsible for this confounding is "negative affectivity" and that the impact of this confounding is so great that self-reports of job work conditions are essentially a measure of negative affectivity [21].

However Bosma has demonstrated, using the demand/control model and data from the Whitehall study, "an absence of consistently stronger effects of job control in participants with reported negative personal characteristics [which] also indicates that a neurotic tendency to complain cannot explain the job control-CHD association" [24, p 406]. These and other recent findings have demonstrated that it may not be useful to measure and control for negative affectivity in studies using self-reports of psychosocial work conditions [25].

CONCLUSIONS

In summary task-level control and effort-reward imbalance were independently associated with self-reported health status and effort reward imbalance was associated with self-reported presence of any chronic condition. Modeled in combination, effort/reward imbalance and task-level control was more predictive for both outcomes than the effort/reward imbalance and demand/control models alone. The predictive power of the full effort/reward imbalance model was only marginally greater than for the partial model using both health outcome measures. Future work should explore the combined effects of these two models of psychosocial stress at work on health more thoroughly.

COMPETING INTERESTS

None.

Authors' Contribution

AO conducted the research, organized data gathering, and wrote the paper.
SK carried out data cleaning tasks.
PD provided guidance in study design.
CM provided writing help and conceptual design.
CH provided conceptual help.

Acknowledgments

I'd like to thank Dr. Johannes Siegrist and Dr. Micky Kerr for their help in reviewing this paper. Acknowledgments to the Canadian Institute of Health Research and Micheal Smith Foundation for Health Research for Dr. Ostry's salary support. As well, acknowledgments to the Canadian Population Health Initiative, the Institute of Work and Health, the Canadian Institute of Advanced Research, the Center for Health Services and Policy Research, and Forest Renewal British Columbia for their financial and intellectual support for this project.

References

[1] Karasek R. Job demands, job decision latitude, and mental strain: Implication for job redesign. *Admin Sci Quart* 1979;24:285-308.

[2] Landsbergis P A, Schnall P, Schwartz J, Warren K, Pickering TG. Job strain, hypertension, and cardiovascular disease: Recommendations for further research. In *Organisational risk factors for job stress*, ed. S. L. Sauter and L. R. Murphy. 97-112. Washington: American Psychological Association, 1995.

[3] North F, Syme L, Feeney A, Shipley M, Marmot M. Psychosocial work environment and sickness absence among British civil servants: The Whitehall II study. *Am J Public Health* 1996;86:332-340.

[4] Frese M, Zapf D. Methodological issues in the study of work stress: Objective vs subjective measurement of work stress and the question of longitudinal studies. In: Cooper C, Payne R, editors. *Causes, coping, and consequences of stress at work*. New York:John Wiley & Sons Ltd, 1988:375-411.

[5] Siegrist J, Peter R, Junge A, Cremer P, Seidel D. Low status control, high effort at work and ischemic heart disease: Prospective evidence from blue-collar men, *Soc Sci & Med* 1990;31(10):1127-1134.

[6] Karasek R, Theorell T. *Healthy work*. New York: Basic Books, 1990.

[7] Siegrist J. Adverse health effect of high-effort/low-reward conditions. *J Occupat Hlth Psychol* 1996;1:27-41.

[8] Bosma H, Peter R, Siegrist J, Marmot M. Two alternative job stress models and the risk of coronary heart disease. *Am J Public Hl*th, 1998; 88(1): 68-74.

[9] Hertzman C, Teschke K, Ostry A, Dimich-Ward H, Kelly S, Spinelli J, et al. Cancer incidence and mortality in sawmill workers exposed to chlorophenols. *Am J Public Health* 1996;87:71-79.

[10] Ostry A, Marion SA, Green L, Demers PA, Hershler R, Kelly S, et al. Technological change in relation to changes in psychosocial conditions of work in BC sawmills (1950 -1996). *Scand J Work Environ Health* 2000;26(3):273-277.

[11] Ostry A, Marion SA, Green L, Demers PA, Hershler R, Kelly S, et al.. A comparison of expert-rater methods for assessing psychosocial job strain. *Scand J Work Environ Health*, 2001;27(1):1-6.

[12] Statistics Canada. *Standard occupational classifications*, 1980, Ottawa.

[13] Pineo P. *Revisions of the Pinio-Porter-McRoberts socioeconomic classification of occupations for the 1981 census*, QSEP Research Report No. 125, Program for Quantitative Studies in Economics and Population, McMaster University, Hamilton, Ontario, February 1985.

[14] Karasek R, Gordon G, Pietrokovsky C, Frese M, Pieper C, Schwartz J, et al. *Job content instrument: questionnaire and users' guide*. Lowell(MA): University of Massachusetts, 1985.

[15] Johnson J, Hall E, Theorell T. Combined effects of job strain and social isolation on cardiovascular disease morbidity and mortality in a random sample of the Swedish male working population. *Scand J Work Environ Health* 1989;15:271-279.

[16] Stansfeld S, Bosma H, Hemingway H, Marmot M. Psychosocial work characteristics and social support as predictors of SF-36 health functioning: the Whitehall II study *Psychsom Med* 1998;60:247-255.

[17] Kelly S. Self-reported Health: Stitching together a picture from the fabric of life. P.h.D. Thesis, University of British Columbia, 2003.

[18] de Jonge J, Bosma H, Peter R, Siegrist J. Job strain, effort-reward imbalance and employee well-being: a large scale cross-sectional study. *Soc Sci & Med.* 2000;50:1317-1327.

[19] Kasl S. Measuring job stressors, and studying the health impact of the work environment: an epidemiologic commentary. *J Occupat Hlth Psychol* 1998;3(4):390-401.

[20] Kristensen T. Job stress and cardiovascular disease: a theoretic critical review. *J Occupat Hlth Psychol* 1996;1(3):246-260.

[21] Chen P Y, Spector PE, Jex S M.. Effects of manipulated job stressors and job attitude on perceived job conditions:A simulation. In: Sauter SL, Murphy LR, editors. *Organizational risk factors for job stress*. Washington D.C.: American Psychological Association, 1995..

[22] Spector P, Dwyer D, Jex S. Relation of job stressors to affective, health, and performance outcomes: a comparison of multiple data sources. *J Applied Psychol* 1988; 73:11-19.

[23] Spector P, Jex S. Relations of job characteristics from multiple data sources with employee affect, absence, turnover intentions, and health. *J Applied Psychol* 1991;76: 46-53.

[24] Bosma H, Stansfeld S, Marmot M. Job control, personal characteristics, and heart disease. *J Occupat Hlth Psychol* 1998;3(4):402-409.

[25]	Spector P, Zapf D, Chen P, Frese M. Why negative affectivity should not be controlled in job stress research: don't throw out the baby with the bath water. *J Org Behaviour* 2000; 21:79-95.

In: Psychology of Stress
Editor: Kimberly V. Oxington, pp. 129-144

ISBN 1-59454-246-5
©2005 Nova Science Publishers, Inc.

Chapter VIII

STRESS AND SOMATIZATION: A SOCIOCULTURAL PERSPECTIVE

Rachel A. Askew[1] and Corey L. M. Keyes[1,2]
[1] Department of Sociology, Emory University
[2] Department of Behavioral Sciences
and Health Education, Rollins School of Public Health, Emory University

ABSTRACT

Somatization is the translation of emotional distress into physical symptoms that have no identifiable physical cause. Somatization is widespread: clinical, historical, and anthropological studies have demonstrated its prevalence in different historical periods and across cultures. The majority of literature on somatization conceptualizes it as maladaptive, effectively complicating diagnosis and treatment.

This chapter reviews research literature on somatization and summarizes the findings from an empirical study of somatization in the United States and South Korea. Findings from the empirical study support a sociocultural model of somatization and mental health that posits that the negative association of somatization and mental health is mitigated by culture. Put another way, in loose, individualistic societies such as the U.S., where value is placed on the direct expression of distress and physicians are trained to search for physical rather than psychogenic sources of disease, somatization does indeed hinder diagnosis and treatment. Conversely, somatization is potentially functional in cultures where somatization indirectly expresses, and is interpreted by others as, emotional distress. In tight, collectivistic cultures such as South Korea, where overt expression of psychic distress is seen as deviant, somatization acts as a buffer against the deleterious effects of psychosocial stressors.

INTRODUCTION

Hans Selye's (1956) discovery of stress was motivated by the unanticipated patho-physiological outcomes in his animal studies. Today, stress is a notorious concept because it is commonplace, widespread, and undoubtedly the leading explanation of the genesis of a variety of health outcomes. Since Selye, where the outcome of stress was critical, most research on stress has placed more emphasis on the causes, the nature, the mediators, and the moderators of stress (see e.g., Taylor & Aspinwall, 1996; Thoits, 1995). This shift from stress outcomes was developmental, in part, because little was known about the nature and origins of stress. However, a less obvious and less practical reason for this shift was the belief, only partially supported by research, that stress was connected with deterioration in some health outcomes.

Indeed, there is a universe of possible outcomes of stress. First, stress can cause physical disease, which can occur singularly or, as is often the case, multiply. Second, stress can cause mental disorder, which also can occur singularly or multiply. Third, stress can cause comorbidities between physical disease and mental disorder. Fourth, and for a variety of interesting reasons, stress may not cause physical disease or mental disorder.[1] Individuals may remain healthy or unchanged because they have experienced "eustress," or what has been called "just manageable difficulties" that sometimes result in growth and positive change (see e.g., Brim, 1992; Csikszentmihalyi, 1990). Individuals may remain unchanged by stress because they have coped successfully with negative stress (see e.g., Turner & Avison, 1992). Individuals' health status may remain unchanged after stress because they have accrued allostatic load, or sustained wear-and-tear (see e.g., McEwen & Stellar, 1993), but their health problems have yet to reach a diagnostic threshold. Finally, rather than causing any clear patho-physiological outcome, stress can and often does result in somatization, a significant, culturally-mediated outcome of stress, and the topic of this chapter.

Somatization is the translation of emotional or psychic distress into physical symptoms that have no identifiable organic cause. Despite the traditional belief that somatization is only the province of non-Western, developing countries (Lambo, 1956; Neki, 1973), decades of epidemiologic research (e.g., Kroenke & Price, 1993; Simon & VonKorff, 1991) suggest that somatization is ubiquitous and common in all societies. As Kirmayer noted: "Somatization has been found wherever it has been sought and, worldwide, somatic symptoms are more common than emotional complaints as a way of presenting psychosocial distress" (1984). Within the general population, less severe forms of somatization are common (Escobar, Burnam, Karno, Forsythe, & Golding, 1987; Kroenke & Price, 1993), and Rief, Hessel, & Braehler (2001) estimate that, depending on diagnostic criteria used, between 0.3% and 23.6% of the general population meet the criteria for a somatoform disorder. Furthermore, within primary care populations, researchers estimate that one-fourth to two-thirds of primary care visits are prompted by somatic complaints for which no physical cause is found (Bridges & Goldberg, 1985; Cummings & VandenBos, 1981; Goldberg, 1979; Katon, Ries, & Kleinman, 1984; Kroenke & Mangelsdorff, 1989; Kroenke & Price, 1993).

---

[1] As obvious as this universe of stress outcomes may appear, there is surprisingly little theorizing or research on the universe of outcomes. For instance, how or why does stress sometimes cause physical disease or mental disorder but not both? How or why does stress sometimes cause comorbidities within but not between physical disease and mental disorders? How or why does stress sometimes cause comorbidities between but not within physical disease and mental disorders? Last, how or why does stress sometimes not result in health deterioration of any kind?

Thus, somatization is a common method of presentation worldwide, and its prevalence has profound implications for the way that health care is provided. Studies on somatization in Western health care systems point to the high cost of somatization (e.g., Barsky, Ettner, Horsky, & Bates, 2001; Escobar, Golding, Hough, Karno, Burman, & Wells, 1987; Shaw and Creed, 1991; Smith, 1994). Somatizers in Western health systems use more services, engender more diagnostic tests, switch doctors more frequently, and, from a doctor's point of view, generally prove to be more difficult to treat than are patients who present in a more straightforward manner (Barsky & Borus, 1995; E. H. Lin et al., 1991; Mayou & Sharpe, 1995; Hahn et al., 1994). The majority of the literature on somatization (e.g., Allen, Gara, Escobar, Waitzkin, & Silver, 2001; Barsky & Borus, 1995; Smith, 1994) presents it as a problem to solve. Yet is somatization maladaptive everywhere and in all situations?

Nichter (1981), C. D. F. Parsons (1984), and other cultural anthropologists (e.g., Good, 1977; Kleinman, 1982; K. M. Lin, 1983; Parsons & Wakeley, 1991) consider somatization in certain contexts as a cultural idiom of distress: a nonverbal, symbolic, and *recognizable* method of expressing psychic or emotional distress through physical manifestations that differs by culture. To the extent that somatizers effectively communicate the underlying cause of their symptoms to others through a somatic presentation, the complications generally associated with somatization (namely misdiagnosis leading to over-utilization of health services) should not apply. This chapter addresses the question of whether somatization is maladaptive everywhere by examining somatization in various cultural contexts.

This chapter argues that the degree to which a somatic presentation is adaptive or maladaptive is a function of culture. Within cultures that accept a separation of body and mind, and view somatic presentations of psychic distress as masking a 'true' mental disorder, a somatic idiom of distress will be maladaptive. Conversely, within cultures that view the body and mind as interconnected and favor the indirect expression of emotions, somatization will be an effective coping mechanism. The ubiquity of somatization means this conclusion has important implications for the provision of health care in Western societies.

Somatization as Western Cultural Construct

Fabrega (1990) argues that the concept of somatization—psychic distress 'inappropriately' expressed as somatic ailment(s)—is a Western cultural construction embedded in a medical system that views the body and mind as separate and distinct entities rather than as an interconnected whole. Put another way, the concept of somatization is a cultural consequence of the Western biomedical model of disease. The Western biomedical model of disease considers the body and mind as separate entities and views physical symptoms of disease as emanating from anatomic, chemical, or physiologic changes in the body. This model of disease projects a 1:1 causal correspondence between anatomical changes or dysfunctions and physical symptoms, and sees any psychic distress that patients display when presenting to a doctor as secondary to the physical disorder. As a consequence, Western medicine relies on technical examinations and laboratory procedures that aim to pinpoint the anatomical or chemical disturbance. Western doctors tend to read patients' illness behavior as a sign of a *physical* imbalance, and patients' illness narratives are used primarily as a roadmap to find the biological cause of the sickness. It is implicitly assumed that once the anatomical cause of disease is pinpointed and eradicated, the patient's illness behavior will disappear.

In direct refutation of the biomedical notion of a 1:1 correspondence between physical disease and illness behavior, Angel and Thoits (1989) note that many studies (e.g., Fabrega, 1974; Kleinman, 1980) report only an imperfect correspondence between disease and the patients' experience of the disease (i.e., patients' illness behavior). Furthermore, as Fabrega (1990) notes, outside of Western medicine, the Cartesian split between body and mind does not resonate. Instead, in non-Western societies, body and mind are seen as inextricably intertwined. Non-Western societies do not conceive of disembodied mental illnesses. For this reason, diagnostic systems of disease in non-Western countries such as China and Korea contain ailments such as neurasthenia or hwa-byung that contain both physical and psychological components (Kleinman, 1982; K. M. Lin, 1983). Moreover, in non-Western societies, a patient's illness presentation is seen not just as a reflection of anatomical disorder, but also as a reflection of social disorder and understood to emanate from the interactions between patients and their reference groups (e.g., family, friends, employers, physicians) (Fabrega, 1990; Kirmayer, Dao, & Smith, 1993). The concept of somatization is only comprehensible in a culture that conceives of physical illness as separate from mental illness and equates physical disease with illness behavior.

SOMATIZATION AND SOCIAL STRUCTURE

Among societies high in social solidarity, where the social glue between individuals stems from individuals' similar lifestyles, beliefs, and roles (societies that Durkheim would characterize as high in mechanical solidarity) (1984 [1933]), symbols tend to be implicit (Cerulo, 1995). Such societies are characterized by cultural homogeneity, a wealth of shared understandings and experiences that enable members to communicate meanings indirectly through social symbols whose meanings are not understood by outsiders. Triandis (1995) characterizes such societies as tight. Within tight societies, group norms are transparent and adherence to group norms is critical; deviation from normative behavior tends to bring swift punishment. Tight societies tend also to be collectivistic. Collectivistic societies (Triandis, 1995) are characterized by a focus on communal or collective goals and collective well-being over the personal goals and well-being of individuals. Individuals within collectivistic societies maintain strong in-group ties, meaning that individuals are interdependent and heavily involved with those in their in-groups (Hui & Triandis, 1986). In collectivistic societies, an individual's well-being is bound to the welfare of other members of their in-groups. The direct expression of distress within tight, collectivistic societies, then, directly implicates and reflects poorly on members of one's in-groups. As a result, tight, collectivistic societies favor the indirect expression of psychic distress. Asian, African, and Latin American societies tend to be tight and collectivistic (Hofstede, 1980).

In contrast, loose societies are characterized by cultural heterogeneity and complexity (Triandis, 1995). Such societies are held together by organic solidarity (Durkheim, 1984 [1933]), meaning that social solidarity is a result of individuals' complementary (rather than similar) functions within society. The cultural heterogeneity within loose societies corresponds to greater heterogeneity of proper behavior, and thus more ambiguity about how to sanction individuals who break norms. Loose societies tend to be individualistic (Triandis, 1995), valuing creativity, individual achievement, and a focus on individual goals. In-groups in loose, individualistic societies are more flexible, more easily permeated, and individuals' identities are less tied to any one in-group than are individuals' identities in tight, collectivistic societies. Within loose, individualistic societies characterized by cultural complexity, a focus on the individual, and ambiguity with respect to appropriate behavior, symbols must be more explicit and direct if they are to be understood by in-group members (Cerulo, 1995). As a result, loose societies tend to favor the direct expression of meaning, or expressive individualism (Bellah, Madsen, Sullivan, Swidler, & Tipton, 1985). North American and Western European societies tend to be loose and individualistic (Hofstede, 1980).

SOMATIZATION IN COLLECTIVISTIC SOCIETIES

Within tight, collectivistic societies characterized by homogeneity, where emphasis is placed on proper behavior, group solidarity, and conformity, overt expressions of distress are seen as a breach of decorum and as a poor reflection on one's in-groups (Hofstede, 1983). As a result, individuals in tight, collectivistic societies tend to express their discontent in indirect ways. One method of conveying suffering is through sublimating personal and social distress into identifiable physical symptoms. Expressing distress through culturally-appropriate physical symptoms is a somatic idiom of distress (Katon, Ries, & Kleinman, 1984; Kleinman, 1982; Nichter, 1981). In tight, collectivistic cultures, somatic idioms of distress can function as a coping mechanism for the sufferer by eliciting social support from friends and family, by relieving the sufferer from overwhelming social responsibilities, by sanctioning failure, and by sparing sufferers the intense stigma attached to mental illnesses in such cultures, while a psychological presentation may result in shame for the sufferer and her family (Kirmayer, Dao, & Smith, 1998; Kirmayer & Young, 1998; Raguram, Weiss, Channabasavanna, & Devins, 1996).

The functionality of somatic idioms of distress in tight, collectivistic cultures does not mean that somatizers are malingerers or hypochondriacs who intentionally somatize in order to reap the benefits of the sick role (Epstein, Quill, & McWhinney, 1999). Their distress, physical symptoms, and pain are very real, and the majority of somatizers are not aware of a connection between their psychic distress and their physical symptoms (Kleinman, 1982; K. M. Lin, 1983), or if they are aware, they do not consider their psychological distress the "real" problem. Instead, due to the non-Western holistic view of the body, mind, and soul as intertwined, illness in the body or mind reflects a general imbalance. As a result, many disorders in non-Western societies involve both physical and psychological symptoms, and both types of symptoms are treated as equally valid (Fabrega, 1990), although emphasis is generally placed on somatic symptoms, perhaps because of the debilitating stigma attached to mental illness in many non-Western cultures.

Anthropologists studying health and illness behavior in China (Kleinman, 1982), Korea (Lin, 1983), and Puerto Rico (Guarnaccia, 1989), among other tight, collectivistic areas, have identified somatic idioms of distress that highlight the culturally-shaped and potentially adaptive nature of such illness behaviors. One such idiom is the condition of neurasthenia in China. The expression of dysphoric emotion in China has traditionally been regarded as shameful to individuals and their families (Kleinman & Kleinman, 1985). Furthermore, the expression of distress was thought to engender illness (Tseng, 1974). Neurasthenia is characterized by headaches, insomnia, dizziness, and dysphoria (depression, sadness, and irritability). Using standard North American assessment techniques, Kleinman (1982) confirmed that neurasthenia patients in China would be diagnosed with depression or other psychiatric disorders were their evaluations done in North America. Nevertheless, all patients in the study *and their physicians* considered their problems as primarily physical; all rejected the label of depression. This focus on physical symptoms held despite the fact that virtually all patients had recently undergone stressful life events or were involved in tense interpersonal relationships, and despite the fact that all were attending a psychiatric clinic in addition to receiving a great deal of general medical services each month. Kleinman (1982) noted that for a large majority of the patients, the chronic neurasthenia symptoms communicated otherwise unexpressed personal and social distress, and increased control over difficult social relationships.

K. M. Lin (1983) and Lin and colleagues (1992) studied a Korean idiom of distress known as hwa-byung. The label hwa-byung is given to patients with a plethora of psychological and somatic symptoms such as tightness or constriction of the chest, headaches, heat sensations, and dysphoric symptoms such as depression and irritability. Persons self-labeled with hwa-byung consider their illness somatic in nature, but believe that interpersonal and psychological factors are critical in its onset (Lin, 1983). Hwa-byung literally means "anger syndrome" (Lin et al., 1992), and is understood by Koreans and Korean Americans as the result of the suppression of anger at being trapped in an inescapable situation or at facing a lack of opportunities. Thus, hwa-byung functions as an indirect expression of anger at distressing social circumstances that could otherwise not be expressed.

Ataques de nervios or "attacks of nerves" in Latino communities refers to a culturally-sanctioned idiom of distress that conveys psychic suffering due to familial conflict, grief, or fear (Angel & Guarnaccia, 1989; Guarnaccia, 1989). Physical symptoms that may accompany ataques de nervios include trembling, heart palpitations, loss of consciousness, heat sensations, dizziness, and difficulty moving limbs. The person may strike out at others, swear, or collapse, and the attacks tend to take place at opportune moments such as during funerals and family fights (Guarnaccia, 1989). The culturally-appropriate response to a family member or friend undergoing an ataques de nervios is to rally around, pray over the sufferer, and attempt to resolve the conflict that triggered the ataque. Often such ataques can be alleviated through social support, and medical help need not be sought. Thus, an ataques de nervios serves to quell conflict and direct attention to the sufferer. While Latinos appreciate that an ataque is generated by an emotional reaction to an interpersonal relationship, the ataque is understood as a legitimate physical ailment over which the sufferer has no control, and is treated with due seriousness.

Somatization in Individualistic Societies

Somatizers in tight, collectivistic societies such as Asia, Africa, and Latin America are able to voice their psychic distress through physical symptoms, simultaneously communicating otherwise inexpressible distress over social circumstances while reaping the benefits of social support that physical illness engenders. Somatizers in loose, individualistic societies, however, are sufferers in search of a disease. Or, more accurately, they are sufferers in search of the meaning behind their pain.

Due to the emphasis on indirect expression of distress in tight, collectivistic societies (Triandis, 1995), a medical system that conceives of disease as affecting both body and mind (Fabrega, 1990), and a culturally-homogeneous environment that allows for symbols to be implicit (Cerulo, 1995), somatizers in such societies are expressing their psychic anguish in culturally-appropriate and recognizable ways. Their idioms of distress are adaptive because they are shared and accepted by others in their social worlds (physicians, friends, family, employers). Conversely, within loose, individualistic societies, due to an emphasis on the direct expression of feelings and thoughts (Bellah et al., 1985), a medical system that conceives of the body and the mind as separate and distinct entities (Fabrega, 1990), and a cultural heterogeneity that mandates symbols be explicit if they are to be understood (Cerulo, 1995), somatizers in such societies are unintelligible. Somatizing patients in such societies are seen as intractable patients that drain the medical system of resources, are unproductive members of society, have a penchant for suffering, and are deluding themselves that they are sick when there is no "real" organic disease. One Western physician summed up the medical profession's view of somatizers as pariahs in the following way:

> "The chronic somatizer plays the medical game but will not play by the rules...Somatizers are a burden on society, not only because of the medical costs, but also because their social productivity is reduced when they do not work or engage in other useful roles. Further, we hope that we can learn to help these people because their own suffering seems endless and they impose it on those with whom they interact" (Brodsky, 1984, p. 674).

Furthermore, family and friends of chronic somatizers in loose, individualistic societies may originally offer the same social supports that their counterparts do in tight, collectivistic societies, but as time moves on and the somatizers' physicians systematically rule out evidence of likely organic diseases, the somatizer may increasingly be looked on as suspect, and resented for their drain on emotional, social, and monetary resources (Epstein, Quill, & McWhinney, 1999).

Perhaps the most maladaptive aspect to somatizing in loose, individualistic societies is the impact that such illness behavior has on the somatizers themselves. Somatizers are in pain and attribute their pain to organic disease (as they are *also* embedded in a culture that expects a 1:1 correspondence between organic disease and physical symptoms). Yet when they present to primary care doctors, they are led through a long and costly series of medical exams, procedures, and, in some cases, unnecessary surgeries (Ziporyn, 1992) that potentially exacerbate their symptoms, and tend to lead only to more questions about their condition. Even more disconcerting, after their doctors exhaust the range of diagnostic tests available, somatizers are literally confronted by medical staff, friends, and family with the possibility that their pain may be all in their heads. Due to a biomedical epistemology that views mental disorders as less important than and separate from physical disorders (as evidenced by the less generous or nonexistent health insurance coverage available for mental illnesses in the U.S. and other individualistic societies), the assertion that one's illness may be psychologically generated is often seen by somatizers as equivalent to a questioning of the validity of their pain and their mental faculties. Somatizers generally do not accept the label of mental illness since their physical pain suggests to them an organic cause (Shorter, 1992; Stewart, 1990). Feeling threatened, misunderstood, and still in search of the meaning behind their pain, somatizers often go on to seek help from other medical providers, and the cycle of misdiagnosis, excessive testing, and confrontation begins anew.

Still in pain, and finding medical professionals of little help in treating their symptoms, some somatizers in the U.S. and other loose, individualistic societies become attracted to and convinced that they have the latest fashionable disease to which the media has drawn the public's attention (Shorter, 1997; Stewart, 1990). Somatizers are ineluctably drawn to recently "discovered," ill-defined, amorphous conditions such as chronic fatigue syndrome, multiple chemical sensitivity disorder, and environmental hypersensitivity disorder, in an effort to find a reason for their pain that the medical establishment will certify as a "real" disease (Shorter, 1992). These conditions tend to endorse such symptoms as chronic pain, exhaustion, and allergic reactions, symptoms that occur regularly in the general population.

From a production-of-culture perspective (Petersen & Anand, forthcoming), this "disease-of-the-month" (Shorter, 1995) phenomenon in the U.S. is due to a number of converging factors. Somatizers who feel misunderstood and ill-treated by the medical establishment are in the market for a disease to bring meaning to their suffering. Doctors have lost authority and money due to the change in the industry structure from fee-for-service care to managed care (Starr, 1982), and in search of job security and prestige, many doctors build occupational careers by endorsing certain new diseases. Shorter (1995) notes that "physician advocacy is essential in launching an epidemic of nondisease" (235). Physicians' loss of professional authority is also tied to the proliferation of media outlets (e.g., television commercials advertising new drugs, WebMD on the Internet) that offer health information to patients and their families. These outlets serve to educate the public about the latest "new" diseases, and somatizers respond by forming advocacy groups that proclaim the validity of the new syndrome as a legitimate organic disease.

Ultimately, however, the cultural production of new diseases does not end somatizers' search for meaning. The Western biomedical paradigm drives scientists to look for the organic causes of these new "fashionable" diseases (Fabrega, 1990). When no organic cause is found for the new conditions, or when an organic cause is found and then ruled out (as with the Epstein Barr virus thought to cause chronic fatigue syndrome, until it was discovered that the majority of the population had the virus in their system) (Shorter, 1992), somatizers are again labeled as malingerers or mentally ill. Unwilling to accept these stigmatizing labels, somatizers in loose, individualistic societies are destined to chronically inhabit the sick role (T. Parsons & Fox, 1952) as they wait for the next "disease-of-the-month" to surface (Shorter, 1995).

AN EMPIRICAL STUDY OF SOMATIZATION IN THE U.S. AND SOUTH KOREA

A study by Keyes and Ryff (2003) directly tested the sociocultural model of somatization and mental health. In this study, the authors used data from a cross-cultural study of midlife parenting consisting of random probability samples of 215 U.S. and 220 South Korean (S.K.) non-institutionalized adults between the ages of 39 and 65. These data provided an excellent basis for testing the sociocultural model, as the U.S. is a loose and individualistic society and South Korea is a tight and collectivistic society.

In each sample, adults completed self-administered questionnaires. Mental health was measured with the Center for Epidemiological Studies Depression (CESD) scale (Radloff, 1977) and Ryff's six scales of psychological well-being (Ryff & Keyes, 1995). Respondents were also presented with a standard list of physical illnesses and common physical symptoms in order to identify somatizers. Respondent in this study were presented with a list of 16 physical illnesses, and then self-reported whether a medical professional had ever diagnosed the illness, and whether that illness had been present during the past month. The respondents were also given a list of 22 physical symptoms and asked how frequently during the past month they experienced each symptom on a scale from "never," "1 to 2 times per month," "weekly," or "daily." Somatization was operationalized as the self-report of one or more physical symptoms experienced during the past month in the absence of any diagnosed physical illness.

The measurement structure of physical health and mental health were comparable in both South Korea and the U.S. First, the measurement structures, reliabilities, and the correlation of depressive symptoms (CESD scale) and psychological well-being were comparable in the U.S. and S.K. Second, the rank order of self-reported physical illnesses and physical symptoms were comparable between samples. Moreover, somatization and symptom reporting were similar between cultures. The prevalence of somatization was 28.8% in the U.S. sample and 25.5% in the South Korean sample. There were minor differences in symptom-reporting frequency between samples, but no differences in the quantity of symptoms reported. U.S. somatizers experienced particular symptoms more frequently than the South Korean somatizers, yet somatizers in each sample reported an average of 4 physical symptoms.

Although the mental and physical health structures were comparable between samples and, by extrapolation, between cultures, the sociocultural model hypothesis predicted a distinctive correlation between somatization and mental health outcomes. The authors hypothesized that the usual correlation between somatization and mental health (positively correlated with mental illness and negatively correlated with positive mental health) would be mitigated in the South Korean sample, a collectivistic culture in which somatization should be adaptive. Findings strongly supported the sociocultural model of somatization.

First, the zero-order correlations showed that somatization was negatively correlated ($r = -.42, p < .01$) with psychological well-being and positively correlated ($r = .59, p < .01$) with the CESD depressive scale among the U.S. somatizers. Thus, as U.S. adults somatized more (i.e., manifested more physical symptoms), psychological well-being tended to decrease and depressive symptoms tended to increase. However, there was no correlation between somatization and either psychological well-being or the CESD scale among the South Korean somatizers. On the other hand, among South Koreans with at least 1 or more diagnosed physical illnesses, there was a modest correlation between increased physical symptoms and the mental health outcomes.

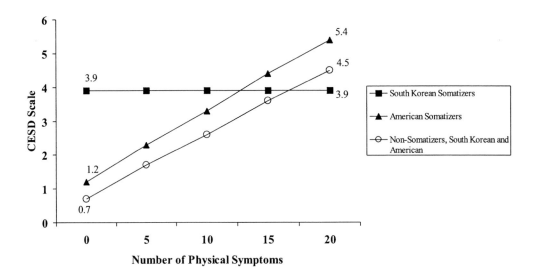

Figure 1. Mean Level of Depressive Symptoms by Number of Physical Symptoms For Individuals Who Reported No Physical Illness (ie., Somatizers) and Those Who Had a Physical Illness (i.e., Non-Somatizers)

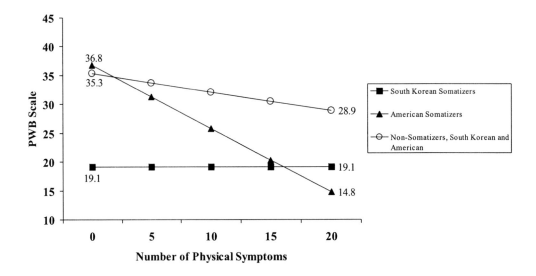

Figure 2. Mean Level of Psychological Well-Being (PWB) by Number of Physical Symptoms For Individuals Who Reported No Physical Illness (i.e., Somatizers) and Those Who Had a Physical Illness (i.e., Non-Somatizers)

The results of the multivariate regressions depicted in Figures 1 and 2 reveal the relationship between the level of physical symptoms and the mental health outcomes for

South Korean and American somatizers and non-somatizers. Among non-somatizers (adults with 1 or more diagnosed physical illnesses and no unexplained physical symptoms), the relationship between the number of physical symptoms and respondents' mental health was the same for South Koreans and Americans; more physical symptoms corresponded to diminished mental health. The only marked cultural differences in the relationship between physical symptoms and well-being occurred among the somatizers. At low levels of somatization, American somatizers reported higher physical well-being and lower depressive symptoms than the South Koreans. At high levels of somatization, the South Korean somatizers reported higher psychological well-being and less (or about equal) depressive symptoms than the Americans.

Is Somatization Maladaptive Everywhere?

Given the devastating effect (demonstrated above) that chronic somatization has on somatizers, their families, their physicians, and the health care systems in individualistic societies, the fact that somatization is widely considered dysfunctional is understandable. Nevertheless, as demonstrated by the adaptive nature of somatic idioms of distress in China, Korea, and Puerto Rico, the negative association of somatization and mental health is mitigated by culture. Put another way, in loose individualistic societies such as the U.S., where value is placed on the direct expression of distress and physicians are trained to search for physical rather than psychogenic sources of disease, somatization does indeed hinder diagnosis and treatment. Conversely, somatization is potentially functional in cultures where somatization indirectly expresses, and is interpreted by others as, emotional distress. In tight collectivistic societies such as China and Korea, where overt expression of psychic distress is seen as deviant, somatization acts as a buffer against the deleterious effects of psychosocial stressors.

CONCLUSION AND IMPLICATIONS

The widespread belief in Western culture that somatization is always dysfunctional (see, for example, Allen et al., 2001) leads researchers and health care professionals to search for solutions to help chronic somatizers break their cycle of chronic ill health. Among clinicians' suggestions for improving care to somatizers is early detection of psychiatric problems (Katon & Roy-Byrne, 1988; Mayou & Sharpe, 1995), cognitive-behavioral therapy (Salkovskis, 1989), having physicians schedule regular, routine appointments with somatizers so that emergency care is avoided (Smith, Monson, & Ray, 1986), and helping somatizers change their attributions of etiology so that they will eschew primary care in favor of psychological help (Bridges & Goldberg, 1985).

Each of the above suggestions may have promise in alleviating the burden that somatizers place on Western health care systems. Yet will any of these suggestions help somatizers find the meaning of their symptoms? Will any of these suggestions help somatizers in loose, individualistic societies find a way to communicate to others the psychic distress that is at the root of their physical symptoms, and thus help them elicit important social support and understanding?

Each of the clinical suggestions above accepts the cultural construction of somatization; each suggestion reifies the split between body and mind, and treats somatizers as isolated individuals, rather than as members of familial and other social groups. The ubiquitous nature of somatization is a direct challenge to the cultural assumption embedded in biomedicine that body and mind are separate and distinct. Furthermore, somatization is widely believed to be the result of psycho*social* stressors. Rather than developing treatment plans that focus solely on the individual and exclude families from involvement in treatment, and rather than attempting to persuade patients of the psychogenic nature of their pain, we suggest medical professionals adapt the way they practice medicine in order to fully incorporate the patient and her family into her own treatment and consider the patient's health holistically, body and mind.

Simon and VonKorff (1991) found that somatization within the NIMH Epidemiologic Catchment Area Study was not associated with masked psychiatric morbidity. Instead, respondents who reported high levels of somatic symptoms also tended to report high levels of psychic distress. The authors suggest that the oft-held belief that somatizers are unwilling or unable to express their emotional distress is inaccurate. Instead, somatizers focus on physical symptoms in part because physical symptoms are "the appropriate problems to present to doctors" (1498). By extension, should physicians focus both on the health of patients' bodies *and* minds, patients would do so as well. The result would likely be a more complete and accurate picture of somatizers' problems and more effective and expeditious medical care for these patients.

In "Somatization Reconsidered: Incorporating the Patient's Experience of Illness" (Epstein, Quill, & McWhinney, 1999), Epstein and colleagues propose a biopsychosocial model of care whereby practitioners assess all patients' mental, emotional, and physical health upon entering care, rather than first attempting to rule out organic disease. They go on to advocate involving patients' families in their care. Finally, with respect to somatizers, they advocate a focus on care rather than cure of somatic symptoms; a modest goal they assert will alleviate undue pressure on physicians and somatizers alike. Studies have shown that somatizers whose physicians communicate empathy for their patients and attempt to incorporate the patient's understanding of their condition into therapy are more satisfied with their care, less likely to change physicians, and more likely to adhere to treatment regimens (Downes-Grainger, Morriss, & Faragher, 1998; Salmon, Peters, & Stanley, 1999). These clinical findings, coupled with the adaptive nature of somatization in certain contexts, suggest that if Western physicians are to help somatizers they must first attempt to understand them.

REFERENCES

Allen, L. A., Gara, M. A., Escobar, J. I., Waitzkin, H., & Silver, R. C. (2001). Somatization: A debilitating syndrome in primary care. *Psychosomatics, 42,* 63-67.

Angel, R. & Thoits, P. (1987). The impact of culture on the cognitive structure of illness. *Culture, Medicine, and Psychiatry, 11,* 465-494.

Angel, R., & Guarnaccia, P. J. (1989). Mind, body, and culture: Somatization among Hispanics. *Social Science and Medicine, 28*, 1229-1238.

Barsky, A. J., & Borus, J. F. (1995). Somatization and medicalization in the era of managed care. *Journal of the American Medical Association, 274*, 1931-1934.

Barsky, A. J., Ettner, S., Horsky, J., & Bates, D. W. (2001). Resource utilization of patients with hypochondriacal health anxiety and somatization. *Medical Care, 39*, 705-715.

Bellah, R. N., Madsen, R., Sullivan, W. M., Swidler, A., & Tipton, S. M. (1985). *Habits of the heart: Individualism and commitment in American life.* Berkeley, CA: University of California Press.

Bridges, K. W., & Goldberg, D. P. (1985). Somatic presentation of DSM-III psychiatric disorders in primary care. *Journal of Psychosomatic Research, 29*, 563-569.

Brim, O. G. (1992). *Ambition: How we manage success and failure throughout our lives.* New York: Basic.

Brodsky, C. M. (1984). Sociocultural and interactional influences on somatization. Psychosomatics, 25, 673-680.

Cerulo, K. A. (1995). *Identity designs: The sights and sounds of a nation.* New Brunswick, NJ: Rutgers University Press.

Csikszentmihalyi, M. (1990). *Flow: The psychology of optimal experience.* New York: Harper & Row.

Cummings, N. A., & VandenBos, G. R. (1981). The twenty years Kaiser-Permanente experience with psychotherapy and medical utilization: Implications for national health policy and national health insurance. *Health Policy Quarterly, 1*, 159-175.

Downes-Grainger, E., Morriss, R., Gask, L., & Faragher, B. (1998). Clinical factors associated with short-term changes in outcome of patients with somatized mental disorder in primary care. *Psychological Medicine, 28*, 703-711.

Durkheim, E. (1984 [1933]). The division of labor in society. Translated by W. D. Halls. New York, NY: Free Press.

Epstein, Ronald M., Quill, Timothy E., & McWhinney, Ian R. (1999). Somatization reconsidered: Incorporating the patient's experience of illness. *Archives of Internal Medicine, 159*, 215-222.

Escobar, J. I., Burnam, M. A., Karno, M., Forsythe, A., & Golding, J. M. (1987). Somatization in the community. *Archives of General Psychiatry, 44*, 713-718.

Escobar, J. I., Golding, J. M., Hough, R. L., Karno, M., Burman, M. A., & Wells, K. B. (1987). Somatization in the community: Relationship to disability and use of services. *American Journal of Public Health, 77*, 337-340.

Fabrega, H. Jr. (1974). *Disease and social behavior: An interdisciplinary perspective.* Cambridge, MA: MIT Press.

Fabrega, H. Jr. (1990). The concept of somatization as a cultural and historical product of Western medicine. *Psychosomatic Medicine, 52*, 653-672.

Goldberg, D. P. (1979). Detection and assessment of emotional disorders in a primary care setting. *International Journal of Mental Health, 8*, 30-48.

Good, B. J. (1977). The heart of what's the matter: The semantics of illness in Iran. *Culture, Medicine, and Psychiatry, 1*, 25-58.

Guarnaccia, P. J. (1989). The multiple meanings of ataques de nervios in the Latino community. *Medical Anthropology, 11*, 47-63.

Hahn, S. R., Thompson, K. S., Wills, T. A., Stern, V., & Budner, N. S. (1994). The difficult doctor-patient relationship: Somatization personality and psychopathology. *Journal of Clinical Epidemiology, 47*, 647-657.

Hofstede, G. (1980). *Culture's consequences*. Beverly Hills, CA: Sage.

Hofstede, G. (1983). National cultures revisited. *Behavior Science Research, 18*, 285-305.

Hui, C. H. & Triandis, H. C. (1986). Individualism and collectivism: A study of cross-cultural researchers. *Journal of Cross-Cultural Psychology, 17*, 225-48.

Katon, W., & Roy-Byrne, P. P. (1988). Antidepressants in the medically ill: Diagnosis and treatment in primary care. *Clinical Chemistry, 34*, 829–836.

Katon, W., Ries, R. K., & Kleinman, A. (1984). The prevalence of somatization in primary care. *Comprehensive Psychiatry, 25*, 208-215.

Keyes, C. L. M., & Ryff, C. D. (2003). Somatization and mental illness: A comparative study of the idiom of distress hypothesis. *Social Science and Medicine, 57*, 1833-1845.

Kirmayer, L. J. (1984). Culture, affect, and somatization. *Transcultural Psychiatry Research Review, 21*, 159-188.

Kirmayer, L. J., & Young, A. (1998). Culture and somatization: clinical, epidemiological, and ethnographical perspectives. *Psychosomatic Medicine, 60*, 420-430.

Kirmayer, L. J., Dao, T. H. T., & Smith, A. (1998). Somatization and psychologization: Understanding cultural idioms of distress. In S. O. Okpaku (Ed.), *Clinical Methods in Transcultural Psychiatry* (pp. 233-265). Washington, DC: American Psychiatric Press, Inc.

Kleinman, A. M. (1980). *Patients and healers in the context of culture*. Berkeley, CA: University of California Press.

Kleinman, A. M. (1982). Neurasthenia and depression: A study of somatization and culture in China. *Culture, Medicine, and Psychiatry, 6*, 117-189.

Kleinman, A., & Kleinman, J. (1985). Somatization: The interconnections in Chinese society among culture, depressive experiences, and the meanings of pain. In A. Kleinman and B. Good (Eds.), *Culture and Depression: Studies in the Anthropology and Cross-Cultural Psychiatry of Affect and Disorder* (pp. 429-490). Berkeley, CA: University of California Press.

Kroenke, K. & Mangelsdorff, A. D. (1989). Common symptoms in ambulatory care: Incidence, evaluation, therapy, and outcome. *American Journal of Medicine, 86*, 262-266.

Kroenke, K. & Price, R. K. (1993). Symptoms in the community. Prevalence, classification, and psychiatric comorbidity. *Archives of Internal Medicine, 153*, 2474-2480.

Lambo, T. A. (1956). Neuropsychiatric observations in the Western Region of Nigeria. *British Medical Journal, 2*, 1388-1394.

Lin, E. H., Katon, W., VonKorff, M., Bush, T., Lipscomb, P., Russo, J., & Wagner, E. (1991). Frustrating patients: Physician and patient perspectives among distressed high users of medical services. *Journal of General Internal Medicine, 6*, 241-246.

Lin, K. M. (1983). Hwa-byung: A Korean culture-bound syndrome? *American Journal of Psychiatry, 240*, 105-107.

Lin, K. M., Lau, J. K. C., Yamamoto, J., Zheng, Y. P., Kim, H. S., Cho, K. H., & Nakasaki, G. (1992). Hwa-byung: A community study of Korean Americans. *Journal of Nervous and Mental Disease, 180*, 386-391.

Mayou, R. & Sharpe, M. (1995). Patients whom doctors find difficult to help. *Psychosomatics, 36*, 323-325.

McEwen, B. S., & Stellar, E. (1993). Stress and the individual. *Archives of Internal Medicine, 153*, 2093-2101.

Neki, J. S. (1973). Psychiatry in South-East Asia. *British Journal of Psychiatry, 123*, 257-269.

Nichter, M. (1981). Idioms of distress: Alternatives in the expression of psycho-social distress: A case study from South India. *Culture, Medicine, and Psychiatry, 5*, 379-408.

Parsons, C. D. F. (1984). Kinship and sickness among the people of the kingdom of Tonga. *Culture, Medicine, and Psychiatry,8*, 71-93.

Parsons, C. D. F. & Wakeley, P. (1991). Idioms of distress: Somatic responses to distress in everyday life. *Culture, Medicine, and Psychiatry, 15*, 111-132.

Parsons, T., & Fox, R. (1952). Illness, therapy, and the American family. *Journal of Social Issues, 8*, 31.

Petersen, R. A., & Anand, N. (in press). The production of culture perspective. *Annual Review of Sociology.*

Radloff, L. S. (1977). A self-report depression scale for research in the general population. *Applied Psychological Measurement, 1*, 385-401.

Raguram, R. D. P. M., Weiss, M. G., Channabasavanna, S. M., & Devins, G. M. (1996). Stigma, depression, and somatization in South India. *American Journal of Psychiatry, 153*, 1043-1049.

Rief, W., Hessel, A., & Braehler, E. (2001). Somatization symptoms and hypochondriacal features in the general population. *Psychosomatic Medicine, 63*, 595-602.

Ryff, C. D., & Keyes, C. L. M. (1995). The structure of psychological well-being revisited. *Journal of Personality and Social Psychology, 46*, 1097-1108.

Salmon, P., Peters, S., & Stanley, I. (1999). Patients' perceptions of medical explanations for somatisation disorders: Qualitative analysis. *British Medical Journal, 318*, 372-376.

Salkovskis, P. M. (1989). Somatic problems. In K. Hawton, P. M. Salkovskis, J. W. Kirk, & D. M. Clark (Eds.), *Cognitive-Behavioral Approaches to Adult Psychiatric Disorders: A Practical Guide* (pp. 235-276). Oxford, England: Oxford University Press.

Selye, H. (1956). *The stress of life.* New York: McGraw-Hill.

Shaw, J. & Creed, F. (1991). The cost of somatization. *Journal of Psychosomatic Research, 35*, 307-312.

Shorter, E. (1992). *From paralysis to fatigue: A history of psychosomatic illness in the modern era.* New York, NY: Free Press.

Shorter, E. (1995). The borderland between neurology and history. Conversion reactions. *Neurologic Clinics, 13*, 229-239.

Shorter, E. (1997). Somatization and chronic pain in historic perspective. *Clinical Orthopaedics and Related Research, 336*, 52-60.

Simon, G. E., & VonKorff, M. (1991). Somatization and psychiatric disorder in the NIMH Epidemiologic Catchment Area Study. *American Journal of Psychiatry, 148*, 1494-1500.

Smith, G. R. (1994). The course of somatization and its effects on utilization of health care resources. *Psychosomatics, 35*, 263-267.

Smith, G. R., Monson, R. A., Ray, D. C. (1986). Psychiatric consultation in somatization disorder: A randomized controlled study. *New England Journal of Medicine, 314*, 1407-1413.

Starr, P. (1982). *The social transformation of American medicine*. New York: Basic Books.

Stewart, D. E. (1990). The changing faces of somatization. *Psychosomatics, 31*, 153-158.

Taylor, S. E., & Aspinwall, L. G. (1996). Mediating and moderating processes in psychosocial stress: appraisal, coping, resistance, and vulnerability. In H. B. Kaplan (Ed.), *Psychosocial Stress: Perspectives on Structure, Theory, Life-Course, and Methods* (pp. 77-110). San Diego, CA: Academic Press.

Thoits, P. A. (1995). Stress, coping, and social support processes: Where are we? What next? *Journal of Health and Social Behavior,* (Extra Issue), 53-79.

Triandis, H. C. (1995). *Individualism and collectivism*. Boulder, CO: Westview Press.

Tseng, W. S. (1974). The development of psychiatric concepts in Chinese medicine. *Archives of General Psychiatry, 29*, 569-575.

Turner, R. J., & Avison, W. R. (1992). Innovations in the measurement of life stress: Crisis theory and the significance of event resolution. *Journal of Health and Social Behavior, 33*, 36-50.

Ziporyn, T. (1992). *Nameless diseases*. New Brunswick, NJ: Rutgers University Press.

In: Psychology of Stress
Editor: Kimberly V. Oxington, pp. 145-163

ISBN 1-59454-246-5
©2005 Nova Science Publishers, Inc.

Chapter IX

CHILDREN AND ADOLESCENTS' PSYCHOPATHOLOGY AFTER TRAUMA: NEW PREVENTIVE PSYCHOTHERAPEUTIC STRATEGIES

Ernesto Caffo and Carlotta Belaise[*]

Department of Psychiatry and Mental Health, University of Modena
and Reggio Emilia, Italy

ABSTRACT

Each year millions of children are exposed to traumatic experiences. The body of literature related to children and their responses to disasters and trauma is growing. Mental health professionals are increasing their understanding about what factors are associated with increased risk (vulnerability) or decreased risk (resilience) for developing psychopathology after exposure to traumatic experiences. Most of the victims, children included, develop adaptation processes and react positively, both if they have been experiencing trauma directly or indirectly. It exists, however, a significant proportion of children who develop high levels of psychological distress after traumatic events, which interfere with child's social and family life and his/her developmental and learning processes. PTSD, anxiety and mood disorders, sleep disorders, conduct disorders, learning and attention disorders (ADHD) are the most common psychiatric problems following traumatic experiences, including physical injuries. In terms of providing treatment, CBT emerges as the best validated therapeutic approach for children and adolescents who experienced trauma-related symptoms, particularly symptoms associated with anxiety or mood disorders. Family support also may be necessary to help the family through this difficult period. Research on resilience in development reveals that extraordinary resilience and recovery power of children depend on basic human protective systems operating in their favour. This finding has produced a fundamental

[*] Carlotta Belaise, Psy.D Dept. of Psychiatry and Mental Health University of Modena and Reggio Emilia Largo del Pozzo, 71, Modena, Italy Ph. +39-348-8276620 Fax. +39-051-6766974 E-mail: carlottabelaise@libero.it

change in the framework for understanding and helping children at high risk or already in trouble. This shift is evident in a changing conceptualization of the goals of prevention and intervention that currently address competence and psychological well-being. This article reviews some strategies fostering resilience and describes the main characteristics and technical features of a novel psychotherapeutic strategy, Well-Being Therapy. This psychotherapeutic technique should be tested in future child psychiatry controlled psychotherapy trials to verify its efficacy on children's protective factors.

INTRODUCTION

Children and adolescents are frequently direct victims or witnesses of traumatic stresses. These include natural disasters (e.g., tornadoes, floods, hurricanes), motor vehicle accidents, life-threatening illnesses and associated painful medical procedures (e.g., severe burns, cancer, limb amputations), physical and sexual abuse, witnessing domestic or community violence, sudden death of a parent, kidnapping, war and terrorist attacks. Most of such children do organize, adapt and rebound in a surprising way despite the horrific and frightful experience they experienced or witnessed [1]. It exists, however, a significant proportion of children who develop high levels of psychological distress after traumatic events, which interfere with child's social and family life and his/her developmental and learning processes. Acute Stress Disorder (ASD), Posttraumatic Stress Disorder (PTSD), anxiety and mood disorders, sleep disorders, conduct disorders, learning and attention disorders (ADHD) are the most common psychiatric problems following traumatic experiences, including physical injuries [2-17]. There is also growing evidence that children who have subthreshold ASD or PTSD symptoms have impairments similar to those who meet full diagnostic criteria [18]. Traumatized children have also increased risk for a series of difficulties in adolescence and adulthood such as suicide attempts, delinquent behavior, substance abuse and personality disorders [19-22]. These findings outline the increasing need for child mental health professionals to investigate effective therapeutic strategies in hopes of preventing or treating PTSD and trauma related symptoms. This article shortly reviews current empirical findings about psychological interventions after trauma and suggests future research directions in terms of preventive psychotherapeutic strategies fostering resilience and psychological well-being.

CURRENT PSYCHOTHERAPEUTIC STRATEGIES FOR PTSD AND TRAUMA RELATED SYMPTOMS

Psychological Debriefing (PD) and *Cognitive Behavioral Therapy (CBT)* are the two main psychological therapeutic strategies that have been investigated.

There is substantial evidence to state that single sessions of Psychological Debriefing after trauma are not effective in preventing or treating post-traumatic stress disorder (PTSD) and trauma related symptoms both in adults and children [23-26]. Some data show this technique may have even harmful effects and may exacerbate subsequent symptoms [27, 28]. During Psychological Debriefing participants are encouraged to provide a full and detailed account of the trauma, included facts, cognitions and emotions. After disclosure, individuals are reassured that "they are reacting normally to an abnormal event", told to be prepared to further emotional responses, instructed in how to manage them and where to ask for help and support [25]. Individuals are invited to attend PD regardless of the degree of their acute symptoms or functional impairment [29]. PD main assumption is, in fact, that everyone exposed to a potentially traumatizing event is at high risk for a stress reaction or PTSD and that everyone can take advantage from sharing their experiences and learn about trauma and how to deal with it [30].

Psychological Debriefing lack of efficacy may be summarized as follows:

> By including both victims at risk and not into sessions, this model completely ignores current epidemiological findings showing that not everyone is equally vulnerable to PTSD and other trauma-related symptoms after exposure to a traumatic experience [31, 32]. Most of the victims, included youths, develop adaptation processes and react positively, both if they have been experiencing trauma directly or indirectly [33].

> PD may interfere with alternation of intrusive thoughts and avoidant behavior typical of the natural processing of a traumatic event [34] by increasing awareness of distress after trauma and not allowing victims adequate time for habituation. In this way it might sensitize victims to these stimuli [35] and cause retraumatization.

> This technique might lead victims ignoring social support provided by families and friends that might be sufficient for a complete recovery [26].

Cohen (2003) reached the same conclusions after a recent review of pediatric literature on early intervention after trauma. Also in pediatric field, there is evidence to suggest that treatment should start several months after the traumatic event rather than been offered shortly after [36].

CBT protocols have been shown to effectively reduce the subsequent development of PTSD and trauma-related symptomatology. Particularly Exposure Therapy (ET) and Anxiety Management Training (AMT) techniques are considered as two of the most effective strategies for PTSD patients. According to the most CBT protocols currently used, *in vivo* exposure consists of returning to the site of the traumatic event to reduce patient's avoidance behavior and to get control on the situation. On the other hand, *imaginal* exposure is used for treating PTSD when *in vivo* exposure is not possible (e.g. returning to a very distant location or an earlier time in life) [37]. It mainly consists of reliving traumatic cues in imagery, describing the event in details from the perspective of stimulus, response and meaning propositions linked to the event. There is evidence [38- 43] supporting the combination of treatment packages including these techniques.

March and his colleagues (1998) evaluated the efficacy of a group-administered CBT 18-week protocol for a single-incident stressor. The sample was made up of a peer group of children, treated in the school setting with individual sessions that dealt with issues related to each participant's traumatic experience. A parallel group design, with random assignment to different treatments, was not employed. Nevertheless, authors found that children and adolescents treated with CBT showed significant improvement on all main dependent measures and that these findings, which were both clinically and statistically significant, persisted for the duration of the study [44]. Similarly, Goenjian et al. (1997) provided a brief trauma/grief-focused psychotherapy to early adolescents exposed to the 1988 Armenian earthquake. This treatment included both school based and individual treatments, using several techniques beyond those typical of CBT. By the end of the study, adolescents who received psychotherapy showed significant improvements in intrusion, avoidance, and arousal symptoms of PTSD [45]. Deblinger et al. (1990) evaluated the efficacy of a cognitive-behavioral treatment program in a group of sexually abused children with PTSD. The results of this study revealed significant improvements across all PTSD subcategories, externalizing and internalizing behaviors, anxiety, and depression [46].

All of these treatments have demonstrated efficacy for PTSD in children, but they have not been specifically tested for children who have experienced injuries. Stoddard and Saxe (2001) reported that the three different models described above might be effective for PTSD related to different kind of injuries [9]. There have been also seminal randomized controlled psychotherapy trials which have examined efficacy in groups of sexually abuse children. Pine and Cohen [3] extensively described six of them and summarized their data [47-54]. All six psychotherapy trials used cognitive behavioral therapy (CBT) to target symptoms of PTSD or anxiety among children exposed to sexual abuse. The trials targeted children in a wide age range, from 3 to 17 years, and a relatively wide range of symptoms, from specific symptoms of PTSD to symptoms of various mood, anxiety and behavioral disorders. The results of each study showed relatively strong evidence of the efficacy of CBT in children exhibiting psychiatric symptoms after sexual abuse. In all five studies that compared CBT to either a non-CBT active comparison or a wait-list condition, clear success of CBT emerged on at least one clinical measure but usually on many measures. These data, obviously, pertain only to victims of sexual and/or physical abuse, who show meaningful differences from victims of other traumas in terms of exposure lengths and degrees of other social or contextual risk factors for psychopathology [55- 58]. Similar studies, for example, have not been applied to child victim of other traumatic events, such as natural disasters or wars. This suggests the need for researchers to focus future randomized controlled trials on children's symptoms associated with diverse stressors, different from physical or sexual abuse, such as grief or potential loss of loved ones, interpersonal conflicts with peers, separation fears, or social concerns [3].

Strong clinical consensus among experts in the field suggests essential components of treatment for children with PTSD such as direct exploration of the trauma, use of specific stress management techniques, exploration and correction of inaccurate attributions regarding the trauma, and inclusion of parents in treatment [59, 60].

However, some clinicians avoid directly discussing the event for fear of transiently re-traumatizing the child or because of their own desire to avoid the negative feeling that arise from such discussion [61]. In most CBT protocols currently used with children, discussing about the trauma means encouraging the child, through relaxation and desensitization procedures, to describe the event with diminished hyperarousal and negative affect. Authors vary in the degree to which they advocate explicit exposure techniques. While Deblinger and Heflin (1996) [62] and March et al. [44] generally use gradual exposure to increasingly upsetting aspects of the trauma, other protocols do not include hierarchical exposure. Thus, strong clinical consensus as well as limited empirical evidence [48, 62, 45] support trauma-focused interventions for these children.

Persistent talking about traumatic memories with children who are very embarrassed or highly resistant may not be useful and may in fact worsen symptoms. Indirect methods of addressing traumatic issues might be more helpful in these situations and even less traumatizing for the child. Children exposed to trauma who are asymptomatic may not require treatment but may need monitoring for emergence of delayed or "sleeper" symptoms [63, 64].

Stress management techniques frequently are used before the direct discussion of the traumatic event. Progressive muscle relaxation, thought-stopping, positive imagery, and deep breathing are taught to the child prior to detailed discussions of the trauma [65, 62, 66-69]. Mastering these skills gives the child a sense of control over thoughts and feelings rather than feeling overwhelmed by them, and it allows the child to approach the direct discussion of the traumatic event with more confidence.

Another element common to most interventions for traumatized children includes cognitive ingredients such as evaluation and reconsideration of cognitive assumptions the child has made with regard to the traumatic events [59, 65, 62, 70-72]. Faulty attributions regarding the trauma (e.g., "It was my fault," "Nothing is safe anymore") should be investigated and challenged.

Expert consensus also indicates that inclusion of parents and/or supportive others in treatment is important for resolution of PTSD and trauma related symptoms. Parental emotional reaction to the traumatic event may have a strong influence on children's response. Helping parents resolve their emotional distress related to the trauma can help them be more perceptive of and responsiveness to the child's emotional needs [73, 74]. Including parents in treatment helps them learn appropriate behavior management techniques and how to reinforce the child both in the intervals between treatment sessions and after therapy is terminated. Most authors describing treatments for children with PTSD recommend including one or more parent-directed components [59, 60, 62, 65, 66, 73, 75-83].

Data on the efficacy of group versus individual therapy for children with PTSD are scarce. A meta-analysis of treatment outcome studies for PTSD in adult women survivors of childhood sexual abuse demonstrated a larger effect size for individual therapy than group treatment across a variety of therapeutic approaches [84]. Although most treatment protocols recommend individual child therapy, several authors have focused on the efficacy of offering crisis intervention to parents, teachers, and/or children in groups at school, in the hospital, or in other community settings [75, 78, 45, 81, 85-90]. Many of these interventions used convenience samples of schools or towns exposed to a common traumatic event. Group interventions in such situations gives the advantage of providing the most timely intervention to the largest possible number of exposed children. Intervention approaches for children and adolescents after disasters have been developed and designed for each particular phase of the traumatic event (preimpact, impact and recoil disaster phase, postimpact phase and recovery and reconstruction phase) [91].

THE CONCEPT OF RESILIENCE

Not all children exposed to traumatic events develop PTSD or trauma related symptoms. A major research area has been identifying factors (mediating factors) that are associated with increased risk (vulnerability) or decreased risk (resilience) for developing PTSD following exposure to traumatic stress [92]. As discussed by Perry (1999), each of these mediating factors can be related to the degree to which they either prolong or attenuate the child's stress-response activation resulting from the traumatic experience. Factors that increase stress-related reactivity (e.g., family chaos, lack of support) will make children more vulnerable, whereas factors that provide structure, predictability, care and sense of safety will decrease vulnerability. "Persistently activated stress-response neurophysiology in the dependent, fearful child will predispose to "use-dependent" changes in the neural systems mediating the stress response, thereby resulting in posttraumatic stress symptoms" [93]. Pelcovitz et al. (1998) discovered that adolescents with cancer who developed PTSD rated their families as more chaotic than adolescents with cancer who did not develop PTSD. In addition, 85% of mothers of the PTSD group also developed PTSD related to their child's cancer [94]. The capacity to provide a consistent, predictable and supporting environment is compromised if the family is disorganized and the child's primary caregiver is traumatized by an event [93].

The concept of resilience in development has been extensively discussed by Masten and Reed (2002) in a recent book on Positive Psychology [95]. During the seventies, the systematic study of resilience in psychology emerged from the study of children at risk for problems and psychopathology [96, 97]. Some investigators were surprised to discover that there were children at high risk for problems who were reacting and developing quite well. Subsequent researchers defined these high-risk children as "invulnerable", "stress resistant" and finally labeled them as "resilient". The concept of resilience generally refers to a "class of phenomena characterized by patterns of positive adaptation in the context of significant adversity or risk" [95]. But why do some people fare better than others in the context of adversity? The answer requires the analysis of individual and environmental factors. In order to explain the phenomena of resilience, Masten and Reed (2002) provided definitions of concepts such as *assets, resources* and *protective factors*. Assets have been defined as the opposite of risk factors and it has been demonstrated that their presence predicts better outcomes for one or more domains of good adaptation, regardless of level of risk. Resource stands for the human, social and material wealth used in adaptive processes. Protective factor is a measurable characteristic of individuals or their situation that predicts positive outcome in the context of high risk or adversity. Protective processes explain how protective factors work when development is threatened. The most common potential protective factors against developmental hazard found in studies measure differential attributes of the child, the family, other relationships and the major context in which the child grows up and develops, such as school and neighborhood. As protective factors within the child, Masten and Reed (2002) reported good cognitive abilities, including problem solving and attentional skills; positive self-perceptions and self-efficacy; faith and self meaning in life; talents valued by self and society, etc.. As protective factors within the family, the authors indicated a close relationship with care giving adults; authoritative parenting including high/warmth, structure/monitoring and expectations; organized home environment; parents involved in child's education, socioeconomic advantages, etc.. Close relationship to competent, pro-social and supportive adults and connections to pro-social and rule-abiding peers were described as important protective factors within family or other relationships. Within the community, factors like effective school, high level of public safety, good public health and health care availability seem to protect the child against developmental hazard across a wide variety of situations [95].

The findings on resilience suggest that the greatest threats for children are those unfavourable conditions that weaken the basic human protective systems for development. Consequently, efforts to promote competence and resilience in children at risk should focus on strategies that prevent damage to, repair or compensate for threats to these basic systems [95]. A novel well-being enhancing psychotherapeutic strategy, Well Being-Therapy, will be described in the next section together with other strategies fostering resilience in children and adolescents.

THE ROAD TO POSITIVE PSYCHOLOGY

The work on resilience suggests that we need to move towards positive goals. "*Promoting healthy development and competence is at least as important as preventing problems and will serve the same end*" [95]. Recent orientation in child psychiatry suggests detaching from viewing the psychological and behavioral deficits in a developmental perspective. As an alternative, it has been proposed to focus on child's and his/her own family competencies and enhancing growth in psychological domains.

Issues such as the building of human strength in different psychotherapeutic strategies and the characteristics of subjective well-being have become increasingly important in psychological research [98, 99]. A recent review by Ryan and Deci (2001) examines the concept of well-being and describes two main approaches adopted by researchers: the hedonic one and the eudaimonic one. According to the former, well-being consists of subjective happiness, pleasure and pain avoidance. Thus, the concept of well-being is equated with the experience of positive emotions versus negative emotions and with satisfaction in various domains of one's life. According to the eudaimonic perspective, well-being consists of fulfilling one's potential in a process of self-realization. Under this umbrella some researchers describe concepts such as fully functioning person, meaningfulness, self-actualization and vitality. These two approaches are quite different and have lead to different areas of research, but they complement each other in defining the construct of well-being [100]. However, in clinical psychology the eudaimonic view has found much more feasibility because it concerns human potential and personal strength [101]. In particular, Ryff's model of psychological well-being, encompassing autonomy, personal growth, environmental mastery, purpose in life, positive relations and self-acceptance has been found to fit specific impairments of patients with affective disorders [102-105].

Johnson and Roberts suggested that "looking at strengths rather than deficits, opportunities rather than risks, assets rather than liabilities is slowly becoming an increasing presence in the psychotherapy, education and parenting literature" [106]. In a positive psychology orientation, the main goal is to focus on the child when he/she is in development by promoting competence, functioning, psychological well-being, skills and coping strategies. In addition, working with children requires a developmental perspective in line with a process of ongoing change over time in the psychology of children [107].

As reviewed by Maddux et al. (1986) [108], two main elements are important for a developmental approach:

(1) A future orientation in terms of intervention which is considered important in view of its relationship to improving health status later in life
(2) Attention must be given to particular problems evident in childhood particular phases.

In line with this developmental perspective is the idea that childhood may be the optimal time in life to enhance healthy behaviors, adjustments and prevention of problems for many skills such as language, social abilities or self-efficacy beliefs. As stated by Roberts (1991), "Prevention is basically taking action to avoid development of a problem and/or identify problems early enough in their development to minimize potential negative outcomes" [109].

Well-Being Therapy

In this conceptual framework, improvement of psychological well-being by means of a specific psychotherapeutic model defined as Well-being Therapy [110] could be an effective strategy for clinicians dealing with child and adolescent victims of trauma, in view of the protective effects of well-being as to life adversities [111].

Well-Being Therapy is a short term well-being enhancing psychotherapeutic strategy, that extends over eight sessions of 30 to 50 minutes duration. It is structured, directive, problem-orientated and based on an educational model. It is based on Ryff's cognitive model of psychological well-being (PWB) [112]. In the first sessions, patients are asked to report in a structured diary the circumstances surrounding the episodes of well-being, rated on a scale from 0 to 100, with 0 being absence of well-being and 100 the most intense well-being that could be experienced. When patients are assigned this homework, they often object that they will bring a blank diary, because they never feel well. It is helpful to reply that these moments do exist but tend to pass unnoticed. Patients should therefore monitor them anyway.

Once the instances of well-being are properly recognized, the patient is encouraged to identify thoughts and beliefs leading to premature interruption of well-being by using Ellis and Becker rational-emotive therapy and Beck and colleagues cognitive therapy techniques [113-114] (following 3 treatment sessions). This phase is crucial, since it allows the therapist to identify which areas of psychological well-being are unaffected by irrational or automatic thoughts and which are saturated with them. The therapist refrains from suggesting conceptual and technical alternatives, unless a satisfactory degree of self-observation (including irrational or automatic thoughts) has been achieved. This intermediate phase may extend over 2 or 3 sessions, depending on the patient's motivation and ability, and it paves the way for the specific well-being enhancing strategies.

The monitoring of the course of episodes of well-being allows the therapist to realize specific impairments in well-being dimensions according to Ryff's conceptual framework. Ryff's six dimensions of psychological well-being are progressively introduced to the patients, as long as the material which is recorded lends itself to it. For example, the therapist could explain that autonomy consists of possessing an internal locus of control, independence and self-determination; or that personal growth consists of being open to new experience and considering self as expanding over time, if the patient's attitudes show impairments in these specific areas. Errors in thinking and alternative interpretations are then discussed. The goal of the therapist is to lead the patient from an impaired level to an optimal level in the Ryff's six dimensions of psychological well-being.

Well-being therapy could not necessarily be used on its own; it might become a part of a more complex, symptom-orientated cognitive behavioral strategy or as a new treatment protocol to be applied both in school and psychotherapeutic setting in order to prevent and reduce psychological distress after traumatic events. Well-being promotion could actually represent the key element for a major resistance to external stressful events and for getting through negative effects linked to anxiety and depression [110]. Ryff and Singer remark that, historically, mental health research is dramatically weighted on the side of psychological dysfunction and that health is equated with the absence of illness rather than the present of wellness. They suggest that the absence of well-being creates a condition for vulnerability to possible future adversities and that the route of recovery lies not exclusively in alleviating the negative, but in engendering the positive [101]. There is substantial evidence [115-117] that psychological well-being plays a buffering role in coping with stress, has a favorable impact on disease course and has important immunological and endocrine connotations [118]. It also plays a fundamental role for a complete definition of recovery. It is conceivable that well-being therapy may yield clinical benefits in improving quality of life, coping style and social support in chronic and life-threatening illnesses such as depression, PTSD and anxiety disorders, as was shown for cognitive behavioral strategies [119]. It is also conceivable, even though yet to be tested, that well-being therapy may be particularly valuable in patients whose disease has determined a loss. In this context, loss refers not just to body parts (limb or other amputations) and functions actually lost, but also to deprivations of personally significant needs and values, such as self-esteem, security and satisfaction [120].

A Will to Meaning

Viktor Frankl, a proponent of the existentialist movement in psychology, has argued that a crucial, motivating force in people's behavior is a *"will to meaning"* [121-122]. This topic has been extensively discussed by Nolen-Hoeksema and Davis [123] in a recent book on Positive Psychology. The authors report that experiencing loss in general can lead people to change how they see themselves, how they perceive the world around them and where they are going with their lives. Loss events, especially those that are sudden and unexpected, often appear to initiate a personal evaluation or stocktaking of the meaning of one's life. Frankl challenged his clients who had experienced a loss to create new life meanings as a means of defeating the feelings of loss and suffering. "It is the attitude one adops to adversity that is critical for adjustment" [121]. This challenge includes the process of finding something positive in the trauma by the use of positive coping strategies. Seeking something positive following a loss is not simply a form of denial or defensiveness but it belongs to a package of positive and active coping strategies [123]. Positive coping strategies are searching for positive reappraisal of events, engaging in active problem solving, seeking social support and engaging in constructive expression of emotions [124]. Three benefits commonly reported across studies are that the experience with the event led to a growth in character, a gain in perspective and a strengthening of relationships. The most consistent and strong predictor of finding benefit in a trauma is dispositional optimism [125- 129]. Further studies regarding treatment for children with amputations or other severe injuries, should evaluate the role of these positive coping strategies in the child's complete recovery process in order to create new and effective psychotherapeutic models for this specific population.

Optimism

An upsurge of research has been carried out on the benefits of optimism and the costs of pessimism.

As discussed by Roberts and colleagues (2003) [130], optimists tend to have more success in college than pessimists. They also perform well in sports and at work and they may even live longer than pessimists [131]. Seligman (1991) stated that optimism has 4 different sources:

(1) Genetics [132-133].
(2) Child's environment (parental influence) [133]
(3) Environmental influence (criticism received from parents, teachers, coaches and adults)
(4) Life experiences that may promote either mastery or helplessness.

In this conceptual framework, Jaycox and collegues (1994) [134] and Gillham and collegues (1995) [135] developed an intervention program to prevent depressive symptoms in children at high risk for this disorder. It addressed the child's explanatory style and social problem solving skills. Children were taught to identify negative beliefs, to evaluate them (evidence for and against) and to generate more realistic alternatives. They were also asked to identify pessimistic explanations for events and to substitute them with more optimistic ones. At the end of the prevention program, children had half of depressive symptoms as the control group.

Hope

Also the concept of *hope* as a cognitive element able to improve an individual's capability to achieve goals has been the object of several studies [136-138]. Pilot projects by Lopez (2000) [139] and McDermott et al (1996) [140] report promising results concerning changing in children's hope. Future research is needed to demonstrate what specific experiences are related to high/low hope and under what circumstances children's level of hope could lead to positive/negative outcomes. Further research may also determine what types of intervention may help children to increase their hope and optimism [130].

Other Strategies Fostering Resilience

Still focused on protective factors, Masten and Reed (2002) [95] described three major kinds of strategies for promoting resilience in children and adolescents:

(1) Risk-focused strategies (prenatal care to prevent premature births, school reforms to reduce young adolescents' stress due to transitions, community efforts to prevent homelessness) with the aim to remove or reduce child's threat exposure.

(2) Asset-focused strategies (providing tutors, building recreation centers, strengthening the social or financial position of the child by establishing job programs for parents, programs to reinforce parental and teachers' skills) with the intent to increase (or increase access to) child's resources necessary for developing competence.

(3) Process-focused strategies (programs to improve attachment relationships and efforts to activate the mastery motivation system in order to enable the child to be self-sufficient and motivated to succeed in life) aim to influence processes that will change a child's life.

CONCLUSIONS

The main conclusion that arises from the research on resilience in development is that extraordinary resilience and recovery power of children depend on basic human protective systems operating in their favour. This finding has produced a fundamental change in the framework for understanding and helping children at high risk or already in trouble. There is increasing interest in the road to positive psychology and to a new conceptualization of the goals of prevention and intervention that currently address competence and psychological well-being.

Well-being therapy is obviously at a very preliminary stage. Adequate validation studies should elucidate its specific role in child psychiatry, psychiatry and psychosomatic medicine.

REFERENCES

[1]   Salzer MS, Bickman L. The short and long.term psychological impact of disasters: implication for mental health interventions and policy. In: Gist R, Lubin B, editors. *Response to disaster: psychosocial, community and ecological approaches.* Philadelphia: Brunner/Mazel; 1999. p. 63–82.

[2]   Caffo E, Belaise C. (2003) Psychological aspects of traumatic injury in children and adolescents. *Child Adolesc Psychiatric Clin N Am* 2003;12:493-535.

[3]   Pine DS, Cohen JA. Trauma in children and adolescents: risk and treatment of psychiatric sequelae. *Biol Psychiatry* 2002;51:519–31.

[4]   Shaw JA, Applegate B, Schorr C. Twenty-one-month follow-up study of school-age children exposed to hurricane Andrew. *J Am Acad Child Adolesc Psychiatry* 1996;35:359–64.

[5]   Yule W. Posttraumatic stress disorder in the general population and in children. *J Clin Psychiatry* 2001;62:23– 8.

[6]   Breslau N, Davis GC, Andreski P, et al. Traumatic events and posttraumatic stress disorder in an urban population of young adults. *Arch Gen Psychiatry* 1991;48:216–22.

[7]   Pfefferbaum B. Posttraumatic stress disorder in children: a review of the past 10 years. *J Am Acad Child Adolesc Psychiatry* 1997;36:1503– 11.

[8]   Briere J, Elliott DM. Prevalence and psychological sequelae of self-reported childhood physical and sexual abuse in a general population of men and women. *Child Abuse & Neglect* 2003;27:1205-1222.

[9]   Stoddard FJ, Saxe G. Ten-year research review of physical injuries. *J Am Acad Child Adolesc Psychiatry* 2001;40:1128– 45.

[10] Mertin P, Mohr PB. Incidence and correlates of posttrauma symptoms in children from backgrounds of domestic violence. *Violence Vict.* 2002;17:555-567.

[11] Kilpatrick DG, Ruggiero KJ, Acierno R, Saunders BE, Resnick HS, Best CL. Violence and risk of PTSD, major depression, substance abuse/dependance, and comorbidity: results from the National Surve Adolescents. *J Consult Clin Psychol* 2003;71:692-700.

[12] Shalev AY, Tuval-Mashiac R, Hadar H. Post traumatic stress disorder as a result of mass trauma. *J Clin Psychiatry* 2004;65:4-10.

[13] Vogel JM, Vernberg EM. Children psychological responses to disaster. *J Clin Child Psychol* 1993;22:464–84.

[14] Silverman WK, La Greca AM. Children experiencing disasters: definitions, reactions and predictors of outcomes. In: La Greca AM, Silverman WK, Vernberg EM, Roberts MC, editors. *Helping children cope with disasters and terrorism.* 1st edition. Washington, DC: American Psychological Association; 2002. p. 11– 33.

[15] Pearn J. Children and war. *J Paediatr Child Health* 2003;39:166-172.

[16] Rousseau C, Drapeau A, Rahimi S. The complexity of trauma response: a 4-year follow-up of adolescent Cambodian refugees. *Child Abuse and Neglect* 2003;27:1277-1290.

[17] Reijneveld SA, Crone MR, Verhulst FC, Verloove-Vanhorick SP. The effect of a severe disaster on the mental health of adolescents: a controlled study. *Lancet* 2003;362:691-696.

[18] Carrion VG, Weems CF, Ray R, Weiss AL. Toward an empirical definition of pediatric PTSD: the phenomenology of PTSD symptoms in youths. *J Am Acad Child Adolesc Psychiatry* 2002;41:166-173.

[19] Johnson JG, Cohen P, Brown J, Smailes EM, Bernstein DP. Childhood maltreatment increases risk for personality disorders during early adulthood. *Arch Gen Psychiatry* 1999;56:600-606.

[20] Lipschitz DS, Winegar RK, Hartnick E, Foote B, Sauthwick SM. PTSD in hospitalized adolescents: psychiatric comorbidity and clinical correlates. *J Am Adac Child Adolesc Psychiatry* 1999;38:385-392.

[21] Nelson EC, Heath AC, Madden PAF, Cooper ML, Dinwiddie SH, Bucholz KK, et al. Association between self-reported childhood sexual abuse and adverse psychosocial outcomes. *Arch Gen Psychiatry* 2002;59:139-145.

[22] Ruchkin VV, Schwab-Stone M, Koposov R, Vermeiren R, Steiner H. Violence exposure posttraumatic stress and personality in juvenile delinquents. *J Am Acad Child Adolesc Psychiatry* 2002;41:322-329.

[23] Bisson JI, McFarlane AC, Rose S: Psychological Debriefing; in Foa EB, Keane TM, Friedman MJ (eds): *Effective treatments for PTSD*. New York, Guilford Press 2000.

[24] Gist R, Woodal S: There are no simple solutions to complex problems; in Violanti JM, Douglas P (eds): *Posttraumatic stress intervention: challenges, issues and perspectives*. Springfield, IL, Charles C. Thomas 2000, pp.81-95.

[25] Rose S, Bisson J, Wessely S: A systematic review of single session psychological interventions ("debriefing") following trauma. *Psychother Psychosom* 2003;72:176-184.

[26] Van Emmerik AA, Kamphuis JH, Hulsbosch AM, Emmelkamp PM: Single session debriefing after psychological trauma: a meta-analysis. *Lancet* 2002;360:766-71.

[27] Bisson JI, Jenkins PL, Alexander J, Bannister C: Randomized controlled trial of psychological debriefing for victims of acute burn trauma. *Br J Psychiatry* 1997;171:78-81.

[28] Bisson JI. Single session early psychological interventions following traumatic events. *Clin Psychol Review* 2003;23:481-499.

[29] Hokanson M, Wirth B: The critical incident stress debriefing process for the Los Angeles County Fire Department: automatic and effective. *International Journal of Emergency* 2000;2:249-257.

[30] Litz BT, Gray MJ, Byant RA, Adler AB: Early intervention for trauma: current status and future directions. *Clin Psychol Sci Prac* 2002;9:112-134.

[31] Schnyder U and Moergeli H: The course and development of early reactions to traumatic events: baseline evidence from a non-intervention follow-up study; in Orner RJ Schnyder U (eds): *Reconstructing early intervention after trauma. Innovation in the care of survivors.* Oxford, Oxford University Press 2003, pp.106-117.

[32] Schnyder U and Orner RJ: Progress made towards reconstructing early intervention after trauma: emergent themes; in Orner RJ Schnyder U (eds): *Reconstructing early intervention after trauma. Innovation in the care of survivors.* Oxford, Oxford University Press 2003, pp.249-266.

[33] Salzer MS, Bickman L: The short and long term psychological impact of disasters: implication for mental health interventions and policy; in Gist R, Lubin B (eds): *Response to disaster: psychosocial, community and ecological approaches.* Philadelphia, Brunner/Mazel 1999, pp.63-82.

[34] Horowitz MJ: *Stress response syndromes*. New York, Aronson 1976.

[35] Kramer SH, Rosenthal R: Meta-analytic research synthesis; in Bellak AS, Hersen M, Shooler NR (eds): *Comprehensive clinical psychology: research and methods.* Oxford, Pergamon 1998, pp.351-368.

[36] Cohen JA. Treating acute posttraumatic reactions in children and adolescents. *Biol Psychiatry* 2003;53:827-833.

[37]   Keane TM, Barlow DH. Posttraumatic Stress Disorder; in Barlow DH (ed): *Anxiety and its disorders*. New York, The Guilford Press 2002, pp.418-453.

[38]   Frueh BC, Turner SM, Beidel DC, Mirabella RF & Jones WJ. Trauma management therapy: a preliminary evaluation of a multicomponent behavioral treatment for chronic combat related PTSD. *Behav Res Ther* 1996;34:533-543.

[39]   Foa EB, Dancu CV, Hembree EA, Jaycox LH, Meadows EA & Street GP. A comparison of exposure therapy, stress inoculation training and their combination for reducing posttraumatic stress disorder in female assault victims. *J Consult Clin Psychol* 1999;67:194-200.

[40]   Solomon SD, Gerrity ET & Muff AM. Efficacy for treatments for posttraumatic stress disorder. *Journal of the American Medical Association* 1992;265:633-637.

[41]   Otto MW, Penava SJ, Pollack RA & Smoller JW. Cognitive-behavioral and pharmacologic perspectives on the treatment of posttraumatic stress disorder; in: Pollack RA, Otto MW, Rosenbaum JF (eds). *Challenges in clinical practice: pharmacological and psychosocial strategies.* New York, Guilford Press 1996.

[42]   Keane TM, Fisher LM, Krinsley KE and Niles BL. Posttraumatic stress disorder; in: Hersen M, Ammermann RT (eds). *Handbook of prescriptive treatments for adults.* New York, Plenum Press 1994.

[43]   Facteau G, Nicki R Cognitive behavioral treatment of posttraumatic stress disorder after motor vehicle accident. *Behavioral and Cognitive Psychot*herapy 1999; 27:201-214.

[44]   March JS, Amaya-Jackson L, Murray MC, Schulte A. Cognitive-behavioral psychotherapy for children and adolescents with post-traumatic stress disorder after a single-incident stressor. *J Am Acad Child Adolesc Psychiatry* 1998;37:586– 93.

[45]   Goenjian AK, Karayan I, Pynoos RS, et al. Outcome of psychotherapy among early adolescents after trauma. *Am J Psychiatry* 1997;154:536–42.

[46]   Deblinger E, McLeer SV, Henry D. Cognitive behavioral treatment for sexually abused children suffering post-traumatic stress: preliminary findings. *J Am Acad Child Adolesc Psychiatry* 1990;29:747–52.

[47]   King NJ, Tonge BJ, Mullen P, Myerson N, Heyne D, Rollings S. Treating sexually abused children with posttraumatic stress symptoms: a randomized clinical trial. *J Am Acad Child Adolesc Psychiatry* 2000;39:1347–55.

[48]   Cohen JA, Mannarino AP. A treatment outcome study of sexually abused preschool children: initial findings. *J Am Acad Child Adolesc Psychiatry* 1996;35:1402–10.

[49]   Cohen JA, Mannarino AP. Factors that mediate treatment outcome of sexually abused preschool children: six- and 12-month follow-up. *J Am Acad Child Adolesc Psychiatry* 1998;37:44 – 51.

[50]   Cohen JA, Mannarino AP. Interventions for sexually abused children: initial treatment findings. *Child Maltreatment* 1998;3:53–62.

[51]   Deblinger E, Heflin AH. *Treating sexually abused children and their non-offending parents: a cognitive behavioral approach.* Thousand Oaks (CA): Sage; 1996.

[52]   Deblinger E, Steer RA, Lippman J. Two-year follow-up study of cognitive behavioral therapy for sexually abused children suffering post traumatic stress symptoms. *Child Abuse Negl* 1999; 23:1371–8.

[53] Celano M, Hazzard A, Webb C, McCall C. Treatment of traumatogenic beliefs among sexually abused girls and their mothers: an evaluation study. *J Abnorm Child Psychol* 1996;24:1–17.

[54] Berliner L, Saunders B. Treating fear and anxiety in sexually abused children: results of a two-year follow up study. *Child Maltreatment* 1996;1:294–309.

[55] Fergusson DM, Lynskey TL, Horwood LJ. Childhood sexual abuse and psychiatric disorder in young adulthood: I. Prevalence of sexual abuse and factors associated with sexual abuse. *J Am Acad Child Adolesc Psychiatry* 1996;35:1355–64.

[56] Fergusson DM, Lynskey TL, Horwood LJ. Childhood sexual abuse and psychiatric disorder in young adulthood: II. Psychiatric outcomes of childhood sexual abuse. *J Am Acad Child Adolesc Psychiatry* 1996;35:1365–74.

[57] Terr LC. Childhood traumas: an outline and overview. *Am J Psychiatry* 1991;148:10–20.

[58] DeBellis MD. Posttraumatic stress disorder and acute stress disorder. In: Ammerman RT, Hersen M, editors. *Handbook of prevention and treatment with children and adolescents: intervention in the real world context.* New York: John Wiley & Sons, Inc.; 1997. p. 455– 94.

[59] Berliner L. Intervention with children who experience trauma. In: *The Effects of Trauma and the Developmental Process*, Cicchetti D, Toth S, eds. New York: Wiley 1997, pp 491-514.

[60] Friedrich WN. Clinical considerations of empirical treatment studies of abuse children. *Child Maltreatment* 1996;1:343-347.

[61] Benedek E. Children and psychic trauma: a brief review of contemporary thinking. In: *Posttraumatic Stress Disorder in Children*, Eth S, Pynoos RS, eds. Washington, DC: American Psychiatric Press 1985, pp 1-16.

[62] Deblinger E, Heflin AH (1996), *Cognitive Behavioral Interventions for Treating Sexually Abused Children.* Thousand Oaks, CA: Sage.

[63] Mannarino AP, Cohen JA, Smith JA, Moore-Motily S (1991), Six and twelve month follow-up of sexually abused girls. *J Interpersonal Violence* 6:484-511.

[64] Pfeffer CR (1997), *Severe Stress and Mental Disturbance in Children.* Washington, DC: American Psychiatric Association.

[65] Cohen JA, Mannarino AP. A treatment model for sexually abused preschoolers. *J Interpersonal Violence* 1993;8:115-131.

[66] Parson EW. Posttraumatic child therapy (P-TCT). *J Interpersonal Violence* 1997;12:172-194.

[67] Saigh PA. In vitro flooding in one treatment of a six year-old boy's traumatic Stress Disorder Inventory. *Int J Spec Educ* 1986;4:75-84.

[68] Saigh PA, Yule W, Inamdar SC. Imaginal flooding of traumatized children and adolescents. *J Sch Psychol* 1996;34:163-183.

[69] Snodgrass L, Yamamoto J, Frederick C. Vietnamese refugees with posttraumatic stress disorder symptomatology: intervention via a coping skills model. *J Trauma Stress* 1993;6:569-574.

[70] Joseph S, Brewin C, Yule W, Williams R. Causal attributions and posttraumatic stress disorder in adolescents. *J Child Psychol Psychiatry* 1993;34:274-253.

[71] Pynoos R, Eth S. Witness to violence: the child interview. *J Am Acad Child Psychiatry* 1986;25:306-319.

[72] Spaccarelli S. Measuring abuse stress and negative cognitive appraisals in child sexual abuse: validity data on two new scales. *J Abnorm Child Psychol* 1995;23:703-727.

[73] Burman S, Allen-Meares P. Neglected victims of murder: children's witness to parental homicide. *Soc Work* 1994;39:28-34.

[74] Rizzone LP, Stoddard FJ, Murphy JM, Kruger LT. Posttraumatic stress disorder in mothers of children and adolescents with burns. *J Burn Care Rehabil* 1994;15:158-163.

[75] Blom GA. A school disaster: intervention and research aspects. *J Am Acad Child Psychiatry* 1986;25:336-345.

[76] Brent DA, Perper JA, Moritz G et al. Posttraumatic stress disorder in peers of adolescent suicide victims. *J Am Acad Child Adolesc Psychiatry* 1995;34:209-215.

[77] Butler RW, Rizzi LP, Handwerger BA. The assessment of posttraumatic stress disorder in pediatric cancer patients and survivors. *J Pediatr Psychol* 1996;21:499-504.

[78] Galante R, Foa D. An epidemiological study of psychic trauma and effectiveness for children after a natural disaster. *J Am Acad Child Psychiatry* 1986;25:357-363.

[79] Kolko D. Individual cognitive-behavioral treatment and family therapy for physically abused children and their offending parents: a comparison of clinical outcomes. *Child Maltreatment* 1996;1:322-342.

[80] Macksoud MS, Aber JL. The war experiences and psychosocial development of children in Lebanon. *Child Dev* 1996;67:70-88.

[81] Rigamer EF. Psychological management of children in a national crisis. *J Am Acad Child Psychiatry* 1986; 25:364-369.

[82] Simons D, Silveira WR. Posttraumatic stress disorder in children after television programmes. *BMJ* 1994;305:389-390.

[83] Terr LC. Treating psychic trauma in children: a preliminary discussion. *J Trauma Stress* 1989;2:3-19.

[84] Chard KM. *A meta analysis of post traumatic stress disorder treatment outcomes of women survivors*. Dissertation, Indiana University, Bloomington 1994.

[85] La Greca A, Silverman WK, Vernberg EM, Prinstein MJ. Symptoms of posttraumatic stress in children after Hurricane Andrew: a prospective study. *J Consult Clin Psychol* 1996;64:712-723.

[86] Pynoos RS, Nader K. Psychological first aid and treatment approach to children exposed to community violence: research implications. *J Trauma Stress* 1988;1:445-473.

[87] Stallard P, Law F. Screening and psychological debriefing of adolescent survivors of life threatening events. *Br J Psych* 1993;163:660-665.

[88] Stoddard FJ. Care of infants, children, and adolescents with burn injuries. In: *Child and Adolescent Psychiatry*, Lewis M, ed. Washington, DC: American Psychiatric Press 1996, pp. 1016-1033.

[89] Sullivan JM, Evans K. Integrated treatment for the survivor of childhood trauma who is chemically dependent. *J Psychoactive Drugs* 1994;26:369-378.

[90] Yule W, Udwin O. Screening child survivors for posttraumatic stress disorder: experiences from the Jupiter: sighting. *Br J Clin Psychol* 1991;30:131-138.

[91] Vernberg EM. Intervention approaches following disasters. In: La Greca AM, Silverman WK, Vernberg EM, Roberts MC, editors. *Helping children cope with disasters and terrorism.* Washington, DC: American Psychological Association; 2002. p. 55–72.

[92] Kilpatrick KL, Williams LM. Potential mediators of post-traumatic stress disorder in child witnesses to domestic violence. *Child Abuse Negl* 1998;22:319–30.

[93] Perry B. Posttraumatic stress disorder in children and adolescents. *Curr Opin Pediatr* 1999;11: 310–20.

[94] Pelcovitz D, Libov BG, Mandel F, Kaplan S, Weinblatt M, Septimus A. Posttraumatic stress disorder and family functioning in adolescent cancer. *J Trauma Stress* 1998;11:205–21.

[95] Masten AS, Reed MGJ. Resilience in development. In: Snyder CR, Lopez SJ (eds). *Handbook of positive psychology.* New York: Oxford University Press; 2002, pp. 74–88.

[96] Masten AS. Resilience comes of age: reflections on the past and outlook for the next generation of research. In: Glantz MD, Johonson J, Huffman L (eds). *Resilience and development: positive life adaptations.* New York: Plenum; 1999. p. 282–96.

[97] Masten AS, Garmezy N. Risk, vulnerability and protective factors in developmental psychopathology. In: Lahey BB, Kazdin AE, editors. *Advances in clinical child psychology.* New York: Plenum; 1985. p. 1–51.

[98] Diener, E., Suh, E. M., Lucas, R. E., & Smith, H. L. Subjective well-being: Three decades of progress. *Psychological Bulletin* 1999;125:276–302.

[99] Gillham, J. E., & Seligman, M. E. P. (1999). Footstep on the road to a positive psychology. *Behav Res Ther* 1999;37:5163–5173.

[100] Ryan, R. M., & Deci, E. L. On happiness and human potential: A review of research on hedonic and eudaimonic well-being. *Annual Review of Psychology* 2001;52:141–166.

[101] Ryff, C. D., & Singer, B. H. Psychological well-being: Meaning, measurement, and implications for psychotherapy research. *Psychother Psychosom* 1996;65,14–23.

[102] Rafanelli, C., Park, S. K., Ruini, C., Ottolini, F., Cazzaro, M., & Fava, G. A. Rating well-being and distress. *Stress Medicine* 2000;16:55–61.

[103] Rafanelli, C., Conti, S., Mangelli, L., Ruini, C., Ottolini, F., Fabbri, S., Tossani, E., Grandi, S., & Fava, G. A. Psychological well-being and residual symptoms in patients with affective disorders. II. *Rivista di Psichiatria* 2002;37:179–183.

[104] Fava, G. A., Rafanelli, C., Ottolini, F., Ruini, C., Cazzaro, M., & Grandi, S. Psychological well-being and residual symptoms in remitted patients with panic disorder and agoraphobia. *Journal of Affective Disorders* 2001;31:899–905.

[105] Ruini, C., Rafanelli, C., Conti, S., Ottolini, F., Fabbri, S., Tossani, E., Grandi, S., & Fava, G. A. (2002). Psychological well-being and residual symptoms in patients with affective disorders. I. *Rivista di Psichiatria* 2002;37:171–178.

[106] Johnson NG, Roberts MC. Passage on the wild river of adolescence: Arriving safetely. In: Johnson NG, Roberts MC, Worell J (eds.). *Beyond appearances: a new look at adolescent girls.* Washington, DC: American Psychological Association, 1999, pp.3–18.

[107] Roberts MC, Peterson L. Prevention models: Theoretical and practical implications. In: Roberts MC, Peterson L. *Prevention of problems in childhood: psychological research and applications*. New York: Wiley-Inter Science 1984, pp. 1-39.

[108] Maddux JE, Roberts MC, Sledden EA, Wright L. Developmental issues in child health psychology. *American Psychologist* 1986;41:25-34.

[109] Roberts MC. Overview to prevention research: where is the cat? Where is the cradle? In: Johnson JH, Johnson SB. *Advances in child health psychology*. Gainesville: University of Florida Press 1991, pp. 95-107.

[110] Fava GA, Ruini C. Development and characteristics of a well-being enhancing psychotherapeutic strategy: well-being therapy. *J Behav Ther Exp Psychiatry* 2003;34: 45–63.

[111] Ramirez AJ, Craig TKJ, Watson JP, Fentiman IS, North WR, Rubens RD. Stress and relapse of breast cancer. *BMJ* 1989;298:291–4.

[112] Ryff CD. Happiness is everything, or is it? Explorations on the meaning of psychological wellbeing. *J Pers Soc Psychol* 1989;57:1069–81.

[113] Ellis A, Becker I. *A guide to personal happiness*. Hollywood, CA, Melvin Powers Wilshire Book Company, 1982.

[114] Beck AT, Rush AJ, Shaw BF, Emery G. *Cognitive therapy of depression*. New York, Guilford Press, 1979.

[115] Fava GA. The concept of recovery in affective disorders. *Psychother Psychosom* 1996;65:2–13.

[116] Fava GA. The concept of psychosomatic disorder. *Psychother Psychosom* 1992;58:1–12.

[117] Ryff CD, Singer B. The contours of positive human health. *Psychological Inquiry* 1998;9:1–28.

[118] Fava GA, Sonino N. Psychosomatic medicine: emerging trends and perspectives. *Psychother Psychosom* 2000;69:184–7.

[119] Emmelkamp PGM, Van Oppen P. Cognitive intervention in behavioral medicine. *Psychother Psychosom* 1993;59:116–30.

[120] Lipowski ZJ. Psychosocial aspects of disease. *Ann Intern Med* 1969;71:1197–296.

[121] Frankl VE. *Man's search for meaning: an introduction to logotherapy*. Boston: Beacon; 1962.

[122] Frankl VE. *The doctor and the soul: from psychotherapy to logotherapy*. 3rd edition. New York: Vintage; 1986.

[123] Nolen-Hoeksema S, Davis CG. Positive response to loss: perceiving benefits and growth. In: Snyder CR, Lopez SJ, editors. *Handbook of positive psychology*. Oxford: Oxford University Press; 2002. p. 598–607.

[124] Nolen-Hoeksema S, Larson J. *Coping with loss*. Mahwah (NJ): Lawrence Erlbaum Associates 1999.

[125] Affleck G, Tennen H. Construing benefits from adversity: adaptational significance and dispositional underpinnings. *J Pers* 1996;64:899–922.

[126] Davis CG, Nolen-Hoeksema S, Larson J. Making sense of loss and benefiting from the experience: two construals of meaning. *J Pers Soc Psychol* 1998;75:561–74.

[127] Park CL, Cohen LH, Murch RL. Assessment and prediction of stress-related growth. *J Pers* 1996;64:71–105.

[128] Tedeschi RG, Calhoun LG. *Trauma and transformation: growing in the aftermath of suffering.* Thousand Oaks (CA): Sage 1995.

[129] Tennen H, Affleck G. Finding benefits in adversity. In: Snyder CR, editor. *Coping: the psychology of what works.* New York: Oxford University Press; 1999, pp. 279–304.

[130] Roberts MC, Brown KJ, Johnson RJ, Reinke J. Positive psychology for children: Development, Prevention, and Promotion. In: Snyder CR, Lopez SJ, editors. *Handbook of positive psychology.* New York: Oxford University Press; 2002, pp.663-675.

[131] Seligman MPE. *Learned optimism.* New York: Knopf 1991.

[132] Schulman P, Keith D, Seligman MPE. Is optimism heritable? A study of twins. *Behav Res Ther* 1993;31:569-574.

[133] Seligman MPE, Reivich K, Jaycox L, Gillham J. *The optimistic child.* Boston: Houghton Mifflin 1995.

[134] Jaycox LH, Reivich KJ, Gillham J, Seligman MEP. Prevention of depressive symptoms in school children. *Behav Res Ther* 1994;32:801-816.

[135] Gillham J, Reivich KJ, Jaycox LH, , Seligman MEP. Prevention of depressive symptoms in school children: Two year follow-up. *Psychological Science* 1995;6:343-351.

[136] Snyder CR. *The psychology of hope: You can get there from here.* New York: Free Press, 1994.

[137] Snyder CR, Harris C, Anderson JR, Holleran SA, Irving LM, Sigmon ST, Yoshinobu L, Gibb J, Langelle C, Harney P. The will and the ways: The development and validation of an individual differences measure of hope. *Journal of Personality and Social Psychology* 1991;60:570-585.

[138] Snyder CR, Hoza B, Pelham WE, Rapoff M, Ware L, Danovsky M, Highberger L, Rubinstein H, Stahl KJ. The development and validation of the Children's Hope scale. *Journal of Pediatric Psychology* 1997;22:399-421.

[139] Lopez SJ. *Positive psychology in the schools: Identifying and strengthening our hidden resources.* Unpublished manuscript, University of Kansas, Lawrence, KS 2000.

[140] McDermott D, Hastings S, Gariglietti KP, Gingerich K, Callahan B, Diamond K. *Fostering hope in the classroom.* Paper presented at the meeting of the Kansas Counseling Association, Salina 1996.

In: Psychology of Stress
Editor: Kimberly V. Oxington, pp. 165-206

ISBN 1-59454-246-5
©2005 Nova Science Publishers, Inc.

Chapter X

CAREGIVING DISTRESS AND PSYCHOLOGICAL HEALTH OF CAREGIVERS

Martin Pinquart and Silvia Sörensen
University of Jena
University of Rochester Medical Center

ABSTRACT

In the present chapter, we summarize the research on psychological effects of providing care for an older family member. After a brief overview of sources of caregiver stress, we compare psychological and physical health of caregivers and noncaregivers. Then we explore which aspects of caregiving are most stressful to caregivers. Caregivers experience more symptoms of stress and depression, less positive well-being and self-efficacy, and worse physical health than noncaregivers. However, observed differences are moderate to small. Behavioral symptoms of the care recipient and many hours of care provision are the strongest predictors of caregiver distress and depressive symptoms. Caregivers of dementia patients differ from caregivers of physically frail elders. The longer dementia caregivers are in the caregiver role, the more burdened and depressed they become, whereas the reverse is true for caregivers of physically frail older adults. The amount of care provided per day and the care receivers' physical impairments are more strongly related to depression for caregivers of physically frail older adults than for dementia caregivers.

In the final part of our paper, we review the effects of interventions with caregivers. On average, interventions show statistical significant improvements of caregiver knowledge and perceived abilities, caregiver burden, depressive symptoms, and positive well-being. However, only the effects on caregiver knowledge and abilities are of moderate size, whereas other effects are usually small to very small. Psychotherapy and psychoeducational interventions bring about improvements across all outcome variables, whereas supportive interventions, respite/daycare, and training of the care recipient have only domain-specific effects. Despite the fact caregivers of demented older adults report above-average levels of burden and depression compared to caregivers of physically frail older adults, they benefit less from caregiver interventions. On average, interventions reduce only about half of the caregiver symptoms of stress and depression. Recommendations for improving the effects of caregiver interventions and for future research are provided.

In old age, there is an increasing risk for needing personal care and/or help with household tasks. For example, in the U.S. the risk for illness or incapacity increases from 9.2% in older adults aged 65-69 years to 49.5% for those above 85 years (Hobbs & Damon, 1996); in Germany the proportion of older adults in need of assistance is 7.7% for seniors aged 65-69 and 54.4% for those older than 85 (Schneekloth & Potthoff, 1994). Care services to the elderly are provided primarily by informal helpers, such as spouses and adult children (Stone, Cafferata, & Sangl, 1987). For the young-old, care is most often provided by the spouse. Because of age-associated increase in the rates of widowhood and age-associated decline in spouses' ability to provide care due to declining health, adult children, and daughters in particular, are the most important informal caregivers of the oldest old (Schneekloth & Potthoff, 1994).

Due to population aging, the proportion of older adults will increase in the U.S. and in many other countries (United States Census Bureau, 2004). This development will be associated with an increase in the number of older adults in need of care and help with household tasks. Thus, caregiving, and informal caregiving in particular, will become even more important in the future.

Providing care for disabled older adults has been described as stressful experience that may erode the physical and psychological health of the caregiver (e.g., Aneshensel, Pearlin, Mullan, Zarit, & Whitlach, 1995; Fengler & Goodrich, 1979). The negative impact of providing help on caregivers' psychological and physical health has been a concern of researchers and government agencies because it interferes with the caregiver's self-care, and with his or her ability to continue providing adequate care to dependent elders (Vitaliano, Zhang, & Scanlan, 2003).

Many authors distinguish primary and secondary stressors in caregiving (e.g., Bookwala & Schulz, 2000). Primary stressors refer to difficult caregiving demands, such as many hours of care provision per day or being confronted difficult care receiver behaviors. These behaviors may include dependency, sleep disturbance, constant criticism, anger, agitation, and paranoia, verbal and physical aggression, and confusion (e.g., Steinmetz, 1988; Teri, Logsdon, Uomoto, Zarit, & Vitaliano, 1992). Other primary stressors are physical disabilities and cognitive impairments of demented care recipients (Teri et al., 1992). Secondary stressors refer to impairments of other social roles due to caregiving. For example, caregivers may have less time to spend with friends, to fulfill other family obligations, to pursue leisure pursuits, or to work outside the home (e.g., Gilleard, Gilleard, Gledhill, & Whittick, 1984; Kosberg & Cairl, 1986; Zarit, Reever, & Bach-Petersen, 1980).

Despite caregiving stressors, providing care to the older family member may also be associated with positive events, the so-called uplifts of caregiving, such as feeling useful, appreciating closeness to the care recipient, and experiencing pride in one's own abilities to handle crises (Kinney & Stephens, 1989; Wallsten & Snyder, 1990). For example, in qualitative studies, up to 90% of the caregivers report pride in their ability to meet challenges, an enhanced sense of meaning, or a closer relationship with the care recipient (Farran, Keane-

Hagerty, Salloway, Kupferer, & Wilken, 1991). These uplifts have been described as a source of positive well-being for caregivers (Kramer, 1997).

THE PRESENT PROJECT

Starting in the 1960's there has been an increasing scientific interest in the effects of caring for older adults on family members' psychological and physical health. In order to integrate the available research with the help of meta-analysis, we have collected 629 studies on predictors of caregiver burden, depression, positive psychological well-being, and physical health, and 126 controlled intervention studies. Studies were identified from the developmental and gerontological literature through electronic databases (PSYCINFO, MEDLINE, PSYNDEX; search terms: [(caregiving or caregiver or carer or support provider) and (elderly or old age)], cross-referencing, and searching for relevant unpublished studies at scientific conferences. Reports on subsamples of the current data set have been published previously (Pinquart & Sörensen, 2003a, b; Sörensen, Pinquart, & Duberstein, 2002).

About 48% of the studies focus on caregivers of dementia patients, 13% on caregivers of physically frail older adults (e.g., caregivers of patients with cancer or Parkinson's disease), and 39% include caregivers of demented and nondemented older adults in their samples. Most studies were based on convenience samples (82%).

The caregivers under investigation had the following characteristics. They were, on average, 58.9 years old (SD=7.9). Seventy-two percent were women. The majority were adult children (44.9%) and spouses (43.8%). Sixty-five percent shared the household with the care recipient. About half of the caregivers were employed full-time or part time (48.2%), and 72.2 percent had completed high-school. About 22 percent of the respondents were members of ethnic minorities. The caregivers had been providing care on average for 54.9 months (SD = 19.1), and for about 35.6 hours per week (SD = 26.1). Care recipients were, on average, 75.8 years old (SD = 4.9), and 62.8% of them were women.

Meta-analysis is the statistical integration of available studies with the goal of computing reliable average effect sizes and to identify moderating variables that explain at least part of the heterogeneity of effect sizes that was observed between different studies. As heterogeneity was observed between studies and not all sources of heterogeneity may be identified with meta-analysis, random-effect models were used for the present chapter, based on procedures outlined by Hedges and Vevea (1998) and Raudenbush (1994).

COMPARING PSYCHOLOGICAL HEALTH AND PHYSICAL HEALTH OF CAREGIVERS AND NONCAREGIVERS

A common psychological response to caregiving is role overload which results from the physical, psychological, emotional, social, and financial strains that are associated with providing care to an ill family member (George & Gwyther, 1986). This overload is often divided into objective burden and subjective burden. Objective burden involves events and activities associated with negative caregiving experience, practical consequences of physical and behavioral changes of the care receiver; subjective burden is defined as the emotional reactions of the caregiver, such as feelings of entrapment, worry, anxiety, resentment, frustration, and fatigue (e.g., Montgomery, Gonyea, & Hooyman, 1985; Zarit et al., 1980). Because objective and subjective burden are moderately to strongly correlated (e.g., Montgomery et al., 1985 r = .34; Beery, Prigerson, & Bierhals, 1997 r = .70), most researchers use a global burden measure that sums up indicators of objective and subjective burden to a global burden score (e.g., Zarit et al., 1980). Other responses may be depression (Schulz, O'Brien, Bookwala, & Fleissner, 1995), perceived loss of control (Gignac & Gottlieb, 1996), and impaired physical health (Vitaliano, Zhang, & Scanlan, 2003).

A substantial number of studies shows that providing care for an older family member is associated with increased psychological distress (e.g., Donaldson, Tarrier, & Burns, 1998; Schulz et al., 1995). For example, it has been reported that up to 48% of dementia caregivers are at risk for psychiatric symptomatology (Brodaty & Hadzi-Pavlovic, 1990; Draper, Poulos, Cole, Poulos, & Ehrlich, 1992). However, other studies reported that many caregivers experience few symptoms of distress (e.g., Kramer, 1997; Schulz, Newsom, Mittelmark, Burton, Hirsch, & Jackson, 1997). With the help of meta-analysis, Pinquart and Sörensen (2003a) integrated 84 available studies that compared caregivers with noncaregivers. For the present paper, we added 14 studies to that meta-analysis (see, Appendix A).

We had to limit our first analysis to aspects of psychological and physical health that can be measured in both caregivers and noncaregivers. Thus, outcomes that are highly specific to caregiving (e.g., being burdened by the high level of care provided to the older adult) could not be included in our analysis because such questions would not make much sense for noncaregivers. In addition, we had to limit our focus to variables that have been included in a sufficient number of studies. For the present analysis we set a criterion of at least 10 studies for each variable. We were able to analyze differences between caregivers and noncaregivers in perceived stress symptoms (e.g., having not enough time for rest, agitation, sleeping problems), depression, positive subjective well-being (positive affect, life-satisfaction, perceived quality of life), physical health, and self-efficacy.

In order to integrate the results from different studies, a common metric is needed. Based on Glass, McGraw, and Smith (1981), we computed effect sizes for each study as the difference in psychological/physical health between caregivers and noncaregivers divided by the pooled standard deviation. Effect sizes were also derived from t values, F values, and exact p values. In cases where the direction of differences between caregivers and noncaregivers but no effect size was reported, we used vote counts to estimate the effect size, as suggested by Bushman and Wang (1996). This procedure enabled us to include two additional studies in the present meta-analysis. If in one study effect sizes were reported for more than one subsample (e.g., caregivers for cognitively impaired older adults and for physically impaired adults), separate effect sizes were computed for these subsamples rather than computing an average effect size for the whole sample. The effect size estimates were adjusted for biases due to overestimation of the population effect size (common for small samples), based on Hedges (1981). Studies were weighted by the reciprocal of the sum of the between-study variance component and the variance of the particular study, and weighted mean effect sizes were computed. Confidence intervals that include 95% of the effects were computed for each effect size.

As shown in Figure 1, caregivers had higher levels of stress symptoms (e.g., agitation, sleep problems; d=.60 standard deviation units) and depression (d=.53) as well as lower levels of positive subjective well-being (d=.38), self-efficacy (d=.54), and physical health (d=.15) than noncaregivers. As shown by the non-overlap of the 95% confidence intervals, differences in clinician-rated depression (d=.71) were larger than differences in self-rated depression (d=.45). This may indicate that caregivers tend to downplay their depressive symptoms or that clinicians overestimate the level of caregiver depression, given their expectation that caregiving leads to depression. However, the size of differences between caregivers and noncaregivers did not vary for subjective health, as measured with a single-item indicator assessing health on a dimension from poor to very good/excellent, versus objective health, as measured by symptom checklists, number of diagnoses, and medication use.

According to Cohen's guidelines (1992), the size of the differences between caregivers and noncaregivers in stress, depression, and self–efficacy should be interpreted as medium, and the differences in subjective well-being and physical health as small. Rosenthal (1991) suggested the binomial effect size display (BESD) as a tool for interpreting the practical importance of meta-analytic results: If the number of caregivers and noncaregivers is equally divided and based on a median split of the outcome variables, 64% of all caregivers show an above-average level of stress symptoms, as compared with 36% of noncaregivers. The rates are 63% (caregivers) versus 37% (noncaregivers) for depression, 62.5% and 37.5 % for self-efficacy, 59% versus 41% for impaired positive well-being, and 54% versus 46% for impaired physical health.

Differences between caregivers and noncaregivers were smaller than expected by some authors. For example, up to 48% of dementia caregivers have been identified as being at risk for psychiatric symptomatology (Brodarty & Hadzi-Pavlovic, 1990; Draper et al., 1992). However, because many caregivers do not only experience stressors but also uplifts of caregiving (e.g., Kinney & Stephens, 1989; Wallsten & Snyder, 1990), and many caregivers cope well with their role (e.g., Garity, 1997), negative effects of providing care to an older family member should not be overestimated.

As shown by the non-overlap of the 95% confidence intervals, we found that differences between caregivers and noncaregivers were larger for stress symptoms, depression, self-efficacy, and subjective well-being than for physical health. No other differences between caregivers and noncaregivers were statistically significant. This may indicate that effects of caregiving on physical health are mediated by changes in psychological health (e.g., Yates, Tennstedt, & Chang, 2000). For example, high levels of caregiving demands, such as having not enough time for rest, may lead to feelings of distress, and reduce the caregiver's health-promoting behaviors, leading to deterioration of caregiver physical health.

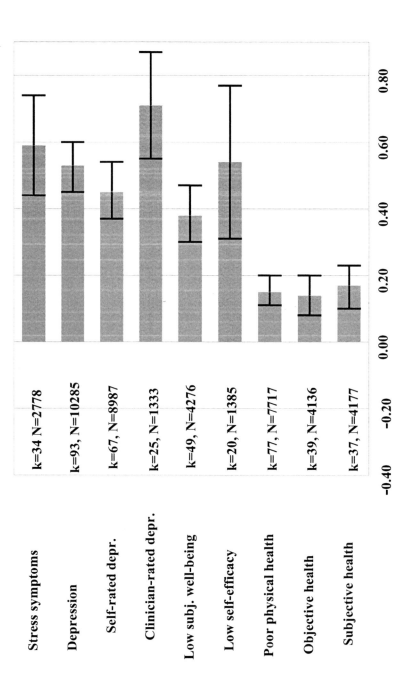

Figure 1. Differences between caregivers' and noncaregivers' psychological and physical health (Mean difference and 95% confidence intervals). Note. Positive values indicate worse psychological and physical health of caregivers compared to noncaregivers. k = number of samples. N = number of caregivers.

Differences between physical health of caregivers and noncaregivers have also been reported in a recent meta-analysis by Vitaliano et al. (2003). In that analysis, the size of differences varied by the measures used. The largest differences in favour of noncaregivers appeared with regard to stress hormones, antibodies, and global self-reported health, whereas differences in the number of chronic illnesses and health care utilization were smaller and nonsignificant. This indicates that chronic illnesses of caregivers are not necessarily related to the caregiving experience. In addition, although caregivers perceive their health as worse than noncaregivers, this does usually not lead to more doctor visits probably because many caregivers do not have enough time for their own health care.

All observed differences between caregivers and noncaregivers in our analysis were heterogeneous. Thus, we analyzed whether the size of differences in psychological and physical health of caregivers and noncaregivers would differ by several moderators: the illness of the care recipient, spousal status, gender and age of the of the caregiver, and by the quality of the study, as indicated by the representativeness of the sample, demographic equivalence of caregiver and noncaregivers, and publication status. Weighted ordinary least squares regression analyses were computed with the following independent variables: illness of the care recipient (1 = dementia, 0 = nondementia/mix of demented and nondemented care receivers), percentage of spousal caregivers, percentage of female caregivers, mean age of the caregivers, the representativeness of the sample (1 = yes, 0 = no), demographic equivalence of caregivers and controls (1 = yes, 0 = no), and quality of the source of publication (1 = peer reviewed journal, 0 = others). The dependent variables were stress, depression, subjective well-being, physical health, and self-efficacy.

Larger differences between caregivers and noncaregivers were found in studies focused on dementia caregiving than in other studies, although this effect was only marginally significant for depression and positive subjective well-being (see Table 1). Caring for demented older adults is probably a more stressful experience than caring for physically frail older adults, because of dementia-related shifts in personality, behavioral problems, the high need for supervision and the associated lack of spare time, the isolation of the caregiver due to the care receiver's behavioral problems, the limited ability of care recipients to express appreciation, and the progressive deterioration of the care receiver, which reduces or eliminates visible positive long-term effects of caregivers' engagement (e.g., Clipp & George, 1993; Ory, Yee, Tennstedt, & Schulz, 2000).

Differences between stress levels of caregivers and noncaregivers were larger for spouses than for other caregivers. Spouses provide up to four times the amount of care provided by nonspousal family caregivers (Tennstedt, McKinlay, & Sullivan, 1988), they are more likely to have age-associated illnesses and disabilities (Schneider, Murray, & Banerjee, 1999), and they are more likely than other caregivers to report a lack of alternative roles and social activities outside the home which might function as buffer against caregiver stress (Barber & Pasley, 1995).

Table 1. Predictors of differences in caregivers' and noncaregivers' psychological and physical health (Weighted ordinary least squares regression analysis)[1]

	Stress		Depression		Low subj. well-being		Poor physical health		Low self-efficacy	
	B	β	B	β	B	β	B	β	B	β
Dementia caregivers (1=yes, 0=no/mix of caregivers)	.464**	.43	.086⁺	.11	.082⁺	.14	.155**	.39	.251*	.36
Percentage of spousal caregivers	.009**	.62	.001	.09	-.001	-.02	.001	.13	-.001	-.13
Percentage of female caregivers	-.000	-.01	.001	.06	.001	.09	.003*	.29	.002	.17
Mean age of caregivers	-.014	-.25	.014*	.28	.003	.09	.008*	.36	.020*	.55
Representative sample (1=yes 0=no)	-.002	-.00	-.186*	-.22	-.250*	-.41	-.050	-.13	-.222	-.31
Demographic equivalence of caregivers and controls	-.159	-.29	.001	.02	-.057	-.16	-.042	-.15	-.010	-.02
Quality of source (1= peer-reviewed journal, 0=others)	.295*	.29	-.086	-.12	.108*	.28	-.018	-.06	.095	.31
Constant	.221		-.228		-.064		.533		-1.127	
R^2	.50		.25		.43		.32		.46	

Note. 1) Dependent variable is the difference between caregivers' and noncaregivers' psychological and physical distress. Higher positive values indicate higher distress of caregivers than noncaregivers. B = unstandardized regression coefficient, β = standardized regression coefficient, R2 = explained variance by the moderators, ** p < .01, * p < .05, + p≤.10

Furthermore, we found significant effects of caregivers' gender: In samples with a higher percentage of female respondents, caregivers reported poorer physical health. Women provide more caregiving assistance in general and personal care tasks in particular; they are also more likely than men to assume the primary caregiver role, are more likely to stay in the caregiver role even if it becomes very stressful, are less likely to obtain informal and formal assistance with caregiving, tend to have fewer psychological coping resources, such as internal locus of control, and are more likely to experience social pressure to become caregivers. In contrast, male caregivers are more likely to feel that they have chosen to assume the caregiving role (e.g., Miller & Cafasso, 1992; Yee & Schulz, 2000).

In addition, age differences emerged. Older caregivers were more likely to report higher levels of depression, lower levels of self-efficacy, and stronger impairments of physical health than younger samples. Older caregivers have lower levels of psychological, physical, and financial resources (e.g., Fitting, Rabins, Lucas, & Eastham, 1986), have fewer stress-buffering roles and activities due to age-associated losses of social roles (e.g., Barber & Pasley, 1995), and may be less likely to use formal support (Hooker, Monahan, Bowman, Frazier, & Shifren, 1998), for example due to a lack of knowledge about available sources. However, because older caregivers are less likely to be employed and to have additional caregiving responsibilities for their independent children, they are not more likely to suffer from high levels of psychological stress.

The quality of the study influenced the size of observed differences between caregivers and noncaregivers: Smaller differences in depression and subjective well-being were found in representative samples than in nonrepresentative samples. Negative effects of caregiving are often overestimated for nonrepresentative samples of highly distressed caregivers, such as people who seek help (Schulz et al., 1995, Schulz, Newsom, Mittelmark, Burton, Hirsch & Jackson, 1997). Nonetheless, population-based studies with representative samples may underestimate effects of caregiving because they do not directly assess whether the respondent provides care, but rather define caregiving as the provision of a minimum level of support to an older adult, or even as merely living with an impaired family member (Schulz et al., 1997). We ensured that the latter source of bias was not the case in our analysis by excluding studies on family members who shared the household with ill older adults without providing support.

Finally, we found larger differences between caregivers and noncaregivers in studies that were published in peer-reviewed journals than in other studies with regard to depression and subjective well-being, reflecting a file-drawer problem (Rosenthal, 1991): Nonsignificant results are less likely to be published. However, the differences with regard to physical health were smaller in published studies. This effect was mainly based on one large study that found only small caregiving effects on physical health (e.g., Schulz et al., 1997).

PREDICTORS OF PSYCHOLOGICAL AND PHYSICAL OUTCOMES OF CAREGIVING

Stress and coping theories, which evolved from Lazarus and Folkman's general model of stress and coping (Lazarus & Folkman, 1984), have dominated the area of research on psychological effects of caregiving. Other theories have mainly been applied for specific aspects of the caregiving process, such as role theories for explaining gender differences in caregiving involvement and outcomes (e.g., Miller & Cafasso, 1992; Stoller, 1992), or social exchange theory for characterizing rewards/cost ratio as a source of caregiver distress and positive well-being (e.g., Carruth, 1996).

Several specific models of predictors of psychological and physical outcomes of caregiving have been suggested in the literature (e.g., Fingerman, Gallagher-Thompson, Lovett, & Rose, 1996; Gallagher-Thompson & Powers, 1997; Kramer, 1997; Pearlin, Mullan, Semple, & Skaff, 1990; Schulz, Thomkins, Wood, & Decker, 1987; Yates, et al., 1999). They usually include background and contextual variables, caregiving stressors, resources, appraisals, and outcomes.

The basic stress model by Pearlin et al. (1990) includes four major aspects of caregivers stress: stressors, mediators, outcomes, and contextual or background factors. The model acknowledges that multiple types of factors can lead to caregiver outcomes and that multiple indicators should be used. Schulz et al. (1987) proposed a five-aspect model of psychological outcomes of caregiving. The first aspect contains conditioning variables (health, income, social support, satisfaction with social contact, nature of previous relationship, personality factors, coping strategies). Conditioning variables are hypothesized to moderate the relationship between (b) conditions conductive to stress (functional status, patient affective status, other manifestations of illness, nature of disability onset, prognosis) and (c) perceived stress. In addition, conditioning variables were suggested to moderate the relationship between (d) responses to stress (psychological, physiological, behavioral) and (e) enduring outcomes (SWB, life satisfaction, depression, physical well-being), and to moderate the relationship between perceived stress and responses to stress. More succinctly, Fingerman et al. (1996) suggested three groups of predictors of caregiver affect: a) internal resourcefulness (skills and behaviors to deal with negative internal experiences), b) caregiving context (task demands, caregivers' reactions to care recipients' behaviors), and c) coping responses to the caregiving situation (different forms of coping).

Stress models have been criticized because positive outcomes of caregiving have rarely been recognized and investigated within this paradigm and because the models do not focus on the dynamic relationship between the care receiver and the caregiver, as characteristics of the care recipient are often considered only as stressors (Yates et al., 1999).

A second group of models puts an emphasis on appraisal processes. The appraisal model by Lawton and associates (Lawton, Kleban, Moss, Rovine & Glicksman, 1989; Lawton, Moss, Kleban, Glicksman, & Rovine, 1991) groups subjective variables together into the category of appraisal, and adds the appraisal factor to the stress model. Appraisals are defined as all cognitive and affectional appraisals and reappraisals of the potential stressor and of the efficacy of one's coping efforts (Lawton et al., 1989). This model expands the stress model to view the caregiving situation as a dynamic process that involves caregivers, care receivers, and other environmental and psychological factors. Another appraisal model (Kramer, 1997) suggests that caregiver characteristics and competing life responsibilities and characteristics of the care receiver influence both caregiver effort (such as the number of daily hours of care provision) and attitudes regarding the caregiver task. Attitudes and effort are expected to determine the types of resources that are available to manage caregiving responsibilities, which are hypothesized to influence the appraisal of role strain and role gain of the caregiving experience. Finally, direct effects of these appraisals and of caregiving resources on indicators of psychological well-being are suggested. Compared to the Lawton model, Kramer differentiates strain and gain as well as of indicators of positive and negative psychological well-being. However, the model is less clear about the role of relevant background and context variables. In addition, no rationale is provided for the model's lack of direct associations between stressors and appraisal of the caregiving experience as strain or gain. Most stress-and-coping paradigms propose that resources moderate the association of stressors and outcomes rather than mediating it as suggested in Kramer's model.

The appraisal models have been criticized because the components of appraisals overlap with components of resources and coping strategies (e.g., Braithwaite, 1996; Gatz, Bengtson, & Blum, 1990). Thus, Yates et al. (1999) have tried to integrate the stress model and the appraisal model. In their approach primary stressors, such as cognitive impairments, functional disability, and problem behavior of the care recipient, are suggested to influence primary appraisal, which is defined as hours of informal care. Yates et al.'s model conceptualizes secondary appraisal as similar to caregiver burden. The effect of the primary appraisal on secondary appraisal (i.e., role overload) is suggested to be, in part, mediated through caregiving resources (e.g., the use of formal services, emotional support, the quality of the relationship with the care recipient, caregiver mastery). In this model psychological outcomes of caregiving are influenced by secondary appraisal, resources, primary appraisals, and primary stressors. However, although it is plausible that caregivers' appraisal of the elder's needs determines the amount of care provision, it is misleading, in our view, to categorize the number of hours of support provision as primary appraisal, rather than as a stressor, as has been suggested in the stress model.

Based on the abovementioned models of predictors of psychological health of caregiving (Fingerman et al., 1996; Kramer, 1997; Schulz et al., 1987; Yates et al., 1999), we propose a six-element model of caregiver burden and depression (Figure 2). The first element contains background variables, namely characteristics of the caregiver that may influence the provision of support and psychological effects of caregiving (age, gender, socioeconomic status, relationship to care receiver, coresidence with the care recipient, employment status, and ethnicity). Elements 2 and 3 contain stressors as main sources of caregiving outcomes. The second element includes care receiver conditions conductive to caregiver stress (functional status, cognitive status, behavioral problems) which may be measured by the experimenter and assessed by ratings of the caregiver. The third element contains amount and quality of caregiving tasks (hours of provided support, types of care, months in the caregiver role, positive and negative experiences of caregiving). High levels of functional deficits, cognitive deficits and behavioral problems have a direct and indirect impact (mediated by the increase of the amount of care provided) on subjective caregiving outcomes. The fourth element contains personal and social resources that may protect well-being of the caregiver, including received informal and formal support, the quality of the relationship between the caregiver and care receiver, caregiver's health, and coping processes (e.g., positive appraisals, attempts to change the situation). We expect that the level of care receiver impairment and the amount of care provided will also influence the availability of resources. High caregiving demands may activate caregivers to obtain resources (e.g., by seeking and receiving informal and formal support), but they may also erode resources (e.g., impairing the quality of the relationship with other relatives and friends due to the lack of time to cultivate these relations). In our model, psychological and social resources have a direct effect on outcome variables and a buffering effect on the relationship of objective stressors with caregiver burden, and the association of burden with general psychological and physical health (see for example, with regard to social support, Li, Seltzer, & Greenberg, 1997).

Two groups of direct outcome variables are considered, variables specific to the caregiving experience (burden and gain; Element 5), and general indicators of psychological and physical health, such as caregiver depression or physical health (Element 6). Stressors are expected to have a direct effect and an indirect effect on caregiver health that is mediated by caregiver burden and gain.

Unfortunately, most caregiving studies are not based on a complex model of caregiving variables, but are focused on selective relationships, such as predictors of caregiver burden and depression. In addition, there is only limited research on interaction effects of stressors and resources on caregiving outcomes. Thus, we had to restrict the focus of the present chapter on selected parts of the present model.

CORRELATES OF CAREGIVER BURDEN AND DEPRESSION

Most existing studies have investigated associations of stressors with caregiver burden and depression. Pinquart & Sörensen, (2003b) summarize the available findings. For the present report 23 additional studies were included in our analysis (see Appendix B). Based on the proposed model, the present study focuses on two classes of primary stressors, type of care receiver impairment and level of caregiver involvement, and on uplifts of caregiving. Too few studies were available on secondary stressors or indirect consequences of providing care (such as caregiving-work-conflicts; Pearlin et al., 1990) to include them in the present meta-analysis. Random effects models were computed (Hedges & Vevea, 1998; Raudenbush, 1994). Because associations of stressors with caregiver burden and depression are usually reported as correlations, the final results are presented in the metric of correlation coefficients.

As shown in Figure 3, at the bivariate level, behavior problems of the care recipient, his or her physical impairments and cognitive impairments, as well as the number of caregiving tasks, and the number of hours of care provision per week were associated with higher levels of caregiver burden and depression. The mean correlations ranged between $r=.17$ and $r=.40$ for burden and between $r=.13$ and $r=.28$ for depression. According to Cohen (1992), correlation coefficients of .10 are interpreted as small, .30 as medium-sized, and .50 as large. Thus, associations of behaviour problems with burden and depression can be interpreted as medium-sized, and the other associations as small. In our previous meta-analysis we also found a weak positive association between the number of years in the caregiver role and caregiver burden and depression (Pinquart & Sörensen, 2003b). This effect did not reach statistical significance in the present study. Because our previous work was based on meta-analytic fixed effects models that estimate smaller confidence intervals, the effect is no longer significant when computing random effects models.

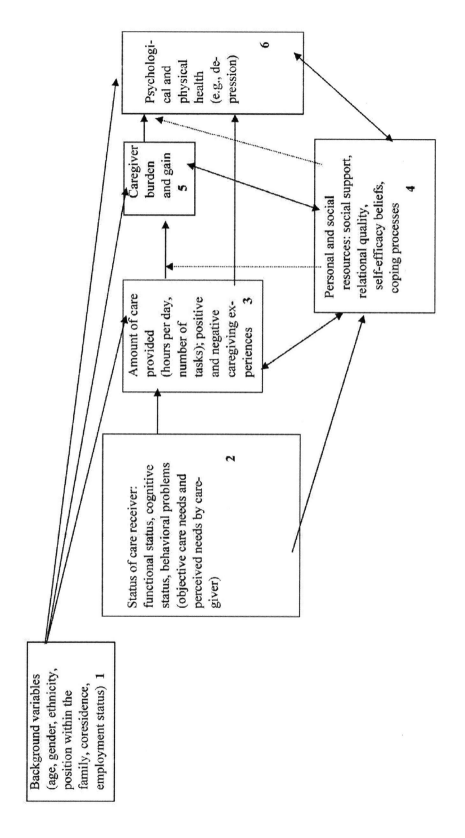

Figure 2. A model of predictors of psychological and physical health of caregivers

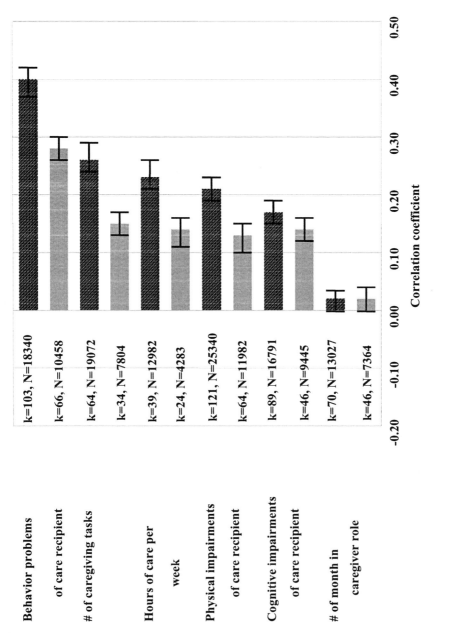

Figure 3. Associations of stressors with caregiver burden and depression. Note. Associations with burden are shown as dark bars and associations with depression as light bars. k = number of samples. N = number of caregivers

We next compared the magnitude of relationships of different stressors with caregiver burden and depression. When 95% confidence intervals do not overlap, the relationships are significantly different from one another (Bushman & Wang, 1995). Of all predictors, care receivers' behavior problems had the strongest relationship to caregiver burden and depression (Figure 3). Duration of caregiving had the weakest association with the two outcomes.

The bivariate analysis of correlates of caregiver burden and depression does not take into account that the aspects of care recipient's impairment and caregiver involvement are correlated. For example, greater care receiver impairments often require more caregiver involvement. To control for such intercorrelations, we computed a weighted multiple linear regression analysis. Because the intercorrelations were based on different sample sizes, the average sample size was used for this analysis. Due to the fact that most bivariate effect sizes showed some heterogeneity, the multivariate results have to be interpreted with caution. As shown in Table 2, more care recipient behavior problems, more care tasks, more caregiving hours per week, and fewer physical impairments of the care recipient were related to greater caregiver burden. In addition, more care receiver behaviour problems and more caregiving hours were associated with higher levels of caregivers depression. The variables explained 22% of the variance of caregiver burden and 10% of the variance of depressive symptoms. More of the variance of burden is explained, compared to depression, because burden assesses outcomes that are specific to caregiving whereas depression is more global and is influenced by many other variables, such as critical life-events, physical illness of the caregiver, and genetic factors (e.g., Blazer, 2002).

Table 2. Associations of caregiving stressors with burden and depressive symptoms (Weighted ordinary least squares regression analysis)

	Caregiver Burden			Caregiver Depression		
	β	C.I.		β	C.I.	
Physical impairments of CR	-.12*	-.23	-.01	-.00	-.11	.11
Cognitive impairments of CR	.02	-.08	.12	.03	-.05	.11
Behavior problems of CR	.35***	.13	.57	.25***	.13	.37
Hours/week provided care	.17***	.09	.25	.09**	.04	.14
Number of care tasks	.24***	.11	.37	.05	-.02	.12
Months in CG role	.05	-.00	.10	.02	-.05	.09
R^2	.22			.10		
N	7,957			5,226		

Note. C.I. = 95% confidence interval. CR = care receiver, *** $p < .001$, ** $p < .01$, * $p < .05$.

The multivariate analysis confirmed the result of the univariate analysis that care receiver behaviour problems and high levels of care provision are the greatest stressors for caregivers. The negative association of physical impairments of the care recipient and caregiver burden should be interpreted as a suppressor effect: High levels of physical impairment are usually associated with higher levels of care provision (e.g., Yates et al., 2000), and in dementia caregiving with high levels of behavior problems (e.g., Majerowitz, 1995). Thus, controlling for these factors eliminates the positive association of physical impairment and burden that has been observed at the bivariate level. In addition Gräßel and Leutbecher (1993) have shown that in the case of severe behaviour problems, such as nightly wandering and disorientation, more care receiver physical impairments may actually reduce behaviour problems and thereby decrease caregiver burden.

The associations of stressors with caregiver burden and depression varied by whether the care recipient has dementia. Caregiver burden was more strongly related to behavior problems among dementia caregivers than among caregivers of physically frail older adults. Whereas dementia caregivers who had provided care over a longer period reported higher levels of burden, the reverse was true for caregivers of physically frail older adults (Figure 4a). For caregiver depression, we found weaker associations with the number of caregiving tasks, the number of caregiving hours per week, and the level of physical impairment of the care recipient among dementia caregivers than among other caregivers. The number of months in the caregiver role was positively associated with depression among dementia caregivers, but negatively among nondementia caregivers (Figure 4b). Thus, for dementia caregivers, care recipient limitations in activities of daily living and caregiver involvement were of lesser importance, whereas behavior problems were of greater importance.

Contradictory hypotheses have been stated in the literature with regard to the association of the duration of caregiving with caregiver outcomes (Haley & Pardo, 1989; Townsend, Noelker, Deimling, & Bass, 1989). On the one hand, the wear-and-tear hypothesis predicts that the longer caregiving is sustained the greater the decline in psychological health of caregivers. Chronic stress and steady progression of a care recipient's illness may erode the caregiver's coping resources. On the other hand, the adaptation hypothesis suggests that caregivers will adapt to the stress of caregiving over time. Negative affect may increase after taking over the caregiver role, with distress being highest at midpoint of care, when behavior problems due to dementia are most frequent. However, negative affect will decline thereafter as a result of adaptational processes or because of a decrease of care receiver's problem behavior. Our results indicate that the wear-and-tear hypothesis is supported for dementia caregivers, whereas the adaptational hypothesis is more likely to be found in caregivers for physically impaired older adults. It may be more difficult to adapt to increasing behavior problems in the care recipient than to care for frail, but mentally intact older adults. However, as dementia caregivers provided, on average, care over a shorter period (M=46.7 months) than caregivers of physically impaired older adults (M=61.8 months), they might also have had less time to adapt to their situation than the other caregivers. We were not able to test for such nonlinear associations between the duration of care provision and caregiving outcomes.

Burden was more strongly related to care recipient's physical impairment and behavior problems for spouses than for adult children. In addition, the duration of caregiving was positively related to burden in spousal but not in child caregivers (Pinquart & Sörensen, 2003b). Spouses may be more distressed by care recipients' symptoms and high levels of care provision because age-associated health problems and functional impairments of the caregiver make the provision of physical care increasingly difficult (Connell, Janevic, & Gallant, 2001; Schneider, Murray, Banerjee, & Mann, 1999).

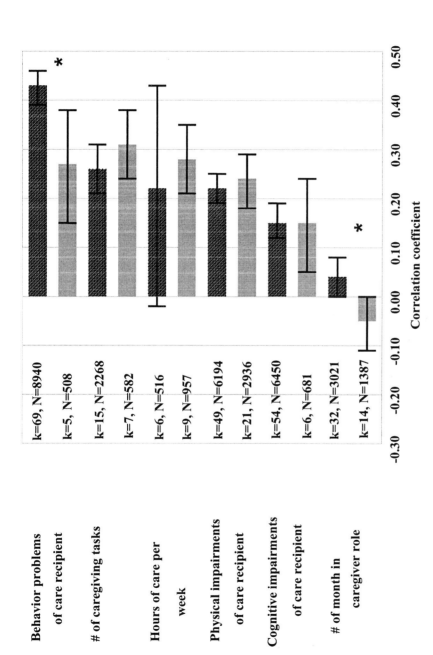

Figure 4a. Associations of stressors with caregiver burden in caregivers of dementia patients versus caregivers of physically frail older adults. Note. Results of dementia caregivers are shown as dark bars and results of other caregivers as light bars. k = number of samples. N = number of caregivers, * indicates significant between-group differences.

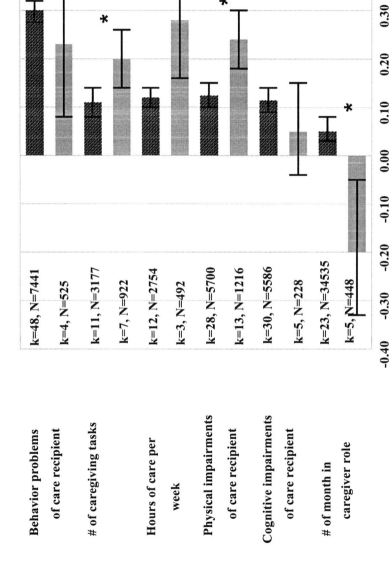

Figure 4b. Associations of stressors with caregiver depression in caregivers of dementia patients versus caregivers of physically frail older adults. Note. Results of dementia caregivers are shown as dark bars and results of other caregivers as light bars. k = number of samples. N = number of caregivers, * indicates significant between-group differences.

Associations of stressors with both caregiver burden and depression were stronger than the associations of stressors with subjective well-being (see Pinquart & Sörensen, 2004). It is possible that caregiver burden measures distress specific to caregiving, whereas positive affect and other indicators of subjective well-being are more general, and are therefore to a larger extend influenced by experiences outside the caregiver role. However, like positive affect, depressive symptoms are not specific to the caregiving experience. Thus, the framework of domain-specificity of sources of positive and negative affect may be the best explanation for our findings: Aspects of negative subjective well-being – such as depressed mood – are mainly influenced by negative experiences, as is the case with caregiving stressors. Positive experiences, however, are more likely to be influenced by positive experiences outside and inside the caregiving experience. In fact, positive experiences of caregiving, such as being appreciated by the care recipient, showed stronger associations with positive well-being than with low levels of depression (Pinquart & Sörensen, 2004).

Very few studies have addressed associations of positive aspects of caregiving with psychological outcome variables. In our meta-analyses, we found only 9 studies that relate depression and subjective well-being of caregivers with perceived uplifts of caregiving, such as perceived gains and benefits and enjoyable aspects of caregiving (Pinquart & Sörensen, 2004). Gains or uplifts of caregiving were correlated with subjective well-being (r=.25, 95% confidence interval (C.I.) .20 to .29) and depression (r=-.16, C.I. -.18 to -.13). The negative association of uplifts and depression may indicate a decline of depressive mood due to a sense of usefulness or improved self-esteem based on perceived abilities to handle difficult situations (e.g., Konstam, Holmes, Wilczenski, Baliga, Lester, & Priest, 2003). Nonetheless, the observed correlations also may indicate that depressed individuals are less likely to perceive positive aspects of caregiving due to their focus on negative aspects of the self and of their daily experience (Ingram, Miranda, & Segal, 1998). Longitudinal studies are needed to test the causal relationships between depression and positive aspects of caregiving.

According to our proposed model, personal and social resources should have direct effects on caregiver psychological outcomes, and buffering effects on the association between stressors and outcomes (Figure 2). Few studies have investigated resource variables, especially with regard to buffering effects. Our analyses show that a more positive relationship with the care recipient is associated with less burden (r=-.26, C.I. -.29 to -.24) and depression (r=-.27, C.I. -.31 to -.23). Similarly, receiving more informal support is related to less caregiver burden (r=-.15, C.I. -.16 to -.14) and depression (r=-.19, C.I. -.21 to -.17). However, the association of the use of formal support with caregiver burden (r=.04, C.I. .03 to .05) and depression is positive, but weak (r=.07, C.I. .05 to .09). Because these analyses are based on correlational data, the causal direction of the associations cannot be interpreted. Presumably, caregivers with higher levels of distress are more likely to seek support. A more direct test of the effects of the use of formal support is provided in the next section. With regard to buffering effects of social resources, too few studies were available to be included in this meta-analysis. Future meta-analyses should focus on the associations of caregiver outcomes with personal resources, such as self-efficacy beliefs.

INTERVENTIONS FOR CAREGIVERS

The results of our meta-analysis have shown that caregivers have higher levels of stress symptoms, depression, lower levels of positive subjective well-being, and reduced self-efficacy beliefs. In addition, sources of psychological distress have been identified. Psychosocial interventions are needed that reduce the levels of objective stressors and of psychological distress. Current caregiver interventions can be divided into two major groups: (1) those aimed at reducing the objective level of stressors, such as the amount of care provided by caregivers (respite, interventions to enhance the competence of the care receiver) and interventions to reduce symptoms of the care recipient, and (2) those aimed at improving the caregiver's coping skills and psychological health (e.g., psychoeducational interventions, support groups).

Respite care is either in-home or site-specific supervision, assistance with activities of daily living, or skilled nursing care designed to give the caregiver time off. It does not imply that activities or programs are offered to the care recipient (e.g., Burdz, Easton, & Bond, 1988). In addition, adult day care programs provide a combination of respite, by engaging the care receiver away from home, and general activity promotion by offering stimulating, disease-appropriate programs (e.g., Guttman, 1991; Zarit, Stephens, Townsend, & Greene, 1998).

Interventions for improving care receiver competence include memory clinics for patients with dementia, and general activity promotion (e.g., LoGiudice, Waltrowicz, Brown, Burrows, Ames, & Flicker, 1999). They may affect caregiver outcomes indirectly by reducing impairments and behavior problems of the care recipient.

The second group of intervention is focused on the caregivers more directly. Psycho-educational interventions have most often been used for supporting informal caregivers. They involve provision of information about the care receiver's disease process, and information about resources and services (e.g., Ostwald, Hepburn, Caron, Burns, & Mantell, 1999), training caregivers in effective response to dementia-related behavior problems, and teaching them how to deal with negative emotions (e.g., Gallagher-Thompson, Lovett, Rose, McKibbin, Coon, Futterman, & Thompson, 2000). They usually include lectures, group discussions, and the provision of written materials.

Supportive interventions subsume both professionally led and peer-led support groups focusing on building rapport among participants and creating a space in which to discuss problems, successes, and feelings regarding caregiving (e.g., Demers & Lavoie, 1996). The exchange between caregivers may provide new information, but information provision is less structured than in psychoeducational interventions.

Psychotherapeutic interventions with caregivers include changing maladaptive beliefs and developing adaptive thinking and behavior, and gaining insight into the development of problems. Most of these interventions with caregivers follow a cognitive-behavioral approach, where therapists may teach self-monitoring, challenge negative thoughts and assumptions that maintain the caregiver's problematic behavior, help the caregiver develop problem solving abilities by focusing on time management, overload, or emotional reactivity, and help the caregiver re-engage in pleasant activities and positive experiences (e.g., Stevens & Baldwin, 1994).

Finally, some intervention studies combine multiple forms of intervention (multicomponent interventions), such as information provision, support, psychotherapy, and respite (e.g. Archbold, Stewart, Miller, & Harvath, 1995). However, not all participants may use all offers.

In a previous paper, we have reported a meta-analysis on 78 controlled intervention studies that were published in peer-reviewed journals (Sörensen, Pinquart, & Duberstein, 2002). For the presen updated meta-analysis, we were able to include an additional 43 papers, amongst others those from the largest multi-site caregiver intervention study (the REACH study, Gitlin, et al., 2003). Because published studies may overestimate the effects of interventions (studies with nonsignificant effects are rarely published; Rosenthal, 1991), 13 unpublished studies were included in the present updated meta-analysis. Similar to the meta-analysis on comparisons of caregivers and noncaregivers, we included burden, depression, and positive subjective well-being as outcome variables. Because the increase in caregiver coping abilities and/or knowledge is a central outcome variable in many interventions, we included this variable as an additional outcome in our meta-analysis. In addition, changes in symptoms of the care recipient (e.g., of memory problems or behavior symptoms) were included as another outcome variable. Too few studies were available for analyzing intervention effects on changes in caregivers' physical health.

Criteria for inclusion of the studies in the meta-analysis were: (1) The care recipients had a mean or median age of $\geq$ 60 years, (2) an intervention condition was compared to an untreated control condition, and (3) at least one of the following outcomes were reported: caregiver burden, depression, measures of psychological well-being (e.g., life-satisfaction, morale, self-esteem, happiness), uplifts of caregiving, knowledge and/or coping abilities of the caregiver, and symptoms of care receivers. We computed effect sizes for each study as the difference in the posttreatment measure between the experimental and control groups divided by the pooled standard deviation (Glass et al., 1981; Hedges, 1981). Effect sizes were also derived from t values, F values, exact p values, and α levels. The effect size estimates were adjusted for bias due to differences in pretests between experimental and control group, based on Mullen (1989), and due to overestimation of the population effect size (common for small samples), based on Hedges (1981). Random-effects models were computed, based on Hedges and Vevea (1998) and Raudenbush (1994).

As shown in Figure 5, all caregiver interventions taken together produced a significant improvement of caregiver burden (d=.22 standard deviation units), depression (d=.30), positive subjective well-being (e.g., positive affect; d=.33), and reported coping abilities/knowledge about disease and caregiving (d=.51). In addition, small but significant reductions in care recipients' symptoms were found (d=.12). According to Cohen's (1992) criteria, improvements of abilities and knowledge can be interpreted as medium-sized, but the other improvements were rather small. According to the Binomial Effect Size Display, 55.5% of the caregivers in the intervention condition as compared to 44.5% of the control group participants show above-average decline in symptoms of burden. The numbers were 57.4% (intervention) and 42.6% (controls) for depression, 58.1% (intervention) and 41.9% (control) for positive subjective well-being, 62.4% (intervention) and 37.6% (controls) for ability/knowledge, as well as 53.0% (intervention) and 47.0% (controls) for symptoms of the care recipient. Immediate posttest intervention effects were significantly larger for ability/knowledge than for caregiver burden and symptoms of the care receiver. In addition, the intervention effects on subjective well-being were larger than the effects on care receivers' symptoms.

Table 3. Comparison of the amount of caregiver distress
relative to the size of effects of caregiver interventions

	Differences between caregivers and non-caregivers (standard deviation units)	Effects of caregiver Interventions (standard deviation units)		Reduction of elevated levels of psychological symptoms of caregiver	
		Immediate effects	Long-term effects	Immediate effects	Long-term effects
All caregivers					
Psychological distress	.60	-.22	-.15	37%	26%
Depression	.53	-.30	-.25	57%	47%
Subjective well-being	-.38	.33	.24	87%	63%
Self-efficacy	-.54	.50	.51	93%	94%
Dementia caregivers					
Psychological distress	.93	-.10	-.11	11%	.12%
Depression	.61	-.15	-.15	25%	.25%
Subjective well-being	-.55	.32	.27	58%	.44%
Self-efficacy	-.73	.50	.34	68%	47%
Caregivers for physically frail older adults					
Psychological distress	.34	-.29	- .14	85%	41%
Depression	.36	-.30	-.33	83%	92%
Subjective well-being	-.22	.34	.15	154%	68%
Self-efficacy	.34	.50	.34	147%	100%

Follow-up measures were assessed, on average, 8 months after the end of the intervention. Improvements of burden ($d=.15$), depression ($d=.25$), and ability/knowledge ($d=.44$) were still statistically significant. However, intervention effects on positive well-being ($d=.24$) and care receiver symptoms ($d=.12$) were no longer significant, presumably due to the small number of available studies that provided follow-up data (Figure 5).

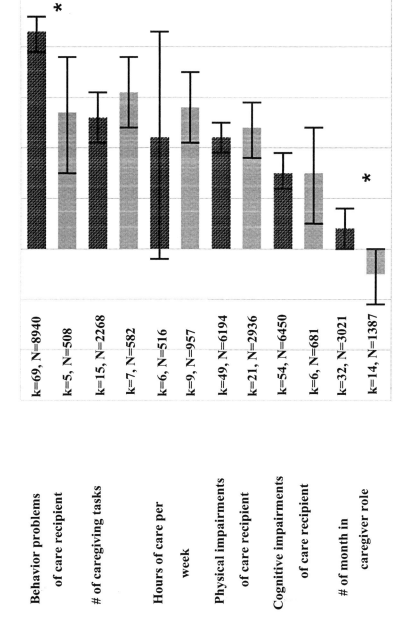

Figure 5. Intervention effects on caregivers' burden, depression, subjective well-being, abilities/knowledge, and symptoms of care recipients. Notes. Positive values indicate improvements. Immediate effects (pretest – posttest) are shown as dark bars and long-term effects (pretest – follow-up) as light bars. k = number of samples. N = number of caregivers.

Other criteria may also be used for evaluating the effects of caregiver interventions. Knowing the percentage of clinically depressed caregivers at the beginning and at the end of the intervention would be of high practical importance. Unfortunately, few caregiver studies have assessed this information. Based on our previous work, we suggest another criterion: The size of the effect of interventions can be compared to the size of difference between caregivers' and non-caregivers' distress. From the meta-analysis on comparisons of caregivers and noncaregivers we know how much caregivers' stress symptoms and depressive symptoms are elevated and how much their well-being and self-efficacy beliefs are impaired. Ideally the effect of an intervention for a specific variable should be as large as the existing difference between caregivers and noncaregivers on that variable. This would indicate a 100% reduction of the elevated levels of caregiver symptoms. Table 3 shows such a comparison:The difference in psychological distress between caregivers and non-caregivers is 0.6 standard deviation units. Interventions reduce this difference by about 37%. Interventions reduced, on average, 57% of caregivers' elevated levels of depressive symptoms, and 87% of their impaired positive well-being. Most impressively, the lower self-efficacy that caregivers typically experience is ameliorated to 93% by caregiver interventions. However, a less optimistic picture emerges when comparing caregivers of dementia patients and caregivers of physically frail older adults. Whereas more than 80% of the elevated levels symptoms of psychological distress and depression in caregivers of physically frail older adults are reduced by the interventions, for dementia caregivers this reduction in psychological distress and depression is only 11% and 25%, respectively. Thus, more efforts are needed for improving the effects of interventions for caregivers of demented older adults.

The intervention effects also varied by the type of intervention. We limit our analysis to immediate intervention effects because data on long-term effects for all outcome variables could only be computed for psychoeducational interventions.

As shown in Figure 6, significant improvements of caregiver burden were found for all interventions except training of the care recipient. Significant effect sizes varied between $d=.38$ (psychotherapy) and $d=.12$ (psychoeducational interventions). With regard to caregiver depression, significant effects emerged for psychotherapy ($d=.53$), psychoeducational interventions ($d=.34$), respite/daycare ($d=.24$), and multicomponent interventions ($d=.22$).

Improvements of psychological well-being were found for 4 out of 5 types of intervention. The strongest effect was found for training of the care recipient ($d=.74$). However, as this effect was based on only one study, this result needs to be replicated in further studies. Significant effects also emerged for psychotherapy ($d=.38$), psychoeducational interventions ($d=.28$), multicomponent interventions ($d=.26$), and respite/daycare ($d=.16$, see also Figure 7). Significant improvements in perceived abilities and caregiver knowledge were found for psychotherapy ($d=.72$), respite/daycare ($d=.62$), psychoeducational interventions ($d=.58$), multicomponent interventions ($d=.48$), and support provision ($d=.34$). As shown in Figure 7, significant reductions of symptoms of the care recipient emerged after training of the care recipient ($d=.45$), psychotherapy ($d=.17$), and psychoeducational interventions ($d=.13$).

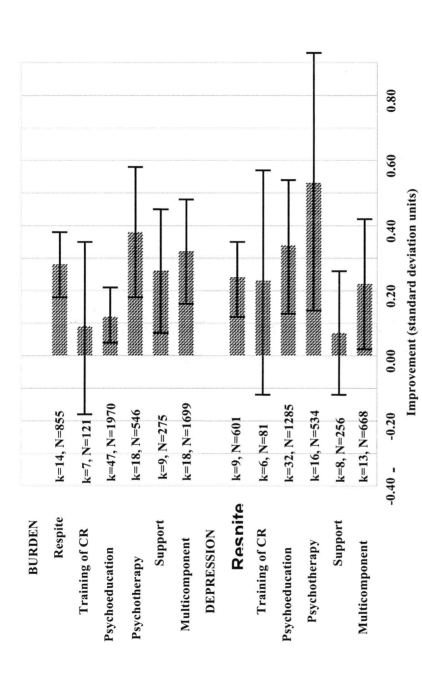

Figure 6. Effects of different forms of intervention on caregiver burden and depression. Notes. Positive values indicate improvements. k = number of samples. N = number of caregivers.

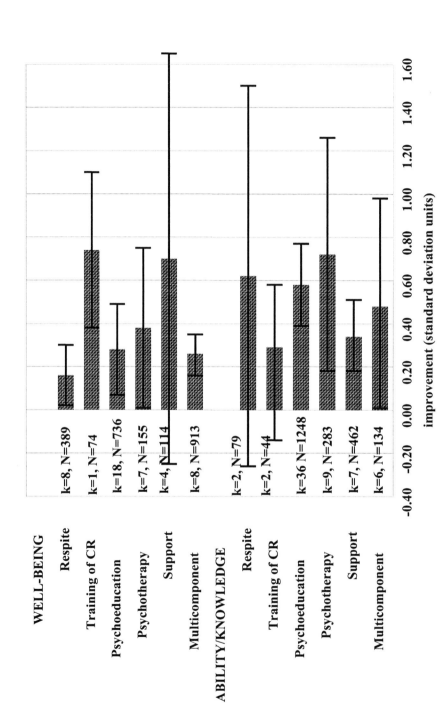

Figure 7. Effects of different forms of intervention on caregiver well-being and ability/knowledge. Notes. Positive values indicate improvements. k = number of samples. N = number of caregivers

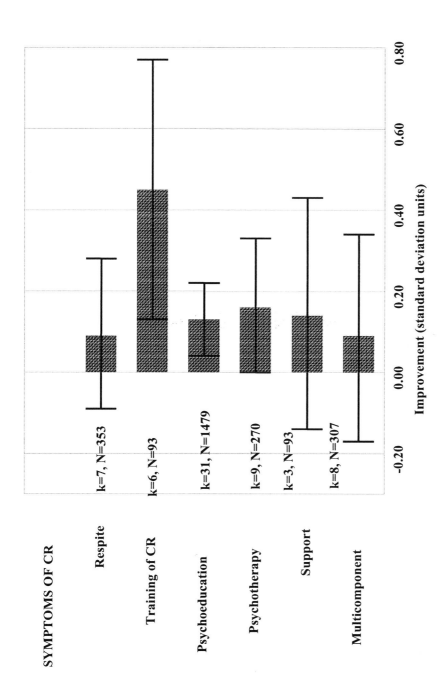

Figure 8. Effects of different forms of intervention on symptoms of the care recipient. Notes. Positive values indicate improvements. k = number of samples. N = number of caregivers.

Table 4. Influence of moderator variables on positive intervention effects (Weighted ordinary least squares regression analysis)

	Improvement of burden		Improvement of depression		Increase of well-being		Increase of ability/knowledge		Improvement of symptoms of care receivers	
	B	β	B	β	B	β	B	β	B	β
Caregiver diagnosis (1=dementia 0=other)	-.133*	-.18	.161	.09	-.167	-.16	.007	.04	.11	.16
Caregiver age (Sample mean)	-.005	-.06	.005	.00	-.002	-.04	.021	.19	.012+	.20
Percent female Caregivers	.006+	.20	.013*	.27	.003	.08	.025***	.52	.004	.14
Group intervention (1=yes, 0=no)	.008	.11	.088	.07	-.148	-.17	.004	.00	.155*	.25
Number of sessions	.003+	.17	-.003	-.09	-.044*	-.28	-.003	-.10	-.002	-.12
Randomization (1=yes, 0=no)	.126+	.17	-.048	-.03	-.339*	-.40	-.197	-.13	-.203+	-.26
Published (1=yes, 0=no)	-.287**	-.24	-.009	-.00	-.149	-.13	-.466	-.12	.190	.15
Year of Publication	-.013*	-.20	-.009	-.07	-.002	-.02	.011	.08	-.001	-.02
(Constant)	26.55*		18.40		3.66		-23.65		1.56	
R²	.18		.08		.25		.23		.25	

Note. + p < .10, * p < .05, **p < .01 *** p < .001

In sum, psychotherapy and psychoeducational interventions showed consistent effects on all outcome measures under investigation. Other interventions had more specific effects. Respite/daycare most affected indicators of caregiver mental health (burden, depression, positive well-being); supportive interventions improved burden, ability/knowledge; training of the care recipient reduced his or her symptoms, such as memory and behaviour problems. Given the limited number of studies for each form of intervention and between-study variability of effect sizes, the size of the observed effects did not differ significantly among different forms of interventions.

We further analyzed whether the size of effects would differ by characteristics of participants and by study characteristics, such as dementia status of the care recipient, mean age and percentage of female caregivers, whether group treatments or individual treatments were used, the number of sessions, randomization, and publication status. Weighted multiple linear regressions were computed for that analysis (Raudenbush, 1994).

Because dementia caregivers showed higher levels of psychological distress than other caregivers, we were interested in whether they would benefit more from caregiver interventions. However, dementia caregivers showed less change in burden than other caregivers (Table 4). We expected larger intervention effects for women than men because of empirical evidence that female caregivers tend to report higher levels of burden and depressive symptoms (Miller & Cafasso, 1992). Female caregivers did report greater improvements in depression and positive well-being, and marginally larger improvements in caregiver burden than did male caregivers.

Interventions in groups were more effective in improving symptoms of the care recipient than other interventions. This contradicts our 2002 findings and may be due to the added studies in the present analysis. In many studies, the group setting may promote the exchange of experiences and techniques in how to influence the care recipient's behavior, thus enabling mutual learning. However, bivariate results suggest that individualized treatment provided by individual interventions is more effective in changing caregiver's psychological health. Additional research is needed to clarify these results.

We found that longer interventions were less effective in improving subjective well-being of the care receiver, probably reflecting the fact that the most effective forms of well-being intervention (psychotherapy, psychoeducational interventions, training of care recipient) were shorter than other forms of intervention.

In randomized studies the interventions appeared to be less effective in improving well-being and symptoms of the care recipient. Individuals with lower subjective well-being and higher motivation are more likely to self-select into the intervention condition in non-random studies and are thus more likely to benefit from the intervention (Gonyea & Silverstein, 1991). Although it has been suggested that nonsignificant results are rarely published and that unpublished studies would show smaller effect sizes than published studies (Rosenthal, 1991), we did not find evidence for such a file-drawer problem. In fact, the intervention effects in published studies for on caregiver burden were smaller than in unpublished doctoral theses or unpublished presentations at conventions (Table 4). A positive explanation may be that doctoral students are highly motivated and have more time to plan and conduct a well-designed intervention study. However, we can not rule out an alternative explanation, that unpublished studies that have not been subjected to peer scrutiny are, in some cases, more likely to contain biased or erroneous data. However, the larger effect of interventions in unpublished studies was limited to one out of five outcome variables, and was mainly based on very few studies focused on caregiver burden. Thus, this finding may need to be treated with some caution. Finally, we found that more recent studies reported smaller effects of the intervention on caregiver burden. Callahan's (1989) and others' criticism of the intervention literature may have initiated a trend toward more careful studies with control groups, higher quality outcome measures, and a greater likelihood for null-results to be published.

SUMMARY AND CONCLUSIONS

In sum, we found that caregivers for older family members show elevated levels of symptoms of stress and depression, lower subjective well-being, lower beliefs in their own abilities to master daily demands, and, to a lesser degree, stronger impairments of physical health. Differences between caregivers and noncaregivers were more pronounced for family members who support dementia sufferers than for caregivers of physically impaired older adults. In addition, we found some evidence that studies with convenience samples tend to overestimate caregivers' levels of impairments of psychological health. Behavior problems of the care recipient and high levels of care provision showed the strongest association with caregiver outcomes. Interventions were most effective in improving caregiver knowledge and perceived abilities to master caregiving demands, but positive effects on burden, depression, and positive well-being of caregivers were also found. Psychotherapy and psychoeducational interventions were effective with regard to all outcome variables, whereas other forms of interventions showed rather specific effects. Finally, interventions with dementia caregivers were less effective than other interventions in reducing the elevated levels of psychological symptoms.

Fewer statistical significant effects emerged in the present random-effects model meta-analysis than in previous meta-analyses that were based on fixed-effects models (Pinquart & Sörensen, 2003b; Sörensen et al., 2002). Random effect models may slightly overestimate the actual between-study variability of effect sizes and make the identification of significant effects more difficult (e.g., Hedges & Vevea, 1998). Nevertheless, this more conservative approach is appropriate for low information situations because it was not possible to control for all sources of heterogeneity and because only very few studies on some types of interventions were available for making statistical inferences (Overton, 1998).

Several conclusions can be drawn from the present study with regard to expected caregiving effects, future research, and needs for intervention. First, given the observed heterogeneity of effects between studies, we need more large studies that are less error-prone. For example, in the correlative caregiver studies, the median number of caregivers was 100, and in intervention studies, the median number of participants in the intervention condition was 29. Studies with small sample sizes do also not allow tests of complex models of the interplay between variables (see, Figure 2). Studies with convenience samples overestimate caregivers' depression and psychological distress. An effective way to obtain representative caregivers samples and less biased estimates of the impact of caregiving may be to use epidemiological studies of physical and mental impairment in elders to reach their caregivers.

Furthermore, since most available studies have focused on bivariate associations between caregiving variables, we need more research on the interaction between variables (e.g., on buffering effects of resources on the association between stressors and psychological outcomes). Also, because most caregiver studies have focused on a limited number of variables (e.g., stressors, social resources, burden, depression), more research is needed on variables that have been neglected. For example, how does the motivation to provide care (e.g., altruistic vs. generic factors) relate to caregiving outcomes (Biegel, Sales, & Schulz, 1991)? Similarly, which forms of coping behaviour are most effective in reducing the negative impact of caregiving?

More efforts are needed to increase the effectiveness of interventions with dementia caregivers. Because multicomponent interventions were, on average, not more effective than simple interventions, we need research on the effects of combining different aspects of intervention in order to find more effective combinations. Our data also suggest that more well-controlled randomized intervention studies are needed to study the effects of respite/daycare as well as the long-term or delayed effects of interventions with caregivers. Finally, because the effects of supportive interventions, respite/daycare, and training of the care recipient were domain-specific, clear intervention goals have to be stated before choosing a form of interventions. For promoting broad effects, psychotherapy and psychoeducational interventions are recommended, at least if the latter is not limited to information provision but includes training of caregivers' coping abilities.

AUTHOR NOTES

Martin Pinquart, Department of Developmental Psychology, Friedrich Schiller University, Jena, Germany; Silvia Sörensen, Geriatrics and Neuropsychiatry, Department of Psychiatry, University of Rochester Medical Center, Rochester NY.

Correspondence concerning this article should be addressed to Martin Pinquart, Department of Developmental Psychology, Friedrich Schiller University, Steiger 3 Haus 1, D-07743 Jena, Germany. Electronic mail may be sent to Martin.Pinquart@uni-jena.de

REFERENCES

Aneshensel, C.S., Pearlin, L.I., Mullan, J.T., Zarit, S.H., & Whitlach, C.J. (1995). *Profiles in caregiving: The unexpected career.* San Diego, CA: Academic Press.

Archbold, P. G., Stewart, B. J., Miller, L. L., Harvath, T. A., et al. (1995). The PREP system of nursing interventions: A pilot test with families caring for older members. *Research in Nursing and Health, 18,* 3-16.

Barber, C.E., & Pasley, B.K. (1995). Family care of Alzheimer's patients: The role of gender and generational relationship on caregiver outcomes. *Journal of Applied Gerontology, 14,* 172-192.

Bass, D.M., Clark, P.A., Looman, W.J., McCarthy, C.A., & Eckert, S. (2003). The Cleveland Alzheimer's Managed Care Demonstration: Outcomes after 12 months of implementation. *The Gerontologist, 43,* 73-85.

Beery, L.C., Prigerson, H.G., & Bierhals (1997). Traumatic grief, depression and caregiving in elderly spouses of the terminal ill. *OMEGA, 35*, 261-279.

Biegel, D.E., Sales, E., & Schulz, R. (1991). *Family caregiving in chronic illness: Alzheimer's disease, cancer, heart disease, mental illness, and stroke.* Thousand Oaks: Sage.

Blazer, D. (2002). *Depression in later life (*3rd. ed.). New York: Springer.

Bookwala, J., & Schulz, R. (2000). A comparison of primary stressors, secondary stressors, and depressive symptoms between elderly caregiving husbands and wives: The caregiver health effects study. *Psychology and Aging, 15*, 607-616.

Braithwaite, V. (1996). Between stressors and outcomes: Can we simplify caregiving process variables. *The Gerontologist, 36*, 42-53.

Brodaty, H., & Hadzi-Pavlovic, D. (1990). Psychological effects on carers of living with persons with dementia. *Australian and New Zealand Journal of Psychiatry, 24*, 351-361.

Burdz, M.P., Eaton, W.O., & Bond, J.B. (1988*)*. Effects of respite care on dementia and nondementia patients and their caregivers. *Psychology & Aging, 3*, 38-42.

Bushman, B. J., & Wang, M. C. (1996). A procedure for combining sample standardized mean differences and vote counts to estimate the population standardized mean difference in fixed event models. *Psychological Methods, 1*, 66-80.

Callahan, J. J. Jr. (1989). Play it again Sam – There is no impact. *The Gerontologist, 29*, 5-6.

Carruth, A K. (1996). Development and testing of the Caregiver Reciprocity Scale. *Nursing Research, 45*, 92-97.

Clipp, E.C., & George, L.K. (1993). Dementia and cancer: A comparison of spouse caregivers. *The Gerontologist, 33*, 534-541.

Cohen, J. (1992). A power primer. *Psychological Bulletin, 112*, 155-159.

Connell, C.M., Janevic, M.R., & Gallant, M.P. (2001). The costs of caring: Impact of dementia on family caregivers. *Journal of Geriatric Psychiatry and Neurology, 14*, 179-187.

Demers, A., & Lavoie, J. P. (1996). Effect of support groups on family caregivers to the frail elderly. *Canadian Journal on Aging, 15*, 129-144.

Donaldson, C., Tarrier, N., & Burns, A. (1998). Determinants of carer stress in Alzheimer's disease. *International Journal of Geriatric Psychiatry, 13*, 248-256.

Draper, B.M., Poulos, C.J., Cole, A.D., Poulos, R.G., & Ehrlich, F. (1992). A comparison of caregivers for elderly stroke and dementia victims. *Journal of the American Geriatrics Society, 40*, 896-901.

Farran, C.J., Keane-Hagerty, E., Salloway, S., Kupferer, S., & Wilken, C.S. (1991). Finding meaning: An alternative paradigm for Alzheimer's disease family caregivers. *The Gerontologist, 31*, 483-489.

Fengler, A.P., & Goodrich, N. (1979). Wives of elderly disabled men: The hidden patients. *The Gerontologist, 19*, 175-183.

Fingerman, K.L., Gallagher-Thompson, D., Lovett, S., & Rose, J. (1996). Internal resourcefulness, task demands, coping, and dysphoric affect among caregivers of the frail elderly. *International Journal of Aging and Human Development, 42*, 229-248.

Fitting, M., Rabins, P., Lucas, M. J., & Eastham, J. (1986). Caregivers for dementia patients: A comparison of husbands and wives. *The Gerontologist, 26*, 248-252.

Gallagher-Thompson, D., & Powers, D.V. (1997). Primary stressors and depressive symptoms in caregivers of dementia patients. *Aging & Mental Health, 1*, 248-255.

Gallagher-Thompson, D., Lovett, S., Rose, J., McKibbin, C., Coon, D., Futterman, A., & Thompson, L. W. (2000). Impact of psychoeducational interventions on distressed family caregivers. *Journal of Clinical Gerontology, 6*, 91-110.

Garity, J. (1997). Stress, learning style, resilience factors, and ways of coping in Alzheimer family caregivers. *American Journal of Alzheimer's Disease, 12*, 171-178.

Gatz, M., Bengtson, V.L., & Blum, M.J. (1990). Caregiving families. In J.E. Biren & K.W. Schaie (Eds.), *Handbook of psychology of aging* (3. ed., pp. 404-426). San Diego, CA: Academic Press.

George, L.K., & Gwyter, L.P. (1986). Caregiver well-being: A multidimensional examination of family caregivers of demented adults. *The Gerontologist, 26*, 253-259.

Gignac, M.A., & Gottlieb, B.H. (1996). Caregivers' appraisals of efficacy in coping with dementia. *Psychology and Aging, 11*, 214-225.

Gilleard, C.J., Gilleard, K., Gledhill, K., & Whittick, J. (1984). Caring for the mentally infirm at home: A survey of the supporters. *Journal of Epidemiology and Community Health, 38*, 319-325.

Gitlin, L.N., Belle, S.H., Burgio, L., Czaja, S., Mahoney, D., Gallagher-Thompson, D., Burns, R., Hauck, W.W., Zhang, S., Schulz, R., & Ory, M.G. (2003). Effect of multi-component interventions on caregiver burden and depression: The REACH multi-site initiative at six months follow-up. *Psychology and Aging, 18*, 361-374.

Glass, G. V., McGraw, B., & Smith, M. L. (1981). *Meta-analysis in social research.* Beverly Hills, CA: Sage.

Gonyea, J. G., & Silverstein, N. M. (1991). The role of Alzheimer's disease support groups in families' utilization of community services. *Journal of Gerontological Social Work, 16 (3/4)*, 43-55.

Gräßel, E., & Leutbecher, M. (1993). *Häusliche Pflege-Skalen HPS zur Erfassung der Belastung bei betreuenden oder Pflegenden Personen* [Home-care scales measuring burden of care providers]. Ebersberg, Germany: Vless.

Guttman, R. (1991). *Adult day care for Alzheimer's patients: Impact on family caregivers.* New York: Garland Publishing.

Haley, W.E., & Pardo, K.M. (1989). Relationship of severity of dementia to caregiving stressors. *Psychology and Aging, 4*, 389-392.

Hedges, L. V. (1981). Distribution theory for Glass's estimator of effect size and related estimators. *Journal of Educational Statistics, 6*, 107-128.

Hedges, L.V., & Vevea, J.L. (1998). Fixed- and random-effects models in meta-analysis. *Psychological Methods, 3*, 486-504.

Hobbs, F. B. & Damon, B. L. (1996). *65+ in the United States.* Washington, DC: U.S. Government Printing Office.

Hooker, K., Monahan, D.J., Bowman, S.R., Frazier, L.D., & Shifren, K. (1998). Personality counts a lot: Predictors of mental and physical health of spouse caregivers in two disease groups. *Journal of Gerontology, Psychological Sciences, 53B*, P73-85.

Ingram, R. E., Miranda, J., & Segal, S. V. (1998). *Cognitive vulnerability to depression.* New York: Guilford.

Kinney, J.M., & Stephens, M.P. (1989). Hassles and uplifts of giving care to a family member with dementia. *Psychology and Aging, 4*, 402-408.

Konstam, V., Holmes, W., Wilczenski, F., Baliga, S., Lester, J., & Priest, R. (2003). Meaning in the lives of caregivers of individuals with Parkinson's disease. *Journal of Clinical Psychology in Medical Settings, 10*, 17-26.

Kosberg, J.I., & Cairl, R.E. (1986). The Cost of Care Index: A case management tool for screening informal care providers. *The Gerontologist, 26*, 273-285.

Kramer, B.J. (1997). Gain in the caregiving experience: Where are we? What next? *The Gerontologist, 37*, 218-232.

Kramer, B.J., & Vitaliano, P.P. (1994). Coping: a review of theoretical frameworks and the measures used among caregivers of individuals with dementia. *Journal of Gerontological Social Work, 23(1/2)*, 151-174.

Lazarus, R., & Folkman, S. (1984). *Stress, appraisal, and coping.* New York: Springer.

Lawton, M.P., Kleban, M.H., Moss, M., Rovine, M., & Glicksman, A. (1989). Measuring caregiver appraisal. *Journal of Gerontology: Psychological Sciences, 44*, P61-71.

Lawton, M.P., Moss, M., Kleban, M.H., Glicksman, A., & Rovine, M. (1991). A two-factor model of caregiving appraisal. *Journal of Gerontology: Psychological Sciences, 46*, P181-189.

Li, L.L., Seltzer, M., & Greenberg, J.S. (1997). Social support and depressive symptoms: Differential patterns in wife and daughter caregivers. *Journals of Gerontology: Social Sciences, 52B*, S200-S211.

Lincoln, N.B., Francis, V.M., Lilley, S.A., Sharma, J.C., & Summerfield, M. (2003). Evaluation of a stroke family support organizer: A randomized controlled trial. *Stroke, 34*, 116-121.

LoGiudice, D., Waltrowicz, W., Brown, K., Burrows, C., Ames, D., & Flicker, L. (1999). Do memory clinics improve the quality of carers? A randomized pilot trial. *International Journal of Geriatric Psychiatry, 14*, 626-632.

Majerowitz, S.D. (1995). Role of family adaptability in the psychological adjustment of spouse caregivers to patients with dementia. *Psychology and Aging, 10*, 447-457.

Miller, B. & Cafasso, L. (1992). Gender differences in caregiving: Fact or artifact? *The Gerontologist, 32*, 498-507.

Montgomery, R.J., Gonyea, J.G., & Hooyman, N.R. (1985). Caregiving and the experience of subjective and objective burden. *Family Relations, 34*, 19-26.

Ory, M.G., Yee, J.L., Tennstedt, S.L., & Schulz, R. (2000). The extent and impact of dementia care: Unique challenges experienced by family caregivers. In R. Schulz (Ed.), *Handbook of dementia caregiving: Evidence-based interventions for family caregivers* (pp. 1-32). New York: Springer.

Ostwald, S. K., Hepburn, K. W., Caron, W., Burns, T., & Mantell, R. (1999). Reducing caregiver burden: A randomized psychoeducational intervention for caregivers of persons with dementia. *The Gerontologist, 39*, 299-309.

Overton, R.C. (1998). A comparison of fixed-effects and mixed (random-effects) models for meta-analysis: Tests for moderator variable effects. *Psychological Methods, 3*, 354-379.

Pearlin, L.I., Mullan, J.T., Semple, S.J., & Skaff, M.M. (1990). Caregiving and the stress process: an overview of concepts and their measures. *The Gerontologist, 30*, 583-594.

Pinquart, M., & Sörensen, S. (2003a). Differences between caregivers and noncaregivers in psychological health and physical health: A meta-analysis. *Psychology & Aging, 18*, 250-267.

Pinquart, M., & Sörensen, S. (2003b). Associations of stressors and uplifts of caregiving with caregiver burden and depressive mood: A meta-analysis. *Journals of Gerontology: Psychological Sciences, 58B*, P112-P128.

Pinquart & Sörensen (2004). Associations of caregiver stressors and uplifts with subjective well-being and depressive mood: A meta-analytic comparison. *Aging and Mental Health* 8, 438-449.

Raudenbush, S.W. (1994). Random effect models. In H. Cooper & L.V. Hedges (Eds.), *Handbook of research synthesis* (pp. 301-321). New York: Sage.

Rosenthal, R. (1991). *Meta-analytic procedures for social research.* Beverly Hills, CA: Sage.

Schneekloth, U. & Potthoff, P. (1994). *Hilfe- und Pflegebedürftige in privaten Haushalten* [Community-dwelling persons in need of support and care]. Stuttgart, Germany: Kohlhammer.

Schneider, J., Murray, J., Banerjee, S., & Mann, A. (1999). Eurocare: A cross-national study of co-residents spouse carers for people with Alzheimer's disease: I - Factors associated with carer burden. *International Journal of Geriatric Psychiatry, 14*, 651-661.

Schulz, R., Thomkins, C.A., Wood, D., & Decker, S. (1987). The social psychology of caregiving: Physical and psychological costs of providing support to the disabled. *Journal of Applied Social Psychology, 17*, 401-428.

Schulz, R., O'Brien, A.T, Bookwala, J., & Fleissner, K. (1995). Psychiatric and physical morbidity effects of dementia caregiving: Prevalence, correlates, and causes. *The Gerontologist, 35*, 771-791.

Schulz, R., Newsom, J., Mittelmark, M., Burton, L., Hirsch, C., & Jackson, S. (1997). Health effects of caregiving: The caregiver health effects study: An ancillary study of the Cardiovascular Health Study. *Annals of Behavioral Medicine, 19*, 110-116.

Sörensen, S., Pinquart, M., & Duberstein, P. (2002). How effective are interventions with caregivers? An updated meta-analysis. *The Gerontologist, 42*, 356-372.

Steinmetz, S.K. (1988). *Duty bound: Elder abuse and family care.* Thousand Oaks, CA: Sage.

Stevens, G. L. & Baldwin, B. A. (1994). Comparative efficacy of didactic versus psychotherapeutic modalities. In E. Light, G. Niederehe, & B. D. Lebowitz (Eds.), *Stress effects in family caregivers of Alzheimer's patients: Research and interventions* (pp. 231-241). New York: Springer.

Stoller, E.P. (1992). Gender differences in the experiences of caregiving spouses. In J.W. Dwyer, & R.T. Coward (Eds.), *Gender, families, and elder care* (pp. 49-64). Newbury Park, CA: Sage.

Stone, R. G., Cafferata, L., & Sangl, J. (1987). Caregivers of the frail elderly: A national profile. *The Gerontologist, 27*, 616-626.

Tennstedt, S.L., McKinlay, J.B., & Sullivan, L.M. (1988). *Informal care for frail elders: The role of secondary characteristics.* Paper presented at the Annual Scientific Meeting of the Gerontological Society of America at San Francisco, CA.

Teri, L., Truax, P., Logsdon, R., Uomoto, J., Zarit, S.H., & Vitaliano, P.P. (1992). Assessment of behavior problems in dementia: The Revised Memory and Behavior Checklist. *Psychology and Aging, 7,* 622-631.

Townsend, A., Noelker, L., Deimling, G., & Bass, D. (1989). Longitudinal impact of interhouse caregiving on adult children's mental health. *Psychology and Aging, 4,* 393-401.

United States Census Bureau (2004). National Population Projections, available at http://www.census.gov/population/www/projections/natsum-T3.html.

Vitaliano, P.P., Zhang, J., & Scanlan, J.M. (2003). Is caregiving hazardous to one's physical health? A meta-analysis. *Psychological Bulletin, 129,* 946-972.

Wallsten, S.M., & Snyder, S.S. (1990). A comparison of elderly family caregivers' and noncaregivers' perceptions of stress in daily experiences. *Journal of Community Psychology, 18,* 228-238.

Yates, M.E., Tennstedt, S., & Chang, B.-H. (1999). Contributors to and mediators of psychological well-being for informal caregivers. *Journal of Gerontology, Psychological Sciences, 54B,* P12-22.

Yee, J.L., & Schulz, R. (2000). Gender differences in psychiatric morbidity among family caregivers: A review and analysis. *The Gerontologist, 40,* 147-164.

Zarit, S.H., Reever, K.E., & Bach-Petersen, J. (1980). Relatives of the impaired elderly: Correlates of feelings of burden. *The Gerontologist, 20,* 649-655.

Zarit, S.H., Stephens, M. A. P., Townsed, A., & Greene, R. (1998). Stress reduction for family caregivers: Effects of adult day care use. *Journals of Gerontology: Social Sciences, 53B,* S267-S277.

APPENDIX A: NEWLY INCLUDED STUDIES THAT COMPARE CAREGIVERS AND NONCAREGIVERS

Beeson, R. & William F. (2003). Loneliness and depression in spousal caregivers of those with Alzheimer's disease versus non-caregiving spouses. *Archives of Psychiatric Nursing, 17,* 135-143.

Broe, G.A., Jorm, A.F., Creasey, H., Casey, B., Bennett, H., Cullen, J., Edelbrock, D., Waite, L., & Grayson, D. (1999). Carer distress in the general population: Results from the Sydney Older Persons Study. *Age and Aging, 28,* 307-311.

Burton, L., Zdaniuk, B., Schulz, R., Jackson, S., & Hirsch, C. (2003). Transitions in spousal caregiving. *The Gerontologist, 43,* 230-241.

Cannuscio, C.C., Jones, C., Kawachi, I., Colditz, G.A., Berkman, L., & Rimm. E. (2002). Reverberations of family illness: a longitudinal assessment of informal caregiving and mental health status in the Nurses' Health Study. *American Journal of Public Health, 92,* 1305-1311.

Caswell, L.W., Vitaliano, P.P., Croyle, K.L.., Scanlan, J. M., Zhang, J., & Daruwala, A. (2003). Negative associations of chronic stress and cognitive performance in older adult spouse caregivers. *Experimental Aging Research, 29,* 303-318.

Castro, C., King, A., Bacak, A., Houseman, R., Gardiner, K., & Brownson, R. (2003). *Rural caregivers and health behaviours: Results from an epidemiological study.* Paper presented at the 56th annual meeting of the Gerontological Society of America, San Diego, CA.

McCann, J.J. (1991). Effects of stress on spouse caregivers' psychological health and cellular immunity. *Dissertation Abstracts International, 52, 4114B.*

McNaughton, M., Patterson, T., Smith, T., & Grant, I. (1995). The relationship among stress, depression, locus of control, irrational beliefs, social support, and health in Alzheimer's disease caregivers. *Journal of Nervous and Mental Disease, 183,* 78-85.

Musil, C.M., & Ahmad, M. (2002). Health of grandmothers: a comparison by caregiver status. *Journal of Aging & Health. 14(1),* 96-121.

O'Reilly, F., Finnan, F., Allwright, S., Smith, G., & Ben-Shlomo, Y. (1996). The effects of caring for a spouse with Parkinson's diesaese on social, psychological, and physical well-being. *British Journal of General Practice, 46,* 507-512.

Sato, R., Kanda, K., Anan, M., & Watanuki, S. (2002). Sleep EEG patterns and fatigue of middle-aged and older female family caregivers providing routine nighttime care for elderly persons at home. *Perceptual and Motor Skills, 95,* 815-829.

Tracy, K., Hochberg, M., & Fredman, L. (2002). *Effects of race and marital status on health of elderly male caregivers.* Paper presented at the 55th Annual Meeting of the GSA at Boston, MA.

Vedhara, K., McDermott, M.P., Evans, T.G., Teanor, J.J., Plummer, S., Tallon, D., Cruttenden, K.A., & Schifitto, G. (2002). Chronic stress in nonelderly caregivers: Psychological, endocrine and immune implications. *Journal of Psychosomatic Research, 53,* 1153-1161.

Wright, L.K., Hickey, J.V., Buckwalter, K.C., Hendrix, S.A., & Kelechi, T. (1999).Emotional and physical health of spouse caregivers of persons with Alzheimer's disease and stroke. *Journal of Advanced Nursing, 30,* 552-563

APPENDIX B: NEWLY INCLUDED STUDIES ON CORRELATES OF CAREGIVER BURDEN AND DEPRESSION

Abe, K., Tsuneto, S., & Kashiwagi, T. (2003). *An adaptation of the two-factor model of caregiving appraisal and psychological well-being to Japanese family caregivers.* Paper presented at the 56th Annual Meeting of the Gerontological Society of America, San Diego, CA.

Anderson, C.S., Linto, J., & Stewart-Wynne, E.G. (1995). A population-based assessment of the impact and burden of caregiving for long-term stroke survivors. *Stroke, 26,* 843-849.

Braungart, E.R., Femia, E.E., Zarit, S.H., & Stephens, M.P. (2003). *The impact of behavioural and psychological symptoms of dementia on primary subjective stress and well-being of the caregiver.* Paper presented at the 56th Annual Meeting of the Gerontological Society of America, San Diego.

Chadiha, L.A., Rafferty, J., & Pickard, J. (2003). The influence of caregiving stressors, social support, and caregiving appraisal on marital functioning among African American wife caregivers. *Journal of Marital and Family Therapy, 29,* 479-490.

Cousins, R., Davies, A.D., Turnbull, C.J., & Playfer, J.R. (2002). Assessing caregiver distress: A conceptual analysis and a brief scale. *British Journal of Clinical Psychology, 41,* 387-403.

Elmstahl, S., Malmberg, B., & Annerstedt, L. (1996). Caregiver's burden of patients 3 years after stroke assessed by a novel caregiver burden scale. *Archives of Physical Medicine & Rehabilitation, 77,* 177-182.

Exel, N.J.v., Reimer, W.S., Brouwer, W.B., Berg, V.v., Koopmanshap, M.A., & Bos, G.v.d. (2004). Instruments for assessing the burden of informal caregiving for stroke patients in clinical practice: A comparison of CSI, CRA, SCQ and self-rated burden. *Clinical Rehabilitation, 18,* 203-214.

Hecht, M.J., Gräßel, E., Tigges, S., Hillemacher, T., Winterholler, M., Hilz, M.J., Heuss, D., & Neundörfer, B. (2003). Burden of care in amyotrophic lateral sclerosis. *Palliative Medicine, 17,* 327-333.

Hinton, L., Haan, M., Geller, S., & Mungas, D. (2003). Neuropsychiatric symptoms in Latino elders with dementia or cognitive impairment without dementia and factors that modify their association with caregiver depression. *The Gerontologist, 43,* 669-677.

Hyer, L., Gould, S., Kannan, H., Coyne, A., & Sohnle, S. (2003*). Predictors of caregiver burden and depression among dementia patients.* Paper presented at the 56th Annual Meeting of the Gerontological Society of America, San Diego, CA.

Kramer, B.J. (1993). Expanding the conceptualization of caregiver coping: The importance of relationship-focused coping strategies. *Family Relations, 42,* 383-391.

Kramer, B.J. (2000). Husbands caring for wives with dementia: A longitudinal study of continuity and change. *Health & Social Work, 25,* 97-107.

Leinonen, E., Korpisammal, L., Pulkkinen, L.M., & Pukuri, T. (2001). The comparison of burden between caregiving spouses of depressive and demented patients. *International Journal of Geriatric Psychiatry, 16,* 387-393.

Moon, A., & Chan, C. (2003). *A comparison of the levels and correlates of depression among Chinese, Japanese, and Vietnamese American caregivers caring for their elderly relatives with Alzheimer's disease.* Paper presented at the 43. Annual meeting of the Gerontological Society of America, San Diego, CA.

Morano, C.L. (2003). Appraisal and coping: moderators or mediators of stress in Alzheimer's disease caregivers? *Social Work Research, 27,* 117-128.

Nagatomo, I., Akasaki, Y., Uchida, M., Tominaga, M., Hashiguchi, W., & Takigawa, M. (1999). Gender of demented patients and specific family relationship of caregiver to patients influence mental fatigue and burdens on relatives as caregivers. *International Journal of Geriatric Psychiatry, 14,* 618-625.

Scholte op Reimer, W.J., de Haan, R.J., Pijnenborg, J.M., Limburg, M., & van den Bos, G.A., (1998). Assessment of burden in partners of stroke patients with the Sense of Competence Questionnaire. *Stroke, 29,* 373-379.

Schulz, R. (2003). *Resources for enhancing Alzheimer's caregiver health 1996-2001* [Computer file]. ICPSR version. Ann Arbor, MI: Consortium for Political and Social Research.

Thornton, M., & Travis, S.S. (2003). Analysis of the reliability of a modified Caregiver Strain Index. *Journal of Gerontology: Social Sciences, 58B*, S127-132.

Turner, W., Butler, S., Johns, E., Kaye, L., & Downey, R. (2003). *Predictors of burden and depressive symptomatology in rural elder caregivers.* Paper presented at the 56th Annual Meeting of the Gerontological Society of America, San Diego, CA.

Walker, A.J., Pratt, C.C., & Wood, B. (1993). Perceived frequency of role conflict and relationship quality for caregiving daughters. *Psychology of Women Quarterly, 17,* 207-221.

White, T.M. (1998). *Comparisons of African American and white women in the parent care role.* Unpublished dissertation, Kent State University.

Yamada, H. (1994). *The effects of social support on the well-being of spouse caregivers of demented elders.* Ann Arbor, Mi. UMI Dissertation Services.

APPENDIX C: NEWLY INCLUDED INTERVENTION STUDIES

Akkerman, R.L., & Ostwald, S.K. (2001). *Managing anxiety in caregivers of persons diagnosed with Alzheimer's disease: A group cognitive-behavioral intervention.* Paper presented at the 54th Annual Meeting of the Gerontological Society of America, Chicago, IL.

Baumgarten, M., Lebel, P., Laprise, H., Leclerc, C., & Quinn, C. (2002). Adult day care for the frail elderly: outcomes, satisfaction, and cost. *Journal of Aging & Health, 14,* 237-59.

Berger, G., Schramm, U., Müller, R., Landsiedel-Anders, S., Peters, J., Kratzsch, T., & Frölich, L. (2004). No effects of a combination of caregivers support group and memory training/music therapy in dementia patients from a memory clinic population. International Journal of Geriatric Psychiatry, 19, 223-231.

Bougard, C.C. (2003). A program evaluation of the Caregiver Assistance Program. *Dissertation Abstracts International, 63(10-A),* 3668.

Buchanan, J., & Fisher, J.E. (2003). The generalization of the effects of a cognitive-behavioral intervention for family caregivers of persons with dementia. *Paper presented at the 56th Annual Meeting of the Gerontological Society of America*, San Diego, CA

Burgio, L., Stevens, A., Guy, D., Roth, D.L., & Haley, W.E. (2003). Impact of two psychosocial interventions on white and African American family caregivers of individuals with dementia. *The Gerontologist, 43,* 568-579.

Caston, C. (1995). Self-directed skills nursing model: Decrease burnout in African-American caregivers. Unpublished dissertation, University of Iowa.

Challis, D., Abendorff, R.v., Brown, P., & Chesterman, J. (1997). Care management and dementia: An evaluation of the Lewinsham Intensive Case Management Scheme. In S. Hunter (Ed.), *Dementia: Challenges and new directions* (139-150). Bristol, PA: Jessica Kingsley.

Challis, D., Abendorff, R.v., Brown, P., Chesterman, J., & Hughes, J. (2002). Care management, dementia care and specialist mental health services: an evaluation. *International Journal of Geriatric Psychiatry*, 17, 315-325.

Coon, D.W., Thompson, L., Steffen, A., Sorocco, K., & Gallagher-Thompson, D. (2003). Anger and depression management: Psychoeducational skill training interventions for women caregivers of a relative with dementia. *The Gerontologist, 43*, 678-689.

Dube, C. & Vezina, J. (2001). *The evaluation of a personalized phone call intervention conducted with family caregivers of individuals suffering from Alzheimer's disease.* Paper presented at the 17th World Congress of the IAG at Vancouver, Canada.

Eisdorfer, C., Czaja, S.J., Loewenstein, D.A., Rubert, M.P., Agüelles, S., Mitrani, V.B., & Szapocznik, J. (2003). The effect of a family therapy and technology-based intervention on caregiver depression. *The Gerontologist, 43*, 521-531.

Farran, C. J. & Keane-Hagarty, E. (1994). Multi-modal intervention strategies for caregivers of persons with dementia. In E. Light, G. Niederehe, & B. D. Lebowitz (Eds.), *Stress effects in family caregivers of Alzheimer's patients: Research and interventions* (pp. 242-259). New York: Springer.

Foster, L. (2003). *Easing the burden of caregiving: The impact of consumer direction on primary informal caregivers in Arkansas.* Paper presented at the 56th Annual Meeting of the Gerontological Society of America, San Diego, CA.

Fritsch, T. (2000). Depression, strain, and health outcomes in caregivers of cognitively impaired, hospitalized patients: Do ACE units help? Unpublished dissertation. Miami University, Ohio, FL.

Fung, W.Y., & Chien, W.T. (2002). The effectiveness of a mutual support group for family caregivers of a relative with dementia. *Archives of Geriatric Nursing*, 16, 134-144.

Gardner, L.A., Buckwalter, K.C., & Reed, D. (2002). Impact of a psychoeducational intervention on caregiver response to behavioral problems. *Nursing Research, 51*, 363-374.

Geddes, J.M., & Chamberlain, J.M. (1994). Improving social outcome after stroke: An evaluation of the volunteer stroke scheme. *Clinical Rehabilitation*, 8, 116-126.

Gendron, C., Poitras, L., Dastoor, D.P., & Perodeau, G. (1996). Cognitive-behavioral group intervention for spouse caregivers: Findings and clinical considerations. *Clinical Gerontologist,* 17, 3-19.

Gitlin, L.N., Belle, S.H., Burgio, L., Czaja, S., Mahoney, D., Gallagher-Thompson, D., Burns, R., Hauck, W.W., Zhang, S., Schulz, R., & Ory, M.G. (2003). Effect of multi-component interventions on caregiver burden and depression: The REACH multi-site initiative at six months follow-up. *Psychology and Aging, 18,* 361-374.

Gitlin, L.N., Winter, L., Corcoran, M., Dennis, M.P., Schinfeld, S., & Hauck, W.W. (2003). Effects of the home environmental skill-building program on the caregiver-care recipient dyad: 6-months outcomes from the Philadelphia REACH initiative. *Gerontologist, 43,* 532-546.

Gray, V. K. (1983). Providing support for home care givers. In M. Smyer (Ed.), *Mental health and aging* (pp. 197-214.). Beverly Hills, CA: Sage.

Guttman, R. A. (1991). *Adult day care for Alzheimer's patients: Impact on family caregivers.* New York: Garland.

Hartiens, J. M. (1995). *The impact of respite on physical health, depression, and marital satisfaction in spousal caregivers of dementia victims*. Unpublished dissertation, Fuller Theological Seminary.

Hartke, R.J., & King, R.B. (2003). Telephone group intervention for older stroke caregivers. Topics in Stroke Rehabilitation, 9(4), 65-81.

Hébert, R., Lévesque, L., Vézina, J., Lavoie, J.P., Ducharme, F., Gendron, C., Préville, M., Voyer, L., & Dubois, M.F. (2003). Efficacy of a psychoeducative group program for informal caregivers of demented persons living at home: A randomized trial. *Journal of Gerontology, Social Sciences, 58B,* S58-67.

Heier, H., Lämmler, G., & Steinhagen-Thiessen, E. (2002). Evaluation eines psychoedukativen Kurses für Angehörige von Schlaganfallpatienten [Evaluation of a psychoeducative program for stroke patients]. *Zeitschrift für Neuropsychologie, 13,* 201-209.

Hung, L.C., Liu, C.C., Hung, H.C., & Kuo, K.W. (2003). Effects of a nursing intervention program on disabled patients and their caregivers. *Archives of Gerontology and Geriatrics, 36,* 259-272.

King, A.C., & Brassington, G. (1997). Enhancing physical and psychological functioning in older family caregivers: The role of regular physical activity. *Annals of Behavioral Medicine, 19,* 91-100.

Kotler, D.L. (1992). *The impact of a psychoeducational support group on caregivers of patients with Alzheimer's disease*. Unpublished dissertation, California School of Professional Psychology, Fresno, CA.

Lewis, M., Hepburn, K., Center, B., Narayan, S., Kindstrom-Bremer, K., Wexler-Sherman, C., & Tornatore, J. (2002). *Distress: A factor-analytically derived composite score of dementia caregiving impact*. Paper presented at the 55th Annual Meeting of the GSA at Boston, MA.

Mahoney, D.F., Tarlow, B.J., & Jones, R.N. (2003). Effects of an automated telephone support system on caregiver burden and anxiety: Findings from the REACH for TLC Intervention Study. *The Gerontologist, 43,* 556-567.

Martindale, J. L. (1993). *The effect of outpatient geriatric evaluation and management treatment on caregiver perception of burden*. Unpublished dissertation, Memphis State University. Memphis, TN.

McCallion, P., Toseland, R.W., & Freeman, K. (1999). An evaluation of a family visit education program. *Journal of the American Geriatrics Society, 47,* 203-214.

McCurry, S.M., Gibbons, L.E., Logsdon, R.G., Vitiello, M., & Teri, L. (2003). Training caregivers to change the sleep hygiene practices of patients with dementia: The NITE-AD project. *Journal of the American Geriatrics Society, 51,* 1455-1460.

Mittelman, M., Ferris, S., Shulman, E., Steinberg, G., Ambinder, A. & Mackell, J. (1997). Effects of a multicomponent support program on spouse-caregivers of Alzheimer's disease patients: Results of a treatment/control study. In L. L. Heston (Ed.), *Progress in Alzheimer's disease and similar conditions* (pp. 259-275). Washington, DC: American Psychiatric Press.

Mittelman, M.S., Roth, D.L., Coon, D.W., & Haley, W.E. (2004). Sustained benefit of suppotive intervention for depressive symptoms in caregivers of patients with Alzheimer's disease. *American Journal of Psychiatry, 161*, 850-856.

Napolitan, S. M. (1999). *An evaluation of the effectiveness of early psychoeducational orientation and home visit intervention for first-time caregivers of stroke patients.* Unpublished dissertation, University of Chicago, Chicago, IL.

Stanley, S.A. (1989). *Impact of a formal education and group support program on the subjective well-being and burden perceptions of primary caregivers for adults with progressive dementia.* Unpublished dissertation: Ohio State University.

Stevens, G. L. & Baldwin, B. A. (1994). Comparative efficacy of didactic versus psychotherapeutic modalities. In E. Light, G. Niederehe & B. D. Lebowitz (Eds.*), Stress effects in family caregivers of Alzheimer's patients: Research and interventions* (pp. 231-241). New York: Springer.

Van den Heuvel, E.T., de Witte, L.P., Stewart, R.E., Schure, L.M., Sandman, R., & Meyboom-de Jong, B. (2002). Long-term effects of a group support program and an individual support program for informal caregivers of stroke patients: Which caregivers benefit the most? *Patient Education and Counseling, 47,* 291-299.

Wood, R.T., Wills, W., Higginson, I.J., Hobbins, J., & Whitby, M. (2003). Support in the community for people with dementia and their carers: A comparative outcome study of specialist mental health service interventions. *International Journal of Geriatric Psychiatry, 18,* 298-307.

Zank, S. (2000). *Chancen und Grenzen der Rehabilitation im Alter [Chances and limits of rehabilitation in old age].* Berlin, Germany: Pabst.

In: Psychology of Stress
Editor: Kimberly V. Oxington, pp. 207-254

ISBN 1-59454-246-5
©2005 Nova Science Publishers, Inc.

Chapter XI

EXPERIENCES OF PAIN, DISTRESS AND QUALITY OF CARE IN RELATION TO DIFFERENT PERSPECTIVES

MarieLouise Hall-Lord and Bodil Wilde Larsson

Division for Health and Caring Sciences Karlstad University SE-651 88 Karlstad Sweden
Marie-Louise.Hall-Lord@kau.se
Bodil.Wilde@kau.se

ABSTRACT

The aim of this chapter is to illuminate pain and distress and quality of care in relation to elderly people, family member, and caregiver perspectives. This chapter is mainly based on previously published studies within the following two areas: pain and distress and quality of care.

INTRODUCTION

The proportion of elderly people is increasing in most countries. Sweden is along with Italy, Greece, and Japan one of the countries in the world with the oldest population (Statistical Yearbook of Sweden, 2003). 8.9 % of Sweden's population in the year 2000 were more than 75 years old, and the oldest part of the population (85+) constituted 2.3% (SCB, 2000). From about the year 2010, the group with individuals over 65 years old will sharply increase (Swedish Institute, 2003). The largest increase is expected during the next 30 years within the group 85+ (Berleen, 2003). It is also within the group of elderly people that most of the caring needs will arise. Although many people today stay healthy longer than previously, the increase of the so-called 'old-old' means a higher level for total need of care systems in most industrialised countries (Steen 2000). Increasing needs and decreasing resources have brought the quality aspect of treatment and care for older people to the foreground. Studies show deficiencies in the quality of care for elderly people (Edberg, 1999) and common problems are pain and distress (Forsell, Jorm & Winblad, 1994; Brattberg, Parker & Thorslund, 1996; Ross & Crook, 1998).

The aim of this chapter is to illuminate pain and distress and quality of care in relation to elderly people, family member, and caregiver perspectives.

This chapter is mainly based on previously published studies within the following two areas: pain and distress and quality of care. MarieLouise Hall-Lord has the main responsibility for the part of the text which highlights pain and distress, while Bodil Wilde Larsson has the main responsibility for the part about quality of care.

PAIN AND DISTRESS - DEFINITIONS AND MODELS

The Taxonomy Committee of the International Association for Study of Pain defines pain as an "unpleasant sensory and emotional experience associated with actual or potential tissue damage, or is described in terms of such damage" (IASP 1979, p. 250). Pain is always a subjective experience, and the meaning of the emotional part in the definition is the unpleasant experience (IASP, 1979). However, pain seems to be a multidimensional phenomenon, and it has been conceptualised in physical, psychological, social, cultural, and existential models (Bonica, 1990; Brattberg, 1995; Haegerstam, 1996). The physical model of explanation has been predominant during the last century but this model does not explain all aspects of pain (Morris, 1991).

Physiological explanation models are based on the assumption that pain can be explained by means of morphological structures in both the peripheral and the central nervous system (Haegerstam, 1996). Psychological factors have an influence on, and are closely linked to, the experience of pain. Worry, fear, depressed mood, and anxiety may increase the pain but pain may also generate these emotions (Brattberg, 1995). These emotions have a great impact on the individual's understanding and control of pain. An individual's reaction to pain is determined by past experiences, personality traits, state of health, level of growth and development, expectations from relatives and friends, and one's current situation (McCready, MacDavitt & O'Sulllivan, 1991). Cultural differences play an essential role in how people perceive and express pain. In cultures where emotional expression is not encouraged, people try to restrain their emotions in connection with pain, while the opposite is true in other cultures (Finer, 1984). Existential pain involves some kind of deeper suffering. When individuals experience different kinds of suffering, they frequently ask questions about life, death, the meaning of life and its lack of meaning (Eriksson, 1991). Seen from the perspective of religion, pain and suffering can be something positive. The needs of the body are ignored, the focus instead being on spirituality, giving life a new meaning (Sternbach, 1987).

No single theory on pain adequately explains all that is known about pain production, pain transmission, pain perception, and pain behaviours (Donovan, 1990). The gate control theory of pain proposed by Melzack and Wall (1965) more than three decades ago, still seems to be the best attempt to integrate the physiological, pathophysiological, and cognitive-emotional interactions of the pain experience. Loeser (1982) and Donovan (1990) proposed models that expand on the basic tenets of the gate control theory. Loeser's model involves nociception, pain, suffering, and pain behaviour. Suffering is a complex affective response generated by pain and other situations that induce negative emotional reactions, and it becomes integrated into a person's life style. Suffering involves functions such as memory, emotion, and meaning (Loeser, 1982). Donovan's (1990) model also involves social factors, for example, family, culture, and care delivery. These factors influence how pain is perceived and interpreted.

A common way to classify pain is into acute and chronic pain. Bonica (1990) defines acute pain as "a complex constellation of unpleasant sensory, perceptual, and emotional experiences and certain associated autonomic, psychological, emotional, and behavioural responses." (p. 19). Acute pain is in general characterised by being related to a specific event as trauma, diseases or treatments (Donovan, 1990). Chronic is described as something that is protracted, lasting, incurable, or constant. This means in practice that an acute pain that lasts longer than three to six months is regarded as chronic pain (Brattberg, 1995). Bonica (1990), on the other hand, argues that the pain has become chronic when "pain that persists a month beyond the usual course of an acute disease or an injury to heal or that is associated with a chronic process that causes continuous pain or the pain recurs at intervals for months or years." (p. 19). The pain is no longer a warning signal when the tissue damage perhaps no longer remains.

Several psychological models have attempted to establish the causes of pain becoming chronic, namely the psychodynamic/personality, behavioural, cognitive-/behavioural, and psycho-physiological models (Adams, Ravey & Taylor, 1996). The first type of model explains the development of pain by emotional and personality characteristics, while the second model is based on the assumption that behaviours are learned and reinforced. The proponents of the third type of model make a statement about the relationship between cognitive processes and behaviour. The last model suggests an interaction of physiological and psychological factors in the development of chronic pain. Gamsa (1994) claims that all these models have both strengths and weaknesses and that none is better than the other is.

In the literature dealing with stress, Selye (1985) denotes the positive aspects of stress 'eustress' and the negative and unpleasant ones 'distress'. Similarly, Frankenhauser (1986) described two components of stress; distress and effort. Effort is probably less damaging than distress. There are various types of distress. Physical distress can be referred to the presence of problems with the body, whereas emotional distress includes for example worry, fear, and dependency (Bergbom-Engberg & Haljamäe, 1989; Elpern, Pattersson, Gloskey & Bone, 1992). Intellectual distress includes for example communication and memory difficulties, disorientation and insufficient information. Existential or spiritual distress may be described as a failure to invest life with meaning, hope, a will to live, belief and faith in oneself (Tillich, 1952; Travelbee, 1971; Frankl, 1974, 1986; Watson, 1985). Being a patient in acute health care, for example in intensive care and postoperative care could be perceived as frightening and stressful (Stanton, 1991; Seers, 1987; Egan, 1989; Boeke, Duivenvoorden, Verhage & Zwaveling, 1991). Also, patients with chronic pain experience distress in various forms (Bonica, 1990; Brattberg, 1995; Walker & Sofaer, 1998).

MODEL AND QUESTIONNAIRE DEVELOPMENT OF PAIN AND DISTRESS

One of the authors (MLHL) of this chapter has, together with colleagues, developed a model of elderly patients' experiences of pain and distress in intensive care, using grounded theory, a qualitative research method (Hall-Lord, Larsson & Boström, 1994). Also, a questionnaire has been developed based on the model (Hall-Lord, Larsson & Steen, 1998; Hall-Lord, Steen & Larsson, 1999a; Hall-Lord, Larsson & Steen, 1999b; Hall-Lord, Johansson, Schmidt & Wilde Larsson, 2003a).

The Model of Pain and Distress

In the study, in where the model was developed, 18 patients between 70 to 85 years were interviewed and observed. Elderly patients' experiences of pain and distress were described in four dimensions formed by 16 categories (Figure 1). The sensory dimension is formed by four categories: *physical pain, physical discomfort, fatigue, and breathing problems.* The intellectual dimension is formed by the categories *not knowing, difficulty in expressing oneself/not being understood, and confused perception of reality.* The emotional dimension is formed by the categories *worry, fear, resignation, bitterness, anger/irritation, and dependency.* Finally, the categories *despair, threat to life, and death acceptance* form the existential dimension. The model is shown in Figure 1.

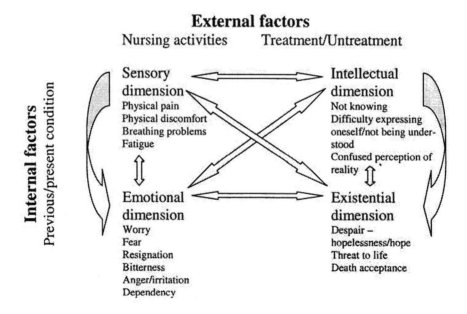

Figure 1. Elderly patients' experiences of pain and distress in intensive care.

The categories may be separate, but they often interact and influence each other in various ways. For example, the categories in the sensory and intellectual dimensions interact with each other. It also emerged that the categories in the sensory and intellectual dimensions may result in forms of pain and distress within the emotional and existential dimensions. Taken together, the categories within the three dimensions sensory, intellectual, and emotional seemed to be able to cause the development of categories in the existential dimension.

External as well as internal factors were found to influence patients' experiences of pain and distress. The external factors could be labelled as nursing activities, treatment and untreatment. Nursing activities refer to when the caregivers were doing things for the patients such as making their beds, turning the patients in the bed and performing various forms of controls. Nursing activities also include activities, which are not immediately directed towards the patients, such as caregivers' talking to each other. Treatment refers to respirator treatment, drug treatment and oxygen treatment. Untreatment means that the patients did not receive the treatment they considered that they ought to have been given, for example surgery or pain killer. Internal factors concern how the patient's previous and present state of health seemed to be influenced by their experiences. Previous state of health refers to various forms of diseases, such as asthma, and complaints, such as level of pain. Present state of health includes the patient's current condition.

The sensory dimension is formed by four categories: *physical pain*, *physical discomfort*, *fatigue*, and *breathing problems*. *Physical pain* was expressed both verbally and non-verbally in terms of intensity, duration, frequency, type, and location. Physical pain was caused by the patients' present or previous condition and could increase by nursing activities and treatment. Physical pain could result in breathing problems and fatigue (sensory dimension), not knowing (intellectual dimension), anger/irritation, dependency, fear, resignation, and worry (emotional dimension). *Physical discomfort* refers to physical problems which could not really be called physically painful caused by the patients' present and previous conditions as well as nursing activities and treatments. Physical discomfort could lead to physical pain and fatigue (sensory dimension), and anger/irritation (emotional dimension). *Fatigue* was described by the patients as hard and painful. Nursing activities such as controls, drug treatment and the patients' present condition were reasons for being tired. The experience of fatigue could result in breathing problems (sensory dimension) and confused perception of reality (intellectual dimension). *Breathing problems* were described by the patients as strained breathing or shortness of breath. Breathing problems were caused by the patient's previous illness as asthma or the patient's present condition, by occurrence of a complication. Also, nursing activities, when a patient was helped to put on his/her clothes, and treatments, such as not getting enough air from the respirator, were other reasons for breathing problems. Breathing problems could lead to physical pain, physical discomfort, and fatigue (sensory dimension).

In the intellectual dimension the categories *not knowing, difficulty in expressing oneself/not being understood*, and *confused perception of reality* emerged. *Not knowing* include the patients' thoughts about where they were, what had happened, and the reasons for being at the hospital. The category also includes the patients' inability to understand the information given by the caregivers. Not knowing was caused by nursing activities, treatment, and the patient's present condition. The category could result in physical pain (sensory dimension), worry (emotional worry), despair and threat to life (existential dimension). *Difficulty in expressing oneself/not being understood* was experienced by patients treated in respirator. The patients' inability to talk and express what they wanted could lead to resignation and anger/irritation (emotional dimension). *Confused perception of reality* was expressed by the patients as not having the ability to distinguish between dream and reality. The patients' present condition, nursing activities and treatment were reasons for the experience. The experience could lead to fear and worry (emotional dimension).

The emotional dimension is formed by the categories *worry, fear, resignation, bitterness, anger/irritation*, and *dependency*. *Worry* was often described as vague and longstanding. Worry appeared in specific situations but was not always directly related to anything specific. Reasons for being worried were the patients present condition, nursing activities, treatment, and untreatment. *Fear* aroused in specific situations and was expressed verbally and non-verbally. Fear was caused by nursing activities such as turning and lifting the patient in the bed, and by treatment. *Resignation* was expressed by the patients as that, that they had given up, they did not seem to bother about what was going on around them and that they did not care at all. The patient's present condition and untreatment were reasons for the experience. *Bitterness* was also expressed when the patients had given up but there was also an element (feature) of anger. Bitterness was caused by untreatment. *Anger/irritation* was expressed by the patients when the nursing staff did not understand what the patients meant or if the nursing activities were not adapted to the patient's needs. *Dependency* aroused when the patients felt that they could not do things by themselves. The patients' previous and present conditions, as well as nursing activities were reasons for this category.

The existential dimension includes the categories *despair, threat to life*, and *death acceptance*. *Despair* implies as a swinging between hope and hopelessness. The patients expressed uncertainty regarding their future existence. The feelings of despair were caused by the relation of patient's present and previous condition, treatment and untreatment. *Threat to life* was expressed by the patients caused by their present condition, how they had been hit by acute illness or an accident. The patients had also felt their lives threatened when waiting for treatment. *Death acceptance* could be noted when a change in the patients condition appeared, in general a complication. The situation in which the patients found themselves could be so hard and painful that they wished to die.

Pain and Distress Instruments

The model and the subsequently constructed questionnaire were developed from a patient perspective and not a personnel perspective. The questionnaire was developed to measure patients' experiences and nurses' assessments of pain and distress in intensive care. The categories in the model except resignation, bitterness, despair, threat to life, and death acceptance were operationalized. The reason for not include the categories in the existential dimension was the risk of causing the patients emotional distress. Resignation and bitterness were difficult to operationalize. As a first step, a questionnaire comprising a large number of items, approximately 100, was constructed by the investigators. This was done in collaboration with experienced intensive care nurses. To make the items as comprehensible as possible for the patients, the wording used for the items was derived from the interview responses obtained in the grounded theory study. As a second step, this pool of items was pilot tested on a small number of patients and nurses in an intensive care unit. Based on the views of the respondents, the items were reduced to 53. Forty-two of the items focused on assessment-oriented issues and 11 items covered intervention aspects. The assessment-oriented part of the questionnaire included the categories: physical pain (2 items), physical discomfort (2 items), breathing problems (10 items), fatigue (6 items), not knowing (7 items), difficulty in expressing oneself/not being understood (3 items), confused perception of reality (1 item), worry (2 items), fear (2 items), dependency (5 items), and anger/irritation (2 items). The intervention aspects were measured with the categories physical pain (2 items), physical discomfort (2 items), breathing problems (2 items), fatigue (1 item), worry (2 items), and fear (2 items). The questionnaire included a Likert-type response scale, using three, four, or five response choices, as well as alternatives 'Do not know' and 'Not applicable'.

The questionnaire was further adjusted to other nursing contexts concerning patients in postoperative care, patients with chronic pain and residents in nursing homes. Furthermore, the categories resignation, bitterness, and despair have been operationalized. The questionnaire has been used on patients, nurses, student nurses, and family members.

EMPIRICAL FINDINGS – ELDERLY PEOPLE

Data from three studies are accounted for in this section. Two of the studies describe patients in postoperative care (Hall-Lord et al., 1999a; Hall-Lord, Wilde Larsson, Bååth & Johansson, 2003b) and the third study describes patients with chronic pain (Hall-Lord et al., 1999b).

Postoperative Patients

Participants and Data Collection

The sample in study I comprised 100 patients, 31 men and 69 women, who had undergone elective surgery at two orthopaedic and two general surgical units in one hospital. Twenty-six patients had undergone hip arthroplasty, 24 knee arthroplasty, 23 had surgery in connection with verified or suspected breast cancer and 27 abdominal surgery. Mean age was 74.3 years (range 65-91). Data was collected through personal interviews at the first and second day after surgery and by telephone ten days after discharge from hospital. A structured questionnaire based on parts of the model of pain and distress was used (see Pain and Distress Instruments section). Sense of Coherence was assessed with nine Likert scale items corresponding to Antonovsky's Sense of Coherence Questionnaire (Antonovsky, interscale correlation with Antonsvsky's scale: 0.70) (Setterlind & Larsson, 1995). Need for Social Support was measured with eight items, constructed for the study.

The sample in study II consisted of 49 patients (12 men and 37 women) with hip fracture with a mean age of 83 years (range 70-92) (Hall-Lord et al., 2003b). The study was undertaken at two hospitals. The patients were interviewed on four occasions at the ward: arrival day, first and third day after surgery, and the day before discharge from hospital. The questionnaire consisted of three items to measure the category physical pain at the three first data collection occasions. At the fourth occasion pain and distress were measured with 20 items. Functional ability was assessed with a questionnaire focused on activities of daily living (ADL) (Sonn, 1995). The questionnaire is included by four defined instrumental activities, I-ADL, (cleaning, shopping, transportation, and cooking) and six defined personal daily activities, P-ADL (bathing/taking a shower, dressing, going to the toilet, transfer, continence, and feeding). Each function is rated as independent, partly independent or dependent.

Overall Findings

The elderly patients' reported experiences in study I varied in some respects between the three interview occasions. The intensity of physical pain and fatigue was reduced on the second day but increased again after discharge. On the first and the second day after operation, 46 and 35% respectively of the patients had physical pain for more than three hours and approximately 25 per cent had moderate or severe pain. Previous studies have shown that patients perceive high levels of postoperative pain (e.g. Closs, Fairtlough, Tierney & Currie, 1993; Sjöström, 1995; Field, 1996; Gillies, Smith, & Perry-Jones, 1999; Zalon, 1993). Normally, postoperative pain decreases gradually from the first to the third day after the operation, but not for all patients (Tittle & McMillan, 1992). Fewer patients reported physical discomfort on the second day compared to the first day after operation. However, after returning home, more patients reported discomfort. Sleep, rest and the ability to manage on one's own were improved after returning home. Six weeks after joint replacement surgery the patients rated their sleep and wound pain as significantly improved (Chamberlein, Petrie, & Azanah, 1992).

In study II the patients experienced physical pain at rest and physical pain with movement as most intense before surgery. Physical pain at rest was lower compared with the pain experience with movement, which is in accordance with the results of another study (Feldt & Oh, 2000). Despite the fact that physical pain decreased during the hospital stay, several of the patients had moderate (at rest, 16.7%; with movement, 26.2%) or severe pain (at rest, 7.1%; with movement, 33.3%) on the day before discharge.

Subgroup Comparisons

In study I a cluster analysis was performed on the basis of the patients' experiences of pain and distress. Profile A, with 43 patients, perceived pain and distress to a minor degree while another profile (C), consisting of twelve patients, reported pain and distress to a great degree. Profile C was significantly less satisfied with pain relief and assistance with physical discomfort and not managing on their own at home. The third patient profile (B) with 36 patients was positioned between the other clusters. The patients in profile C showed a significantly weaker sense of coherence compared with the other two profiles (Table 1).

Table 1. Pain and distress in relation to person and context related aspects

Person-related aspects	Study	Sample	Quality of Care Pain and distress
Age	Study I Hall-Lord et al., 1999a	N = 100 2 types of surgery environment (orthopedic and general surgery units) 65-74 yr (n=57) 75-84 yr (n=34) > 85 yr (n=9)	Patients with higher age had significantly less belief in managing by themselves and were less able to sleep at home ten days after surgery
	Study III Hall-Lord et al., 1999b	N = 42 Chronic pain patients Cluster A M=85.8 SD=4.95 Cluster B M=78.1 SD=7.30 Cluster C M=78.5 SD=7.89	Patients in cluster A were significantly older compared with the other clusters. They were less informed, more resigned, dependent, and had less sufficient pain relief compared with cluster B.

Table 1. Pain and distress in relation to person and context related aspects (Continued)

Person-related aspects	Study	Sample	Quality of Care Pain and distress
Diagnosis	Study I Hall-Lord et al., 1999a	Additional diagnoses (n=56) No additional diagnoses (n=44)	Patients with additional diagnosis were significantly more likely to report fatigue
	Study II Hall-Lord et al., 2003a	Group A Additional diagnoses (55%) Group B Additional diagnoses (90%)	Significantly more persons in group B had additional diagnoses. This group had more physical discomfort and sleeping problems, were more tired, afraid, irritated and had more feelings of meaninglessness. They had less sufficient assistance regarding physical pain, worry and dependency.
Functional ability	Study III Hall-Lord et al., 1999b	N = 42 Cluster A More dependent (n=11) Cluster B More dependent (n=5) Cluster C More dependent (n=7)	Significantly more persons in cluster A and C were dependent compared with cluster B.
Gender	Study I Hall-Lord et al., 1999a	Male (n=31) Female (n=69)	Females had significantly less belief in managing by themselves at home ten days after surgery

Table 1. Pain and distress in relation to person and context related aspects (Continued)

Person-related aspects	Study	Sample	Quality of Care Pain and distress
Sense of coherence	Study I Hall-Lord et al., 1999a	Cluster A M=2.07 SD=0.33 Cluster B M=2.33 SD=0.40 Cluster C M=1.87 SD=0.42	Patients with a weaker sense of coherence had significantly more intense physical pain and were more tired and worried on the first day after surgery. At home, ten days after surgery, patients with a weaker sense of coherence were less able to sleep, had less belief in managing themselves and belief in recovery. Cluster C had significantly lower mean scores on SOC compared with the other clusters. This group had more intense physical pain, fatigue, and worry. They were more dependent and resigned. Cluster C perceived the assistance received regarding pain relief, physical discomfort and with things they did not managed by themselves as less sufficient than cluster A.
	Study III Hall-Lord et al., 1999b	Cluster A M=2.07 SD=0.33 Cluster B M=2.33 SD=0.40 Cluster C M=1.87 SD=0.42	Persons in cluster C had significantly less favorable scores on sense of coherence than the persons in cluster B. The subjects in cluster C had significantly more problems with fatigue, worry, bitterness, and despair than the other clusters. They were significantly less informed, resigned, and dependent than cluster B. The assistance received regarding fatigue and despair was seen as significantly less sufficient than the other clusters.

Table 1. Pain and distress in relation to person and context related aspects (Continued)

	Study	Sample	Quality of Care Pain and distress
Person-related aspects			
Need of social support	Study I Hall-Lord et al., 1999a	No or weak need for social support (n=43) Need for social support (n=47)	Patients with more need of social support had significantly more fatigue and worry first day after surgery
Context related aspects			
Type of surgery	Study I Hall-Lord et al., 1999a	Hip arthroplasty (n=26) Knee arthroplasty (n=24) Breast cancer (n=23) Abdominal surgery (n=27)	Patients who had undergone knee arthroplasty reported significantly more intense physical pain and anger/irritation first day after surgery. 10 days after surgery at home the patients with knee arthroplasty reported more fatigue. Patients who underwent hip arthroplasty reported to a higher extent no belief in managing oneself at home.

Johansson (1998) found that hip fracture patients with a weaker sense of coherence reported significantly more discomfort and less favourable scores in emotional status than the patients with a stronger sense of coherence. More of the patients in profile C and B had a stronger need of social support compared with profile A. Social support has been shown to be related to improvements in mental and physical health (Broadhead et al., 1983; Hinson, Lanford, Bowsher, Maloney & Lillis, 1997). Emotional support, an important factor in nursing care, may lead to feelings of safety and security (Pålsson, Hallberg, Norberg & Björvell, 1996).

In study II the patients were divided into two groups of patients according to the scores of physical pain. Group A (n = 22) suffered from significantly fewer problems compared with the patients in group B (n = 20) in the categories physical discomfort, fatigue, fear, anger/irritation, and despair. Group B perceived the assistance regarding physical pain, physical discomfort, and fatigue as significantly less satisfactory. These findings indicate undertreatment of pain for this group of patients. Carr (1990) showed that the patients' experiences of pain postoperatively were linked to how they perceived their progress and recovery at the hospital. Closs (1992) found that one-third of patients who had undergone surgery felt that pain affected their sleep. In turn, the sleeping problems led to tiredness. More patients in group B had one or more medical diagnoses whereas the patients in group A had no additional medical diagnoses (Table 1). Feldt and Oh (2000) found that the number of chronic illnesses was associated with functional recovery two months after surgery.

Elderly People with Chronic Pain

Participants and Data Collection

This study (III) was carried out in seven primary health care districts in a County Council. The sample consisted of 42 persons with chronic pain and utilising the community health services. The persons were identified by a health care professional (district nurse). Chronic pain was defined as constant pain during at least three months. The subjects had a mean age of 80.1 years (range 66-94) and lived in special housing or in their own homes. Persons with severe heart failure, cancer, and depressive moods were excluded. Interviews were conducted with the elderly persons. A questionnaire based on the model of pain and distress was used. Also, Sense of Coherence and Functional ability were assessed (see above).

Overall Findings

All the persons experienced physical pain, the intensity varied from some pain to excruciating pain. The most intense experience in the sensory dimension, except physical pain, was physical discomfort and thereafter fatigue. The persons with breathing problems perceived the assistance with these problems as insufficient. In the intellectual dimension, information about the persons' condition was perceived as one of the least favourable experiences. Elderly persons are not always informed about the cause of the pain (Walker, Akinsanya, Davis, & Marcer, 1990). The persons' most unfavourable experiences in the emotional dimension were worry, resignation, and dependency. Elderly people may resign to the pain because they do not believe that it can be alleviated (Yates, Dewar, & Fentiman, 1995).

Subgroup Comparisons

In study III a cluster analysis with three profiles was performed on the basis of the persons' scores on pain and distress. The persons in cluster A (n = 15) had significantly less favourable mean scores than the persons in cluster B (n = 18) in three of the categories; not knowing, resignation, and dependence. The subjects in cluster C (n = 12) rated themselves as more tired, worried, bitter, and suffering from despair than did the persons in clusters A and B as well as less informed, more resigned and dependent than did the persons in cluster B. Other studies showed that elderly persons not always felt informed about the cause of the pain (Walker et al., 1990). The persons in cluster C perceived the assistance received regarding fatigue and within the existential dimension as less satisfactory. The subjects in cluster A was less satisfied with pain relief. They were significantly older (Table 1). Elderly people are one such a group to be particularly exposed to undertreatment of pain (Closs, 1994; Yates et al., 1995; American Geriatric Society, 1998). Few elderly people with chronic pain are treated in pain clinics, despite the fact that their problems are at least as severe as those of younger patients (Roy & Thomas, 1987). Yates et al. (1995) found that the most common pain-relieving strategies among older persons, apart from medication, were distraction techniques. However, persons with reduced functional ability may find it difficult to use such techniques on their own. The subjects in cluster C showed a significantly weaker sense of coherence than the persons in cluster B (Table 1). Also, they seemed to be in need of extensive help and support. More persons in cluster A and C were dependent compared with cluster B. This may range from existential and emotional support to help with basic activities of daily living. Older patients with pain place a high value upon caring aspect such as empathy and kindness (Yates et al., 1995; Walker, 1994). A strong sense of coherence has been shown to have positive associations with elderly people's perceived health and functional ability (Sarvimäki & Ojala, 1994; Johansson, 1998).

EMPIRICAL FINDINGS – SIMILARITIES AND DIFFERENCES BETWEEN ELDERLY PEOPLE AND THEIR CAREGIVERS

Data from two studies are presented in this section. Study IV illuminates patients and personnel in intensive care (Hall-Lord et al., 1998) and study V (Hall-Lord, Larsson & Steen, 1999c) describes elderly with chronic pain and assistant nurses in the community.

Intensive Care

Participants and Data Collection

The study (IV) compared patients' reported experiences of pain and distress and to what extent they felt that they had been helped and supported by the assessments of registered nurses and assistant nurses. Comparisons were also made between the two groups of nurses. The sample comprised 51 patients, 44 registered nurses, and 37 assistant nurses. Interviews with a questionnaire based on the model of pain and distress were conducted with the patients on the day before they left the intensive care unit. The nurses filled in a questionnaire included the same questions as the patients' questionnaire; they were asked about their opinion of the patients' experiences.

Overall Findings

The patients' reported experiences of pain and distress did not agree completely with the registered nurses' and assistant nurses' assessments. The registered nurses overestimated some of the patients' experiences, such as breathing problems and difficulty in expressing oneself/not being understood. Previous studies showed that nurses tend to overestimate factors that are stressful to the patients within intensive care (Cochran & Ganong, 1989; Cornock, 1998). One possible reason for the patients perceiving some of their experiences as less stressful compared to the nurses is that they did not remember everything that had occurred during their stay in the ICU. However, results regarding what patients remember from their stay in an ICU vary between different studies (Bergbom-Engberg, Hallenberg, Wickström & Haljamäe, 1988; Puntillo, 1990; Turner, Briggs, Springhorn & Polgieter, 1990; Elpern et al., 1992).

Assistant nurses tended to underestimate the patients' pain and distress, which contrast with the results of another study where personnel perceived that patients in respirators had more problems than perceived by the patients themselves (Riggio, Singer & Hartman, 1982). However, patients' pain has been found to be frequently underestimated (LeVasseur & Calder, 1994).

The patients considered to a lesser extent than assistant nurses that they had received help and support within the sensory dimension with physical pain, physical discomfort and sleep, and within the emotional dimension with fear. Due to assistant nurses' limited training, they are not allowed to make decisions and perform interventions on their own. Consequently, they do not make their own assessments of interventions.

Both registered nurses and assistant nurses judged, to a greater extent than the patients, that the patients could help themselves and that they had been given this possibility. Furthermore, there was a discrepancy between registered nurses' and assistant nurses' assessments regarding breathing problems, sleep, and information about patients' condition and the assistance with sleep, physical discomfort, and fear. This discrepancy may be due to differences in education. It was primarily the assistant nurses who answered "Do not know" to the questions related to the patients' previous experiences in intensive care. However, the nurses also showed a high frequency of "Do not know"-answers within the emotional dimension, which might indicate that communication and documentation between nursing staff do not include assessments of emotional experiences to the same extent as sensory ones.

Community Care

Participants and Data Collection

The sample in study V comprised 38 patients (5 men and 33 women, mean age 81 years, range 65-94 years) and 38 assistant nurses (mean age 37.5 years, range 20-62). The nursing experience ranging from one to 25 years, mean 12.6 years. On average, the nurses had known the patients for 42 months (range 3-128). Interviews were conducted with the patients in their homes, using a questionnaire based on the model. One of the assistant nurses who usually had the responsibility for the care of an older patient with chronic pain filled in a questionnaire. The questions referred to the assistant nurses' perceptions on how the patients usually experienced pain and distress and to what extent they usually received support/help. Assistant nurses also filled in a questionnaire measuring personality. The five-factor personality inventory (FFPI), which measured five factors: extraversion, agreeableness, conscientiousness, emotional stability, and intellect/autonomy, was used (Hendriks, 1997). Also, sense of coherence was measured with Antonovsky's 13-item short version of the sense of coherence questionnaire (Antonovsky, 1987).

Overall Findings

In the sensory dimension the assistant nurses' assessed physical pain, physical discomfort, and breathing problems as less intense compared with the patients' perceptions. The results are consistent with an earlier study of nurses' assessment of chronic pain in elderly patients (Walker et al., 1990). Assistant nurses assessed that the patients received significantly more sufficient information regarding the patients' condition and scheduled events. In the emotional dimension, within the categories resignation and dependency, the patients reported, on the one hand, to a lesser degree than the assistant nurses, that their condition would improve and that they would receive help to get better and, on the other hand, to a greater degree that they were unable to help themselves and had not been given the opportunity to do something on their own.

Only one of the ten help and support variables showed significant differences between patients and assistant nurses. Within the existential dimension, the patients felt that they received sufficient help from the staff to a lesser degree compared to assistant nurses' assessments. The majority of the nurses did not know whether or not the patients received this kind of support from the staff, and most of the patients did not consider the staff able to support them in existential questions. In a study carried out in a rehabilitation clinic, Anderson, Anderson and Felsenthal (1993) found that none of the staff had talked to the patients about existential questions, despite the fact that two thirds of the patients felt this to be important. Elderly patients in hospital and in the community stated that they would welcome nursing involvement and interventions to meet their spiritual needs (Peterson, 1985; Bauer & Barron, 1995).

Subgroup Comparisons

The assistant nurses were divided into two groups according to whether they, in their assessments, had underestimated or overestimated the patients' experiences. The assistant nurses underestimating the patients' experiences showed significantly higher scores on three of five personality dimensions: Agreeableness, Conscientiousness, and Emotional Stability. They also showed a tendency towards higher scores on Extraversion and Sense of Coherence although the differences were not significant. The same pattern emerged regarding another study in which registered nurses who had higher scores on Extraversion, Emotional Stability, Intellect/Autonomy, and SOC seemed to assess pain and distress for acute patients as less intense than the nurses who had lower scores (Hall-Lord & Wilde Larsson, 2003). High scores on the scales Agreeableness and Conscientiousness mean, among other things, that one is helpful, friendly, and kind-hearted, and ambitious and reliable as well as having stamina, factors important in a caregiver. One explanation for the differences between the two groups' assessments could be that it may be easier for assistant nurses with higher scores on the personality scales to cope with patients' problems. Therefore they do not perceive the patient's condition as particularly painful and distressing, in contrast to the assistant nurses with low scores who show greater difficulty in coping with patients' pain and distress. Nurses with more empathy for their patients had higher scores on SOC (Pålsson et al., 1996). Orlando (1990) emphasizes personality as a factor which influences the way in which nurses observe, think, and feel regarding patients' behaviours and reactions in a caring situation. It is important to be able to use, in a conscious way, one's own immediate reactions to be able to understand the meaning of a patient's behaviour. This can in turn lead to nursing interventions of a positive character. However, the present study gives no information on the outcome of the assistant nurses' interventions.

EMPIRICAL FINDINGS - FAMILY MEMBERS' PERCEPTIONS OF PAIN AND DISTRESS

Data from one study is presented in this section. Study VI illuminates family members' perceptions of elderly nursing home residents (Hall-Lord et al., 2003a).

Participants and Data Collection

The sample in study VI consisted of 232 family members (next of kin or guardian) of residents in ten Swedish nursing homes. The mean age of the family members was 62 years (SD = 12.6) and 54% were women. The mean age of the residents was 84 years (SD = 8.3 years) and 68% were women. Drug prescription was analyzed by studying the medication data in the residents' medical records. Dementia was assessed by the head nurse who checked if there was a documented or known diagnosis of dementia. Family members filled in a questionnaire based on the model. Quality of care was measured by the questionnaire Quality from the patient's perspective (QPP) developed from a theoretical model (Wilde, Starrin, Larsson & Larsson, 1993; Wilde, Larsson, Larsson & Starrin, 1994; Larsson, Wilde Larsson Munck, 1998). A modified version of the questionnaire, consisting of 19 factors and 66 items, measuring three of four quality of care dimensions; medical-technical competence, identity-oriented approach and socio-cultural atmosphere, was used. The family members filled out the questionnaires of pain and distress and quality of care.

Overall Findings

Sixty-four percent of the residents were estimated by the family members as having physical discomfort, 67% physical pain, and 82% worry. Sixty-four of 128 residents with physical pain received sufficient pain relief according to the family members. Out of the128 residents reported by family members as suffering from pain, 29 had no analgesics prescribed, while 19 residents reported as not having physical pain had prescribed analgesics.

Cramer, Galer, Mendelson and Thompson (2000) found that the treatment of pain in elderly residents often was inappropriate. They concluded that no pain assessment was conducted for 40% of the residents.

Regarding worry, 53 of 140 family members reported the help/support as sufficient, 71 as sufficient to some extent and 16 as insufficient. Out of the 163 of the residents who felt worry, 144 had psychotropics prescribed. Approximately 68% of the residents were evaluated as suffering from dementia, which could explain the high frequency of worry. A major problem is providing care for demented people, whose activities may seem aimless or meaningless when the caregiver fails to put meaning to it. Elderly people often have complex, varied and rapidly changing needs for nursing care, which in turn, demand a coordinated competence in representatives from various professions. Nowadays it is assistant nurses who meets the elderly person on a daily basis and is most familiar with their needs, wishes, and interests. Supervision is required to guide these staff in meeting the needs of elderly people for nursing care (National Board of Health and Welfare, 2002).

Subgroup Comparisons

The residents were divided into three subgroups (group A = 55, group B = 47, group C = 27) according to the family members scores of pain and distress. The residents in group A showed most favourable scores. The subjects in group B had minor problems. Finally, the persons in group C were perceived as experiencing the most pain and distress. The family members connected to the residents in group C perceived pain relief as more insufficient compared with group A and help/support with physical discomfort as more insufficient compared with group A and B. Group B and C were to a higher degree not satisfied with the support regarding worry.

Significant differences were noted on 16 factors (out of 19 possible) regarding perceived quality of care. Regarding 15 factors the family members in group C were more dissatisfied with quality of care compared with group A. Patients with better health status are often more satisfied with the medical and nursing care provided (Wilde, Larsson, Larsson & Starrin, 1995; Törnkvist, Gardulf & Strender, 2000). The three factors where no significant differences appeared were in the identity-oriented approach (information to the residents before procedures and the residents' participation), and in the social-cultural atmosphere (meaningful occupation) dimensions. All the three groups scored low on these factors. There are no nationally established quality indicators within the care for elderly people in the community. This may lead to contradictory views: that you are generally very satisfied, but at the same time, give very low ratings on certain aspects of health and social care. One important explanation is major deficiencies in the community information for elderly people and their relatives (National Board of Health and Welfare 2002). Group C included more women than the other two groups. Other studies have found that more women than men report severe and persistent pain (Crook, Rideout & Browne, 1984; Brattberg, parker & Thorslund, 1997). Group A had less minor analgesics, antidepressants, anxiolytics, and less than three or more psychotropic drugs prescribed compared with the other groups.

The deficiencies in the use of drugs by elderly people do not only concern underuse, but also overuse of drugs. The use of antidepressants has increased all through the nineties because of the introduction of selective serotonin reuptake inhibitors (SSRIs). In a study from

1989, the number of residents treated with antidepressants was 20% (Andersson, 1989). Another study from 2000, demonstrated that the proportion treated with antidepressants was 31% (Schmidt & Fastbom 2000). The proportion in the present study was 42%.

SUMMARY OF RESULTS AND FURTHER RESEARCH

- Elderly patients' experiences of pain and distress in intensive care may be described in a model including physical, intellectual, emotional, and existential dimensions. In the care of the patients all dimensions should be taken into consideration.
- Several studies showed that there were various profiles/subgroups of elderly people according to their experiences of pain and distress. They showed individual variations in their perception of pain and distress experiences. Their perceptions of the assistance received varied among the groups. This suggests that there is a need to make individual assessments of their needs and to treat elderly people in different ways in the caring situation.
- The profiles/subgroups of elderly people showed variations in age, functional ability, need of social support, sense of coherence, sex, and prescription of drugs. For example the elderly with less favourable scores of pain and distress had a weaker sense of coherence than the elderly with more favourable pain and distress scores. More research is needed about how these and other factors affect elderly peoples' experiences of pain and distress.
- Elderly persons' self-reported experiences of pain and distress did not agree with nurses' assessments. The assessment of patients' pain and distress must be more systematic, and the use of standardised methods is suggested.
- Personality as a nurse characteristic seemed to influence the enrolled nurses' assessment of patients' pain and distress. Nurses need to become aware of possible biases related to pain and distress assessment as a result of personality factors and other variables. Further studies are needed to clarify the effect of personality factors on the assessment of pain and distress. Also, it is of importance to investigate how nurses manage pain and distress in actual caring situations.

QUALITY OF CARE – MODELS AND ASSESSMENT

Quality of care is a multidimensional concept which has been given different meanings in the literature. The concept quality is in theory a neutral one. In everyday speech it is, however, usually associated with something positive and desirable. The concept could consequently be considered emotionally charged. In dictionaries, quality is defined as characteristic, nature, intrinsic value.

A broad and general definition of quality of care was formulated by Lee and Jones (1933), saying that all available scientific medical knowledge should be applied to all those in need of care. This idealistic kind of definition has been criticized by, for instance, Reerink (1990) as being unrealistic in many countries. Also Vuori (1982) is critical and finds it out of the question that all could receive the best possible care. According to Vuori, definitions of this kind cannot possibly be realized. Moreover, they disregard the fact that quality is a continuous variable with some kind of distribution. Vuori is of the opinion that it is feasible to move the whole distribution to the higher quality or to reduce dispersion, and this is the aim of quality assurance. Donabedian (1985) in a similar way recommends "acceptable standards" and stresses the importance of economic realism when working with quality assurance. How care should be (normative aspect) in relation to how it actually is (empirical aspect) is central when working with quality assurance (Donabedian, 1966). He (1966) is of the opinion that the essence of quality definitions is constituted by the balance between benefit and harm in terms of health. He also emphasizes that quality of care is determined by to what extent the care in question agrees with established criteria of good care.

According to Øveretveit (1992), quality of care is to fully meet the demands made by those most in need of care and to achieve this at the lowest possible cost for the organization within the limitations formulated by society. This definition includes quality aspects at different levels; individual, organizational, and societal. It can also be said to include quality from the point of view of different persons involved, e.g., the client/patient, the professional caregivers and the responsible decision-makers. Øvretveit's definition also includes economic aspects plus respect for laws and general demands. Other general definitions have been suggested by WHO (1988) and Williamson (1978).

General definitions of quality of care of the kind mentioned above seem to involved two predominant domains. The first one – which could be called the substance of the concept – include desirable characteristics, criteria, standards, goal documents, policy, and laws. The second domain mainly includes evaluation of the outcome of care (Donabedian, 1966, 1989; Vuori, 1982). Some definitions include both these domains (Donabedian, 1966, 1989) and others only one of them (Reerink, 1990). The latter states that criteria, standards, goal documents, etc., are not synonymous with quality of care. They are intentions to administer care of good quality. Whether the care is of good quality or not will be seen when evaluating the outcome of care (Reerink, 1990). This standpoint could be compared to what Donabedian (1980) describes as "quality level." To sum up, general definitions of quality of care seem first of all to state a rough intention or aim.

Different models and instruments of quality of care specific to elderly people are described in the literature, all designed from the perspective of different parties. For instance, from a professional perspective (see e.g., Bergman & Golander, 1982), or from the perspective of interested parties of patients (see e.g., Lemke & Moos, 1980, 1981, 1986, 1987; Moos & Lemke, 1980). From the perspective of elderly people, Cryns, Nicholos, Katz and Calkins (1989) designed the Older Patient Satisfaction Scale. Other examples of models and instruments from the elderly people's perspective are presented by Bauld, Chesterman and Judge (2000), Boldy and Grenade (1998), Chesterman, Bauld, and Judge (2000), Edebalk, Invad and Lannerheim (1990), Larsen, Attkinson, Hargreaves & Nguyen (1979), Larsson (1996) and McCullough et al. (1993).

Patient satisfaction has increasingly come to be used as an indicator of quality of care (Aharony & Strasser, 1993; Arnetz & Arnetz, 1996; Clerary & Edgman-Levitan, 1997; Cleary & McNeal, 1988; Davies & Ware, 1988; Eriksen, 1995; Geron, 1999; Nettelman 1998, Sitza & Wood, 1997; Smith, 1992; Staniszewska & Ahmed, 1999; van Campen et al., 1995; von Essén & Sjödén, 1991a; 1991b; Vuori, 1991; World Health Organization, 1988;

Williams, 1994). Patient satisfaction can also be looked upon as an assessment of care quality (Donabedian, 1988; Vuori, 1991) and as a result of care. High patient satisfaction is a desirable aim of care, but it can also be seen as a means for parts of the care institutions, as satisfied patients seem to be more willing to follow professional advice and instructions (Aharony & Strasser, 1993), and come back when they need care in the future (see e.g., Donabedian, 1988; Calnan, 1988a; Vuori, 1991). Seeking patients' opinion on quality of care may also be a therapeutic activity; it encourages patients to become active, taking active steps to improve their situation, rather than assuming a passive patient role (Shields, Moris & Hart 1988).

Patients' views on what is important with regard to care can be seen as one aspect of the quality of care (Mahon, 1996). According to Calnan (1988a) and Willians and Calnan (1991), patient satisfaction has been considered valuable for three different reasons. The first one is that care should not only be evaluated with regard to clinical and economic efficiency aspects, but public values, society's, and people's opinions of care should also be considered. A second reason involves political convictions like democratization of care and increased patient influence. A third reason involves ethical and humanitarian aspects. The idea is that the fundamental principle on which the caregiver should base his or her actions is satisfying the patient's wishes and needs (see also Donabedian, 1980; Vuori, 1991; Ware, Davis & Stewart, 1978; Ware & Snyder, 1975).

In sum, quality of care is a relative concept. The meaning of the concept quality of care seems to vary with regard to: (1) the time and culture of the society concerned, e.g., a welfare state or a developing country with limited resources; (2) the level concerned, e.g., individual, organizational, and society level; and (3) who defines the concept, e.g., clients/patients, family members, staff, administrators, or politicians (Donabedian, 1980; Vuori, 1982). The meaning also varies with regard to the care aspects concerned; the structure of the care system, the caring process, or the outcome of care (Donabedian, 1966). It is also obvious that: (1) different definitions could be relevant in different contextual limitations, (2) different responses could be obtained due to the perspective from which the quality of care is studied, and (3) person- as well as situation-specific characteristics must be considered in studies within a given context and from a given perspective (e.g., the patient perspective) in order to understand individual perceptions' of quality of care.

Measuring Patients' Views on the Quality of Care

Patient-Related Problems

Mirror theory. We humans build up our inner image or representation of the objective outside world, based on our sensory impressions – what we see, hear, feel, smell, and taste. This inner image forms the basis of our words and actions. The assumption that a person's subjective statements about a part of reality, e.g., a patient's response in a questionnaire on the quality of health care, is a correct reflection of this reality is often known as the mirror theory (Björkman & Lundqvist, 1981).

This theory has been questioned; particularly regarding surveys conducted using questionnaires. Above all it appears that general (broad) questions on personal and emotionally sensitive factors lead to too "good" answers compared to those asked in in-depth interviews, for example, where specific follow-up questions may be asked.

This tendency seems to apply to a greater extent in "weak groups," e.g., the poorly educated and the elderly (Björkman & Lundqvist, 1981; Blomgren, 1984). A possible reason is that a greater cognitive dissonance occurs – inner imbalance – (Festinger, 1957), for these people when they cannot change their situation as they would like to. This kind of imbalance can be resolved by either reevaluating one's actual situation or by reducing one's demands. In both of these cases "excessively high" values are obtained when measuring satisfaction (Blomgren, 1984). In psychological terms this can be interpreted as when a person "embellishes" his or her inner representation of the external reality through mental defence mechanisms.

Insufficient knowledge and frame of reference. To judge whether something is good or bad a person must possess a minimum level of knowledge of what he or she is to judge. A commonly held view is that certain sections of modern health care are so complicated and advanced that most patients can only understand them on a superficial level. If so, patients' perceptions of quality in complicated sections of health care are of dubious value. However, the results of several studies show that patients can judge medical interventions and doctors' knowledge in an acceptable way (see e.g., Calnan, 1988b).

Patients' dependency on the care providers and the health care system is another feasible source of error (French, 1981). Expressing negative criticism about someone on whom one depends may feel so threatening that one prefers to refrain from doing so. For example, a patient may fear that the care provider might take offence and treat the patient worse if the latter is critcizing. Another possible reason is not wanting to hurt the feelings of the care provider – a risk that probably increases in health care situations where the care provider and the patient know each other well.

Not being able to communicate satisfactorily. Further examples of weaknesses in measuring patients' perceptions of health care quality include the fact that the use of questionnaires and interviews presupposes that the patient is able to communicate. Due to age-related changes and/or the illnesses for which the patients are being treated, many patients cannot communicate at the level required for normal questioning. The same applies to immigrants who cannot understand and answer questions for language reasons. The ability to communicate is therefore an important selection criterion.

The impact of personality on the responses. Surveys of patients' perceptions of the quality of care have also been criticised from a personality psychology perspective. The critics say that the responses tell us more about the people providing the responses than about the issues that are intended to be measured. This affects the responses particularly in cases of negative affectivity; people in a negative frame of mind tend to feel that everything is bad (Watson & Pennebaker, 1989). However, Davies and Wares (1988) conclude that any "distortions" of responses due to personality traits are not sufficiently strong to invalidate the patients' judgements of quality of care.

Reliability-Related Problems

Patient questionnaires have also been called into question due to more technical and reliability-oriented factors. Instructions, the way in which questions are phrased, and the choice of answers may be leading (biased). The language may be on such a high level of abstraction that some patients do not understand the questions – which may be embarrassing to admit. The response alternatives are not always comprehensive, or may overlap. Sometimes more answers are included than most patients can differentiate between. Sometimes dichotomous Yes/No scales are used as answers to questions where a more differentiated scale could be provided.

The length of the questionnaire should also be taken into account. Too many and/or too complicated questions may lead to some patients getting tired of filling in the questionnaire. A "strange" order of questions may have the same effect. Similar effects have been observed when the questionnaire had an unattractive layout or when it was distributed by a bad-tempered, surly care provider in stressed circumstances, etc (see, Rombach 1989).

Interplay also exists between the structure and length of the questionnaire and the personality and intellectual capacity of the respondent. People with a distinctive sense of duty and good verbal ability seem to be able to fill in virtually endless questionnaires and maintain a high level of concentration whilst doing do. However, patients who are more restless and have an aversion to "all sorts of paperwork" often get tired of filling in a questionnaire early on. Other patients like comprehensive questionnaires – they perceive that the person/organisation setting the questionnaire is really interested in their opinions (French, 1981).

Validity-Related Problems

Patient questionnaires have also been criticised as regards validity. Questionnaires are often created that are not based on empirical models of what patients actually include in the concept of quality of care. This entails two possible problems. The first is that questions may be asked on the wrong subjects. The second is that there is no interpretation framework to use as a guide when analysing and evaluating the responses.

Thus, criticism has been raised against various scales designed to measure patients', and family members' satisfaction with, or perception of, quality of care (Calnan, 1988a; LaMonica, et al., 1986; Thomas et al., 1995; van Campen et al., 1995). While several of these scales may be creatively designed, a major criticism against most of them is the lack of a theoretical foundation. The selection of indicators has generally not been related to empirically-based models of patients' or family members' conceptions of the area (Bond & Thomas, 1992; Hall & Dornan, 1988; Rubin, Ware & Mayes, 1990; Thomas & Bond, 1991; Thomas et al., 1995). Consequently, one cannot be sure that the attributes chosen in the scales are the most important with regard to quality of care.

Several questionnaires feature questions about patients' experiences of what health care actually is (really) like. Other questions ask what the patient expects of health care or how subjectively significant various health care attributes are to him or her (ideals). A common way of handling this in operational terms appears to be through calculating differences between expectations or subjective ideals on the one hand and perceived reality on the other (Linder-Pelz, 1982a, 1982b; Parasuraman, Zeithaml & Berg, 1985).

If choosing between estimates of expectations and subjective significance, the latter is preferable. Subjective significance reflects what the person wants health care to be like, whilst estimates of expectations reflect what the person thinks it should be like. Through rumours, reputation, etc, a patient might expect that quality of care at a specific clinic is low. The patient then also perceives that the actual quality of care is low, and a good match is obtained between expectations and perceived outcome. In that case estimates of subjective significance would probably constitute a more valid basis on which to evaluate the quality of health care from the patient's perspective.

Additional Comments

Patients' ability to assess quality of care has been the subject of discussion in the literature. That patient can assess interpersonal aspects - the art of care - and the amenities is relatively unequivocal. Many researchers also consider that the patients are the best judges of these aspects (see e.g., Davies & Ware, 1988; Donabedian, 1980; Vuori, 1991). When it comes to judgments concerning technology of care – the science – Donabedian (1980), for example, thinks that patients only to a certain degree can assess these aspects. However, there are studies which show that patients have clear criteria both for evaluation medical procedures and for judging the capability of the personnel (cf. Calnan, 1988b).

Following a review of studies where patients' and professionals' views on the quality of care have been illustrated, Donabedian (1980) is of the opinion that there are similarities in their views on the general level (see also, Hietanen, Kroll-Paulsby, Schmidt & Wilde, 1993). There are, however, several studies indicating that there could be incongruity between patients', professionals', and family members' views on quality of care (see e.g., von Essen, 1994; McCullough et al., 1993; Windle & Paschall, 1981).

QUALITY OF CARE FROM THE PATIENT'S PERSPECTIVE (QPP) – A SWEDISH MODEL

One of the authors (BWL) of this chapter has, together with colleagues, developed a theoretical model of quality of care from a patient perspective (Wilde et al., 1993) and an instrument aimed to measure quality of care from the patient's perspective (Larsson et al., 1998; Wilde 1994; Wilde Larsson & Larsson 2000, Wilde Larsson & Larsson, 2002; Wilde et al., 1994; Wilde Larsson, Larsson, Larsson & Starrin, 2001).

Model Development

Using a grounded theory approach with a qualitative method of analysis, Wilde et al. (1993) developed a theoretical model of quality of care from a patient perspective. The model was generated from 35 in-depth interviews with patients. Interviews were interpreted in accordance with the advices given in the literature regarding grounded theory on a successively more abstract form of coding (Glaser, 1978; Starrin, Dahlgren, Larsson & Styrborn 1997). As a first step, indicators of quality of care were identified from patients' interview responses (about 900 altogether). A second step, these indicators were grouped into 27 categories. Thirdly, these categories were coded as comprising four dimensions. As a final step, these four dimensions were classified into a model (see Wilde et al., 1993, for further details).

The model stipulates that patients' perceptions of what constitutes quality of care are formed by their encounter with an existing care structure and by their system of norms, expectations, and experiences. From the patients' point of views, quality of care can be seen as a number of interrelated dimensions which, taken together, form a whole. The content of this whole can be understood in the light of two conditions, the resource structure of the care organization and the patients' preferences. The resource structure of the care organization consists of person-related, as well as physical and administrative environmental qualities. The patients' preferences are assumed be rational and human in character. The resourse structure is of two kinds: person-related and physical- and administrative environmental qualities. Person-related qualities refer to the caregivers (the doctor, the nurse, the assistant nurse, etc). Physical and administrative environmental qualities refer to infrastructural components of the care environment, organizational rules, technical equipment, etc.

The patients' preferences are also of two kinds: on the one hand, they have a rational aspect in the sense that the patient strives for some sort of order, a kind of predictability and calculability of care (cf. Weber's (1922) 'instrumental rationality'). On the other hand, they have a human aspect in that the patient expects his or her unique situation to be taken into account. Patients' perception of quality of care may be considered from four dimensions: the medical-technical competence of the caregivers, the physical-technical conditions of the care organization, the identity-orientation in the attitudes and actions of the caregivers, and the socio-cultural atmosphere of the care organization. The contents of the dimensions are summarized below. A diagram of the model is given in Figure 2.

The resource structure of the care organization

	Person-related Qualities	Qualities related to the physical and administrative care environment
The patient's preferences — Rationality	Medical-technical competence	Physical-technical conditions
The patient's preferences — Humanity	Identity-oriented approach	Socio-cultural atmosphere

Figure 2. Model of quality of care from the patient's perspective. Reproduced from Wilde, Starrin, Larsson & Larsson (1993) by kind permission of the Blackwell Science LTD

Medical-technical competence. When the patient's desire for rational care is directed towards the person-related qualities of the care organization, he or she wants those who provide the care to have a high level of 'medical-technical competence.' Rationality implies the availability of qualified personnel with knowledge and proficiency to guarantee that the patient is given a relevant examination, that the correct diagnosis is made, and the necessary measures are taken to effectively treat and alleviate the effects of the disease. Rational care for the patient means that caregivers are available – that one can count on being received and treated by caregivers who are medically-technically competent.

Physical-technical conditions. When the patients' desire for rational care is directed towards the physical and administrative qualities of the care organization, it is a question of the availability of a care organization which can provide the necessary 'physical-technical conditions.' Rationality in this respect means that the patient can count on the hospital, the ward, and the room to provide necessary physical-technical resources for the cure and care he or she is in need of. The rational aspect lies in the fact that the environment is clean, comfortable, and safe, and that good sanitary conditions, food and drink are available, as well as advanced medical-technical equipment.

Identity-oriented approach. Patients' desire for care with a human face in relation to the caregivers is a question of an 'identity-oriented approach.' Humanity in care presupposes that there are qualified caregivers with the knowledge and emphatic skill to meet the patients as unique individuals. The human aspect means that the caregiver shows an interest in and commitment to the patient as a person, i.e., in who the unique person is, what he or she wants and what his or her needs are, and that the caregiver reveals his or her own feelings and sympathy for the patient. Humanity implies a symmetrical relationship between patient and caregiver which is characterized by mutual understanding, respect, trust, honesty, and collaboration.

Socio-cultural atmosphere. Patients' desires for a humane physical-administrative care environment implies requests to what could be labelled the 'socio-cultural atmosphere' of the care environment. A humane environment is one which, as far as possible, resembles a home rather than an institution, one where the patient has the opportunity for self-chosen seclusion and/or self-chosen socializing whenever he or she wishes. Furthermore, it is an environment with a convivial atmosphere.

Operationalization of the Model

The theoretical model mentioned above was operationalized into the questionnaire QPP consisting of 56 items and 17 factors using a conventional factor analytical approach (Wilde et al., 1994). In order to further develop the instrument, a dimensional analysis of all items was performed using structural equation modeling. The result of the dimensional analysis was a model consisting of a general factor and 22 subordinate, residual factors measured by 68 items (some new items were derived from the original patient interviews and pilot tested (Larsson, Wilde Larsson & Munck, 1998). A short version of the QPP consisting of 24 items has also been developed (Wilde Larsson & Larsson, 2002).

Each quality dimension is surveyed with a number of questions expressed in two different ways. Firstly, the person has to assess what quality is actually like with regard to the content of the question, and secondly an assessment is made of how important the content of the question is to him or her.

To measure perceived reality of quality of care, each item is related to the sentence "This is what I experienced...." (for instance, I had good opportunity to participate in decisions regarding my medical care). On this evaluation a 4-point response scale ranging from 1 (Do not agree at all) to 4 (Fully agree) has been used.

The second kind of evaluation concerns the subjective importance the person ascribes to the various aspects of care. Here, each sentence is related to the statement "This is how important it was to me..." (for instance, I had good opportunity to participate in decisions regarding my medical care). A 4-point response scale ranging from 1 (Of little or no importance) to 4 (Of the very highest importance) has been used.

Factor and dimension scores are calculated by summing the raw scores on the items representing the dimension and dividing the sum by the number of items in the scale. Cronbach alphas on the scales have varied across different investigations but tend to range between .70 to .90.

EMPIRICAL FINDINGS - ELDERLY PEOPLE

Quality of care among elderly persons has been studied in several investigations using the QPP-questionnaire. In this section results from four of these studies conducted in Sweden will be presented (Wilde et al., 1995 (Study A); Larsson & Wilde Larsson, 1998 (Study B); Wilde Larsson, 1999 (Study C); Wilde Larsson, Larsson & Starrin, 1999 (Study D). Data were collected by way of personal interviews, structured from the QPP-questionnaire (Study A and B), and questionnaires (Study C and D). In these four studies the QPP-questionnaire consisted of 17 factors covering the four QPP dimensions.

Care Contexts and Participants

In study A, the sample consisted of 428 elderly persons (66-69 years, 70-79 years, 80-89 years, and 90 years or older) in the following four care environments in two Swedish cities: a geriatric department, persons receiving home nursing, nursing homes, and a service home.

In study B the sample consisted of 154 elderly persons (66-75 years 26%, 76-85 years 45%, and 86 years or older 297%) receiving home care in a medium-sized Swedish municipality. All people lived in their own homes or in service homes. The sample in study C consisted of 1056 persons in medical and surgical departments of three county hospitals in Sweden. Their distribution across different age groups was as follows: 16-45 years, 46-65 years, 66-75 years, and 76 year or older. In study D the sample consisted of 831 patients at two Swedish county hospitals. Their distribution across different age groups was as follows: 16-55 years, 56-70 years, and 71 year or older.

Overall Findings

A selection of the results of study A are presented in Table 2.

Highest ratings on the perceived reality scales (in study A and B) were observed for factors designed to measure the medical-technical competence of the caregivers and the physical-technical conditions of the care environment. Factors designed to measure the degree of the identity-oriented in the attitudes and actions of the caregivers received considerably lower ratings. From the perspective of the health care system, the results on the two first mentioned quality of care dimensions seem to be satisfactory, while findings on the interpersonal dimension suggest a need for improvement in the health care and welfare system in these areas. Previous studies indicate that the broad field of care is at least as important as cure for many elderly people (Marshall, 1981; Samuelsson, Ingvad & Edebalk, 1993)

Table 2. Elderly peoples' perception of quality of care (N=428)

Dimension and Factors	Perceived reality [a]		Subjective importance [b]	
	M	SD	M	SD
MEDICAL-TECHNICAL COMPETENCE				
Medical care	3.43	0.91	2.40	0.79
Physical caring	3.34	0.72	2.09	0.68
PHYSICAL-TECHNICAL CONDITIONS				
Care room characteristics	3.30	0.70	2.61	0.46
Care equipment	3.65	0.49	2.68	0.38
Personal necessities	2.83	0.58	2.05	0.46
IDENTITY-ORIENTED APPROACH				
Being personal	3.25	0.79	2.49	0.51
Trust and understanding	3.18	0.79	2.52	0.51
Mental preparation	3.17	0.86	2.26	0.65
Sympathy	2.89	1.10	2.30	0.72
Interest in psychological situation	2.68	1.13	2.30	0.71
Commitment	2.63	1.19	2.33	0.70
Participation	2.46	0.91	2.01	0.67
Interest in view-of-life	1.61	0.98	1.50	0.69
SOCIO-CULTURAL ATMOSPHERE				
Positive treatment of significant other	3.69	0.60	2.32	0.69
General atmosphere and home-like environment	3.21	0.63	2.37	0.41
Meaningful occupation/personal belongings	3.13	0.64	2.21	0.52
Secluded environment not directed by routines	3.13	0.64	2.22	0.43

[a] Scale scores could range from 1 (least favorable evaluation) to 4 (most favorable evaluation).

[b] Scale scores could range from 1 (least importance) to 3 (most importance)

Most of the measured aspects of care were regarded as important (in study A and B). Highest scores on subjective importance were observed on the scales designed to measure care equipment and care room characteristics. This may be due to the fact that physical-technical conditions often have a direct impact on the daily living of elderly people. The results differ slightly from the conclusions drawn by Cryns, Nicholos, Katz and Calkins (1989) who, after reviewing the literature, observed that elderly persons tend to regard the affective components of care as most important. One issue, the caregivers' interest in patients' view-of-life, received much lower subjective importance than the other aspects. A possible reason is that Sweden may be one of the most secularized countries, and most people do not associate these aspects with care.

Subgroup Comparisons

Comparisons between subgroups of participants were made on the following *person-related characteristics*: age, gender, and self-rated psychological well-being, and on one *context-related aspect:* care environment. The results of the subgroup comparisons are presented in Table 3.

In reference to subgroup differences within the group of elderly people (Study A), personal characteristics such as age, gender, and self-rated psychological well-being, were found to have limited effect on reports of what were regarded as highly important care characteristics. Findings on the subjective importance scales suggest that there exists a uniform norm or value hierarchy regarding quality of care among elderly persons across these different personal characteristics.

Age-related comparisons of patients' perceptions of the care they actually received indicated increasingly more positive evaluations with increasing age. This is consistent with most previous studies (Hall & Dornan, 1990; Rosenheck, Wilson & Meterko, 1997). The lack of age-related differences on the subjective importance ratings contradict the popular view that older people make lower demands on care (cf. Rosenheck, Wilson & Meterko, 1997). The result suggests that there exists a transgenerational shared norm on what is, and what is not, important in care settings. The result is in accordance with those presented by Rosenheck, Wilson and Meterko (1997), and by Ross, Steward and Sincore (1993).

Gender-related comparisons on evaluation of actual care received, yielded virtually no differences. This result is consistent with most previous studies (Carmel, 1985; Carr-Hill, 1992; Hall & Dornan, 1990).

A possible explanation for the gender differences in the ratings of the subjective importance is that women tend to rate the importance of health somewhat higher than men do (Cahalnan, Cisnin & Crossley, 1969; Verbrugge, 1982). Women also make more visits to physicians than men (Verbrugge, 1985; Waldron, 1983a; Wyke, Hunt & Ford, 1998) and, for a given physiological condition, tend to rate their own health more unfavourable than men (Waldron, 1983a, 1983b). Given this combination, it seems logical that women assign higher subjective importance ratings to various care conditions than do men.

Table 3. Quality of care in relation to person and context related aspects

Person-related aspects	Study	Sample	Quality of Care	
			Perceived reality [a]	Subjective importance [a]
Age	Study A Wilde et al., 1995	N= 428 4 different care environments (nursing home, home nursing, geriatric department and service home) in 2 cities. 60-69 Yr = 8% 70-79 Yr = 24% 80-89 Yr = 51% > 90 Yr = 17%	Significant differences on 4 scales [a]. Persons in the oldest age group had lower means on three of these scales (2 IO and 1 SC), and persons in the youngest age group had lower on one (PT) scales.	Significant differences on 2 (1 PT and 1 IO) scales [a]. The SI decrease with increasing age.
	Study C Wilde Larsson 1999	N=1056 Medical and surgical departments in 3 county hospitals 16-45 Yr = 15% 46-65 Yr = 32% 66-75 Yr = 30% > 76 Yr = 23%	Significant differences on all 4 quality dimensions (MT, PT, IO and SC). On 3 dimensions (MT, IO and SC) none of the pare-wise comparisons between age groups were statistically significant.	Significant differences on 1 (PT) quality dimension (out of 4). Pair-wise comparisons between age groups on the PT dimension were statistically non-significant.

Table 3. Quality of care in relation to person and context related aspects (Continued)

Person-related aspects	Study	Sample	Quality of Care	
			Perceived reality [a]	Subjective importance [a]
Gender	Study A	$N = 428$ Male = 29% Female =71%	No statistically significant difference	Female participants had significantly higher scores on 1 (SC) scale [a].
	Study D Wilde Larsson, Larsson & Starrin, 1999	N=831 Male = 52% Female =48% Medical and surgical departments in 2 county hospitals 16-55 Yr =30% 56-70 Yr =34% > 71 Yr =36%	Women scored significant higher on 1 (PT) scales [a].	Women scored significant higher on 13 (2 MT, 8 IO and 3 SC) scales [a].

Table 3. Quality of care in relation to person and context related aspects (Continued)

Person-related aspects	Study	Sample	Quality of Care	
			Perceived reality [a]	Subjective importance [a]
Psychological well-being	Study A	N=428 More favorable = 73 % Less favorable = 27 %	Significant differences on 12 scales [a]. These scales representing all 4 dimensions of the model with a dominance of the PT and IO scales. Persons with a more favorable psychological well-being scored higher.	Significant differences on 2 (1 MT and 1 SC) scales [a]. Persons with less favorable psychological well-being scored higher.
Context related aspects				
Care environment	Study A	N= 428 Nursing homes =26% Home nursing = 26 % Geriatric department =12 % Service home = 36%	Significant differences on 14 scales [a]. Participants on service homes and geriatric department tend to score lower. The latter group does this on PT and SC scales particular.	Significant differences on 14 scales [a]. The overall pattern is that persons living in service homes reported lower mea scores, particularly on the scales representing MT dimension.

MT = Medical- technical competence, PT = Physical-technical conditions, IO =Identity-oriented approach, SC =Socio-cultural atmosphere, PR=Perceived reality, SI =Subjective importance, [a] out of 17 scales

Elderly persons with a favourable self-rating of their *psychological well-being* perceived the actual care conditions considerably more positively compared with those with an unfavourable psychological well-being. The result is consistent with previous studies (Samuelsson, Invad & Edebalk, 1993). One possible interpretation is that favourable perceptions of the quality of care caused favourable well-being reports, and vice versa. However, drawing on previous findings, the opposite interpretation seems more likely. Thus, Hall, Milburen and Epstein (1993) conclude that there is no evidence that patients' satisfaction with the care determines later levels of health, while evidence does indicate that health status may influence satisfaction with care. The latter direction of causality was also supported in a study of the relationships between psychiatric symptoms and general life satisfaction on the one hand, and satisfaction with care on the other (LeVois, Nguyen & Atkinson, 1981). If one equates unfavourable psychological well-being with the concept of negative affectivity, these results are consistent with studies showing that low mood state tends to affect a person's perception and ratings of how things are (Golant, 1982; Linn & Greenfield, 1982; Watson & Pennebaker, 1989). In the absence of conclusive prospective studies, however, the door should be left open for a third possible interpretation, where bidirectional causality could exist between ratings of well-being and quality of care.

The type of *care environment* appeared to affect the responses strongly. A possible explanation is that the different types of care environments are connected with different kinds of expectations and needs, and that these differences in turn affect ratings of subjective importance and perceived reality (Samuelsson, Invad & Edebalk, 1993). Through selective perception and socialization processes, such expectations may be strengthened during a person's stay in the particular care environment.

EMPIRICAL FINDINGS – SIMILARITIES AND DIFFERENCES BETWEEN ELDERLY PEOPLE, THEIR FAMILY MEMBERS, AND CAREGIVERS

Similarities and differences between elderly persons, their family members, and caregivers respectively, have been examined in several studies using the QPP-questionnaire. In this section, results from three of these studies, conducted in Sweden, will be presented. Study E (Larsson & Wilde Larsson, 1998) focusing on elderly persons and their caregivers, Study F (Wilde Larsson, Larsson & Rizell Carlson, 2004) focusing on elderly persons and their family members and study G (Wilde, Larsson & Bredberg, 1994) focusing on the elderly person, their family members, and caregivers (contact assistant nurses and assistant nurses). Data were collected by way of personal interviews structured from the QPP questionnaire (elderly persons) and questionnaires (family members and caregivers). In these studies the QPP questionnaire consisted of items covering the four QPP dimensions.

Care Contexts and Participants

In study E the sample consisted of 151 elderly persons and 151 caregivers (assistant nurses) The elderly persons (66-75 years 26%, 76-85 years 45%, 86 years or older 29%) were receiving home care in a medium-sized Swedish municipality. Two-thirds were women. All of these elderly people lived in their own homes or in service homes. The caregivers were employed by the social welfare agency of the municipality. Ninety per cent were women. Their distribution across different age groups was as follows: 25 years or younger 15%, 26-50 years 49%, 51 year or older 36%.

The sample in study F consisted of 67 patients (mean age 66 years, $SD = 13$) receiving advanced home care in Sweden and 82 family members (the person the patient had reported as his or her closest family member) (60 years, $SD = 13$). From these 54 matched pairs of patient and family members were found. Approximately two-thirds of the family members were married to the patient, 15% were children of the patient, and the remaining were other family members. Among the 82 family members, 58 had met the patient every day during the last month, 13 met the patients several times per week, and 11 met him ore her once a week or less often.

The sample in study G consisted of four groups of participants. The first group consisted of 85 elderly persons (69 years or younger13%, 70- 79 years 31%, 80-89 years 45%, and 90 year or older 11%), 60% were women. The second group comprised of 35 family members (the person the patient had reported as his or her closest family member) (69 years or younger 77%, 70-79 years 18%, 80-89 years 6%), 53% were women. The third group consisted of 81 caregivers in charge (contact assistant nurses) and the forth group of 71 caregivers (assistant nurses). The elderly persons were receiving home care in a medium-sized Swedish municipality. The caregivers were employed by the social welfare agency of the municipality.

Overall Findings

Looking at the ratings of perceived reality regarding the quality of care, the elderly persons (study E) reported more favourable scores than the caregivers on most of the scales designed to measure the medical-technical competence of the caregivers, and the physical-technical conditions and socio-cultural atmosphere of the care environment. This is consistent with previous research showing that caretakers or patients generally evaluate care more positively than caregivers (van Campen et al., 1995).

On the scales designed to measure the caregivers' identity-oriented approach, a mixed picture emerged. The elderly persons had significantly more favourable ratings on two of these scales, Being personal and Trust and understanding. However, on two other scales, Commitment and Participation, as well as on the aggregated dimension scale, the caregivers reported significantly higher ratings. The two former scales appear to reflect a more personal warm-cold characteristic of the caregiver. The two latter scales appear to be more action-oriented and reflect more learned characteristics of the caregiver. Comparable research among people with disabilities indicates that caregivers tend to overestimate the caretakers possibility to participate in planning and decision making regarding their care (Ritchardson, 1969).

On ratings on the various items' subjective importance to the elderly person, the caregivers consistently scored higher than the elderly persons. One possible explanation is that caregivers hereby attempt to legitimize their own professional identity and actions (cf. Nygren, 1978). From the elderly persons' point of view, it may be that although the measured care components are important, some of them are not that important and there are many other things in life which are more highly valued.

The elderly persons generally rated the interpersonal aspects of care as being less important than the medical-technical and physical-technical aspects. This is consistent with previous studies (von Essen, 1994, Wilde et al., 1995).

In a context of advanced home care (study F), patients and their close family members perceived the quality of care in a similar way. Regarding evaluation of the subjective importance ascribed to the different aspects of care, close family members appeared to overestimate the importance of medical-technical aspects when compared with the ratings given by the patients themselves. Patients and family members gave the softer side of care almost identical importance ratings.

In study G, the following two conditions emerge in a comparison of responses from the four different groups. The first is that each group demonstrates a similar ranking of the four quality dimensions surveyed. With one exception, satisfaction is greatest within all groups with quality of health care regarding the medical-technical competence of staff and the physical technical conditions in geriatric care. These are followed by evaluations of the socio-cultural atmosphere in health care. Satisfaction scores were lowest for the staff's identity-oriented approach. The second condition that emerges when comparing the four groups are the tangible differences between them. The general pattern is that two groups – the patients receiving treatment and nursing care as well as the contact staff – clearly show great satisfaction with the treatment and nursing care. Members of staff who judged the quality of municipal (local authority) geriatric care generally demonstrated values that are comparable with those of patients' families. However, they tend to be more negative than the contact staff. The differences are statistically significant between the groups.

The results in study G show significant differences between the elderly persons', the family members', and the two groups of staffs' views on quality of care. This raises the questions: Who is right? Who can be trusted?

One reason why patients receiving treatment and nursing care and contact staff's estimates can be seen as right, is that probably no one can judge this better than these two groups. In accordance with this explanation, the lower estimates given by patients' families can also partly be understood as an expression of the families' own sense of guilt that they cannot help the patients themselves – thus, in psychological terms, it is a projection to alleviate feelings of guilt.

One reason why the patients' families, and the staff who have judged geriatric care in general terms, can be regarded as right, is that it is easier for them to make a factual evaluation from their objective (external) position. Patients themselves can be described as being in a dependant position and perhaps do not dare express their opinions freely. Another possible reason for patients keeping their criticism to themselves could be wanting to hurt the feelings of staff – a risk that most likely increases in health care situations where the staff and the patient know each other well. Staff who evaluate their own help may naturally be assumed to be reluctant to award themselves substandard marks.

Summing up, there are clearly arguments for and against the response patterns shown by various groups. Whose perception of reality is true? In a way, perhaps they all are. A common saying in psychology is that "truth is in the eye of the beholder." You can hardly say that one of the groups is right and another is wrong from the surveys conducted. Each group gives evaluations from different starting points – the truth is in the eye of the beholder. The overall interpretation of the results is as follows: seeing as the goal of geriatric care is primarily that the elderly are to be well cared for, the most important and "truest" result is the one obtained from the elderly people themselves.

Subgroup Comparisons

Several subgroup comparisons have been reported in a number of studies. Here, two of them will be described and discussed. The first concerns the amount of help the elderly person received. The second concerns comparisons of elderly persons' ratings and family members' ratings with focus on family members who see the patient daily and family members who see the patient once a week or less often.

Regarding the first issue, separate comparisons were performed within each of the following amount–of–help categories: less often than once a day, once a day and two or more times a day (Study E). Within the subsamples where the elderly person received help once a day or less often, the result fairly similar to the one obtained in the whole sample. However, when comparisons between elderly persons and caregivers were performed within the subset of elderly persons who received help at least twice a day, a different pattern emerged. Compared to the whole sample, considerably fewer differences between elderly persons - caregivers are statistically significant within the subsample consisting of home care users who receive help at least twice a day. One reason for the high similarities could be that these caregiver-caretaker couples see each other often, and therefore get know each other better (Larsson & Wilde Larsson, 1998).

Regarding the second issue, the subgroup analysis shows that family members who saw the patient every day had more favourable scores than family members who saw the patient once a week or less often on all ratings (Study G). On the items measuring the medical-technical competence of the caregivers, family members who saw the patient every day had significantly more favourable scores on 4 items (out of 5) on the perceived reality ratings, and on two items (out of 5) on the subjective importance ratings. The difference was statistically significant for 9 items (out of 16) measuring perceived reality, and for 13 (out of 16) measuring subjective importance on the items designed to map the identity-oriented approach of the caregivers (Wilde Larsson, Larsson & Rizell Carlson) .

In study F, the high degree of perceptual congruence between the caretakers and their family member contradicts most previous research that tends to find more critical voices from family members. The authors suggest that the differences can be attributed to contextual factors. In the advanced home care environment, the patient and his or her close family member typically share the same everyday experiences. The family member may see the caregivers as often as the patient does. Both parties receive the same information on the care process and get to know the caregivers personally. This result can be interpreted in the light of writings on empathic accuracy (Ickes &Tooke, 1988). It has been shown that emphatic precision increases if you know the other person well, including actual length of cohabitation (Bernieri et al., 1994; Marangoni & Ickes, 1995). Shared experiences of the care episode would also appear to be important, particularly in cases where the needs of care vary greatly from day to day. In institutional care settings the opportunities for family members to develop this care domain specific emphatic accuracy is usually limited.

Two additional arguments will be given aiming to support the contextual hypothesis. The first is derived from the outcome of the subgroup analyses in study F. Considerable differences were observed between family members who had met the patient every day during the last month and those who met the patient once a week or less often. The values reported by "the seldom" group are more in accordance with previous research (Wilde Larsson, Larsson, & Rizell Carlson, 2004).

The related argument draws on study G and another study also with the same instrument (adults with learning difficulties; Larsson & Wilde Larsson, 2001). In these studies, one subgroup of caregivers rated the quality of care they gave to a specific care recipient, while another subgroup of caregivers rated the overall quality of care provided in the municipality. The first group of caregivers gave ratings of the quality of care that were very similar to ratings given by their specific care recipient. These caregivers, had detailed knowledge of the care actually given and of the specific patient. The caregivers who made general assessments tended to be more critical.

In conclusion, the reported results suggest that family members as well as caregivers are heterogeneous groups and that generalizations should be done with care. The same holds true for different kinds of care contexts.

SUMMARY OF RESULTS AND FURTHER RESEARCH

- Quality of care is a relative concept.
- Elderly people, their family members, as well as their caregivers, are heterogeneous groups and generalizations should be done with care.
- Patients' views on the quality of care are congruent with the opinions of the family members if they meet every day (live together) and share the same care-related experiences.
- The relationship between quality of care and psychological well-being in elderly people need to be better understood. Further research needs to include a broader spectrum of psychological characteristics, such as personality, sense of coherence, and other instruments designed to measure negative and positive affectivity. From a practical quality enhancement point of view, it seems to be crucial to know if a given quality evaluation mainly reflects the actual conditions of care, or is more an expression of a general psychological state of the person.
- There is a need for further studies illuminating the reasons why men and women tend to assign different subjective importance to different care aspects.

- There is a need for further studies illuminating the reasons why elderly people in various care environments tend to assign different scores on perceived reality scales as well as on the subjective importance scales to different care aspects.

REFERENCES

Adams, N., Ravey, J., & Taylor, D. (1996). Psychological models of chronic pain and implications for practice. *Physiotherapy, 82*, 124-129.

Aharony, L., & Strasser, S. (1993). Patient satisfaction: What we know about it, what we still need to explore. *Medical Care Review, 50*, 49-80.

American Geriatric Society, AGS panel on chronic pain in older persons. (1998). The management of chronic pain in older persons (Clinical practice guidelines). *Journal of American Geriatric Society, 46*, 635-651.

Andersson, M. (1989) Drugs prescribed for elderly patients in nursing homes or under medical home care. *Comprehensive Gerontology* [A], *3*, 8-15.

Anderson, M. J., Anderson, L. J., & Felsenthal, G. (1993). Pastoral needs and support within an inpatient rehabilitation unit. *American Academy of Physical Medicine and Rehabilitation, 74*, 574-578.

Antonovsky, A. (1979). *Health, stress and coping.* San Fransisco: Jossey-Bass Publishers.

Antonovsky, A. (1987). *Unraveling the mystery of health.* San Fransisco: Jossey-Bass Publishers.

Arnetz, J. E., & Arnetz, B. (1996). The development and application of a patient satisfaction measurement system for hospital-wide quality improvement. *International Journal for Quality in Health Care, 8*, 555-566.

Bauer, T. & Barron, C. R. (1995). Nursing interventions for spiritual care. *Journal of Holistic Nursing, 13*, 268-279.

Bauld, L., Chesterman, J., & Judge, K. (2000). Measuring satisfaction with social care amongst older service user: issues from the literature. *Health and Social Care in the Community, 8*, 316-324.

Bergbom-Engberg, I., Hallenberg, B., Wickström, I., & Haljamäe, H. (1988). A retrospective study of patients' recall of respirator treatment (1): Study design and basic findings. *Intensive Care Nursing, 4*, 56-61.

Bergbom-Engberg, I. & Haljamäe, H. (1989). Assessment of patients' experience of discomfort during respirator therapy. *Critical Care Medicine, 17*, 1068-1072.

Bergman, R., & Golander, H. (1982). Evaluation of care for the aged: A multipurpose guide. *Journal of Advanced Nursing, 7*, 203-210.

Berleen, G. (2003). Bättre hälsa hos äldre! Stockholm: Statens folkhälsoinstitut. Rapport nr 41. (In Swedish).

Bernieri, F. J., Zuckerman M., Koestner, R., & Rosenthal R. (1994). Measuring person accuracy: Another look at self other agreement. *Personality & Social Psychology Bulletin, 20*, 367-378.

Björkman, T., & Lundqvist, K. (1981*.) Från MAX till PIA: reformstrategier inom arbetsmiljöområde.* Malmö: Arkiv avhandlingsserie. (In Swedish).

Blomgren, E. (1984). *Är det bra om 54 % tycker att det är bra? Att beskriva levnadsvillkor genom intervju och enkät.* Stockholm: Report from the Swedish National Defence Research Institute C 55065-H3. (In Swedish).

Boeke, S., Duivenvoorden, H. J., Verhage, F., & Zwaveling, A. (1991). Prediction of postoperative pain and duration of hospitalization using two anxiety measures. *Pain, 45,* 293-297.

Boldy, D., & Grenade, L. (1998). *Seeking the consumer view in residential age facilities: A practical guide.* Perth, Australia: Department of health policy and management, Curtin University of Technology.

Bond S., & Thomas L. E. (1992). Measuring patient's satisfaction with nursing care. *Journal of Advanced. Nursing, 17,* 52-63.

Bonica, J. J. (1990). *The management of pain.* Philadelphia: Lea & Febiger,.

Brattberg, G. (1995). *Att möta långvarig smärta.* Stockholm: Almqvist & Wiksell Medicin, Liber utbildning. (In Swedish).

Brattberg, G., Parker, MG. & Thorslund, M. (1996). The prevalence of pain among the oldest old in Sweden. *Pain, 67,* 29-34.

Brattberg, G., Parker, M.G., & Thorslund, M. (1997). A longitudinal study of pain: reported pain from middle age to old age. *The Clinical Journal of Pain, 13,* 144-149.

Broadhead, E., Kaplan, B., James, S., Wagner, V., Schoenbach, V., Grimson, R., Heyden, S., Tibblin, G., & Gehlbach, S. (1983). The epidemiologic evidence for a relationship between social support and health. *American Journal of Epidemiology, 117,* 521-537.

Burke, M. J., Breif, A. P., & George, J. M. (1993). The role of negative affectivity in understanding relations between self-reports of stressors and strains: A comment on the applied psychology literature. *Journal of Applied Psychology, 78,* 402-412.

Cahalnan, D., Cisnin I., & Crossley , H. (1969*). A national study of drinking behaviour and attitudes.* New Haven: College & University Press.

Calnan, M. (1988a). Towards a conceptual framework of lay evaluation of health care. *Social Science & Medicine,* 27, 927-933.

Calnan, M. (1988b). Lay evaluation of medicine and medical practice: A report of a pilot study. *International Journal of Health Sciences, 18,* 311-322.

Carmel, S. (1985). Satisfaction with hospitalization: A comparative analysis of three types of services. *Social Sciences and Medicine, 21,* 1243-1249.

Carmel, S., & Bernstein, J. (1989). Trait - anxiety and sense of coherence: A longitudinal study. *Psychological Reports, 65,* 221-222.

Carr, E. C. J. (1990). Postoperative pain: Patients' expectations and experiences. *Journal of Advanced Nursing, 15,* 89-100.

Carr-Hill, R. A. (1992). The measurement of patient satisfaction. *Journal of Public Health Medicine, 14,* 236-249.

Chamberlein, K., Petrie, K., & Azariah, R. (1992). The role of optimism and sense of coherence in predicting recovery following surgery. *Psychology and Health, 7,* 301-310.

Chesterman, J., Bauld, L., & Judge, K. (2001). Satisfaction with care-managed support of older people: an empirical analyses. *Health and Social Care in the Community, 9,* 31-42.

Cleary, P. D., & McNeal, B. J. (1988). Patient satisfaction as an indicator of quality of care. *Inquiry, 25,* 25-36.

Clearly, P. D., & Edgmam-Levitan, S. (1997). Health care quality. Incorporation consumer perspectives. *Journal of American Medical Association, 278,*1608-1612.

Closs, J. (1992). Postoperative patients' views of sleep, pain and recovery. *Journal of Clinical Nursing, 1,* 83-88.

Closs, S. J. (1994). Pain in elderly patients: a neglected phenomenon? *Journal of Advanced Nursing, 19,* 1072-1018.

Closs, J., Fairtlough, H., Tierney, A. & Currie, C. (1993). Pain in elderly orthopaedic patients. *Journal of Clinical Nursing, 2,* 41-45.

Cochran, J. & Ganong, L. H. (1989). A comparison of nurses' and patients' perceptions of intensive care unit stressors. *Journal of Advanced Nursing, 14,* 1038-1043.

Cornock, M.A. (1998). Stress and the intensive care patient: perceptions of patients and nurses. *Journal of Advanced Nursing, 27,* 518-527.

Cramer, G. W. Galer, B. S., Mendelson, M. A. & Thompson, G. D. (2000). A drug use evaluation of selected opiod and nonopiod analgesics in the nursing facility setting. *Journal of American Geriatrics Society, 48,* 398-404.

Crook, J., Rideout, E., & Browne, G. (1984). The prevalence of pain complaints in a general population. *Pain, 18*: 299-314.

Cryns, A. G., Nicholos, R. F. G., Katz, L. A., & Calkins, E. (1989). The hierarchical structure of geriatric patient satisfaction: An older patient satisfaction scale designed for HMOSs. *Medical Care, 27,* 802-816.

Davies, A. R., & Ware, J. E. (1988). Involving consumers in quality of care assessment. *Health Affairs, 7,* 33-48.

Donabedian, A. (1966). Evaluating the quality of medical care. *Milbank Memorial Fund Quarterly, 44,* 106-206.

Donabedian, A. (1980). *The Definition of Quality and Approaches to its Assessment.* Ann Arbor, Michigan: Health Administration Press.

Donabedian, A. (1985). Twenty years of research on the quality of medical care 1964-1984. *Evaluation & Health Professions, 3,* 243-265.

Donabedian, A. (1988). The quality of care: How can it be assessed? *Journal of Medicine Association, 260,* 1743-1747.

Donabedian, A. (1989). Institutional and professional responsibilities in quality assurance. *Quality Assurance in Health Care, 11,* 3-11.

Donovan, M. I. (1990). Acute pain relief. *Nursing Clinics of North America, 25,* 851-861.

Edberg, A-K. (1999). *The nurse-patient encounter and the patients' state: effects of individual care and clinical group supervision in dementia care.* Doctoral thesis. The Centre of Caring Sciences and Department of Psychogeriatrics, Department of Clinical Neuroscience, Lund: Lund University.

Edebalk, P. G., Ingvad, B., & Lannerheim, I. (1990*). Kvalitetsegenskapernas relativa betydelse i hemtjänsten en pilotstudie.* Lund, Sweden: Gerontologisk centrum. Rapport 90 IV:4. (In Swedish).

Egan, K. J. (1989). Psychological issues in postoperative pain. *Anesthesiology Clinics of North America, 7,* 183-192.

Elpern, E. H., Patterson, P. A., Gloskey, D., & Bone, R. C. (1992). Patients' preferences for intensive care. *Critical Care Medicine, 20,* 43-47.

Eriksen, L. R. (1995). Patient satisfaction with nursing care: Concept clarification. *Journal of Nursing Measurement, 3*, 59-76.

Eriksson, K. (1991). Att lindra lidande. In K. Eriksson & A. Barbosa da Silva.*Vårdteologi* (Eds.), Finland: Reports from the Department of Caring Sciences nr. 3. Åbo Akademi. (In Swedish).

Feldt, K. S., & Oh, H. L. (2000). Pain and hip fracture outcomes. *Orthopaedic Nursing, 19*, 35-44.

Festinger, L. A. (1957). *A theory of cognitive dissonance.* New York: Row & Peterson.

Field, L. (1996). Are nurses still underestimating patients' pain postoperatively? *British Journal of Nursing, 5*, 778-784.

Finer, B. (1984). *Att leva med kronisk smärta.* Stockholm: Bokförlaget Prisma. (In Swedish).

Forsell, Y., Jorm, A. F., & Winblad, B. (1994). Outcome of depression in demented and non-demented elderly: Observations from a three-year follow-up in a community based study. *International Journal of Geriatric Psychiatry, 9*, 5-10.

Frankenhauser, M. (1986). A psychobiological framework for research on human stress and coping. In M. H. Appley & R. Trumbull (Eds.), *Dynamics of stress: Physiological, psychological, and social perspectives.* New York: Plenum.

Frankl, V. (1974). *Livet måste ha en mening.* Stockholm: Aldus Bonniers. (In Swedish).

Frankl, V. (1986). *Viljan till mening.* Stockholm: Natur och Kultur, (In Swedish).

French, K. (1981). Methodological considerations in hospital patient opinion surveys. *International Journal of Nursing Studies, 18*, 7-32.

Gamsa,, A. (1994). The role of psychological factors in chronic pain. *Pain, 57*, 5-15.

Geron, S. M. (1999). *The Home Care Satisfaction Measure (HCSM),* Boston, Massachusetts: Boston University School and Social Work.

Gillies, M. L., Smith, L. N., & Parry-Jones W. L. I. (1999). Postoperative pain assessment and management in adolescents. *Pain, 79*: 207-215.

Glaser, B. G. (1978). *Theoretical sensitivity.* San Francisco: The Sociological Press.

Golant, S. M. (1982). Individual differences underlying the dwelling satisfaction of the elderly. *Journal of Social Issues, 38*, 121-133.

Haegerstam, G. (1996). *Multidimensionell syn..* Södertälje, Sweden: Astra läkemedel. (In Swedish).

Hall, A. & Dornan, M. (1988). Meta-analysis of satisfaction with medical care: Description of research domain and analysis of overall satisfaction levels. *Social Science & Medicine, 28*, 637-644.

Hall, J. A., & Dornan, M. C. (1990). Patient sociodemographic characteristics as predictors of satisfaction with medical care: A meta- analysis. *Social Science & Medicine, 30*, 811-818.

Hall, J., Milburen, M., & Epstein, A. (1993). A casual model of health and satisfaction with medical care. *Medical Care, 31*, 84-94.

Hall-Lord, ML., Johansson, I., Schmidt, I., & Wilde Larsson, B. (2003a). Family members' perceptions of pain and distress related to analgesics and psychotropic drugs, and quality of care of elderly nursing home residents. *Health and Social Care in the Community, 11*, 262-274.

Hall-Lord, ML., Larsson, G., & Boström, I. (1994). Elderly patients' experiences of pain and distress in intensive care: A grounded theory study. *Intensive and Critical Care Nursing, 10*, 133-144.

Hall-Lord, ML., Larsson, G., & Steen, B. (1998). Pain and distress among elderly intensive care unit patients: Comparison of patients' experiences and nurses' assessments. *Heart Lung, 27*, 123-132.

Hall-Lord, ML., Larsson, G., & Steen, B. (1999b). Chronic pain and distress in older people: A cluster analysis. *International Journal of Nursing Practice, 5*, 78-85.

Hall-Lord, ML., Larsson, G., & Steen, B. (1999c). Chronic pain and distress among elderly in the community: Comparison of patients' experiences and enrolled nurses' assessments. *Journal of Nursing Management, 7*, 45-54.

Hall-Lord, ML., Steen, B., & Larsson, G. (1999a). Postoperative experiences of pain and distress in elderly patients. An explorative study. *Aging.Clinical Experimental Research, 11*, 73-82.

Hall-Lord, ML., & Wilde Larsson, B. (2003, June). Nurses' assessments of pain and distress in relation to selected patient and nurse characteristics. Poster session presented at the International Council of Nurses, Geneve, Schweiz.

Hall-Lord, ML., Wilde Larsson, B., Bååth, C., Johansson, I. (2003b, October). Pain and distress in elderly patients with hip fracture. Poster session presented at the 3rd European Nursing Congress, Vulnerable groups in society: a nursing issue, Amsterdam, Netherlands.

Hendriks, A. A. (1997). *The construction of the Five-Factor Personality Inventory.* Groningen, Netherlands: Rijksuniversiteit.

Hietanen, H., Krøll-Paulsby, V., Scmidt, L., & Wilde, B. (1993). Syekplieiekvalitet sett fra de nordiske sykepliernas perspektiv. *Vård i Norden, 13*, 4-10.

Hinson Langford, C..P., Bowsher, J., Maloney, J., & Lillis, P. (1997). Social support: A conceptual analysis. *Journal of Advanced Nursing, 25*, 95-100.

IASP. (1979). Subcommittee on taxonomy: Pain terms. A list with definitions and notes on usage. *Pain, 6*, 249-252.

Ickes, W., & Tooke, W. (1988). The observational method: Studying the interaction of minds and bodies. In S. Duck (Ed.), *Handbock of Personal relationship: Theory, Research, and Interventions.* Chichester: John Wiley & Sons.

Johansson, I. (1998*). Quality of care and assessment of health among elderly in acute care.* Doctoral thesis. Linköping: Department of Medicine and Care, Division of Nursing Sciences, Linköping University.

LaMonica, E. L., Oberst, M. T., Madea, A. R., & Wolf, R. M. (1986). Development of a patient satisfaction scale. *Research in Nursing and Health, 9*, 43-50.

Larsen, D. L. Attkinson, C. C., Hargreaves, W. A., & Nguyen, Y. T. D. (1979). Assessment of client/patient satisfaction: development of a general scale. *Evaluation program Planning, 2*, 197-202.

Larsson, P. (1996). *Hemtjänsten ur tre perspektiv: En studie bland äldre, anställda och ledning.* Doctoral thesis. Department of Sociology. Göteborg: University of Gothenbourg. (In Swedish).

Larsson, G., & Wilde Larsson, B. (1998). Quality of care: Relationships between the perceptions of elderly home care users and their caregivers. *Scandinavian Journal of Social Welfare*, *7*, 262-268.

Larsson, G., & Wilde Larsson, B. (2001). Quality of care and service as perceived by adults with developmental disabilities, their parents, and primary caregivers. *Mental Retardation*, *39*, 249-258.

Larsson, G., Wilde Larsson, B., & Munck, I. M. E. (1998). Refinement of the questionnaire 'Quality of care from the Patient's Perspective' using structural equation modelling. *Scandinavian Journal of Caring Sciences*, 12, 111-118.

Lee, R. I. & Jones, R. W. (1933). *The fundamentals of good medical care. Committee on cost of medical care.* Publication 22. The University of Chicago Press.

Lemke, S., & Moos, R. H. (1980). Assessing the institutional policies of sheltered care settings. *Journal of Gerontology*, *35*, 96-107.

Lemke, S., & Moos, R. H. (1981). The suprapersonal environments of sheltered care setting. *Journal of Gerontology*, *36*, 233-243.

Lemke, S., & Moos, R. H. (1986). Quality of residential settings for elderly adults. *Journal of Gerontology*, *41*, 264-276.

Lemke, S., & Moos, R. H. (1987). Measuring the social climate of congregate residents for older people: Sheltered Care Environment Scale. *Psychology and Aging*, *1*, 20-29.

LeVasseur, S. A. & Calder, W. (1994). A comparative descriptive study of patients admitted to a high dependency unit after major and non-major surgery. *Intensive and Critical Care Nursing*, *11*, 66-70.

LeVois, M., Nguyen, T., D., & Atkinson, C. (1981). Artefact in client satisfaction assessment. *Evaluation Program Planning*, *4*, 139-150.

Linn, L. S., & Greenfield, S. (1987). Patient suffering and satisfaction among the chronically ill. *Medical Care*, *20*, 425-431.

Linder-Pelz, S. (1982a) Towards theory of patient satisfaction. *Social Sciences & Medicine*, *16*, 577-582.

Linder-Petz S. (1982b) Social psychological determinants of patient satisfaction: A test of fine hypotheses. *Social Science & Medicine*, *16*, 583-589.

Loeser, J. D. (1982). *Concepts of pain. Chronic Low Back Pain.* (Eds. Stanton-Hicks M. & Boas R.). New York: Raven Press.

Mahon, P. Y. (1996). An analysis of the concept patient satisfaction as it relates to contemporary nursing care. *Journal of Advanced Nursing, 24*, 1241-1248.

Mashall, V. (1981*).* Physician characteristics and relation with older patients. In M. Haug (ed.), *Elderly patients and their doctors.* New York: Springer Publications Company.

Marangoni, C., Gracias., S., Ickes, W., & Teng, G. (1995). Empathic accuracy in a clinical relevant setting. *Journal of Personality and Social Psychology, 68*, 854-869.

McCready, M., MacDavitt, K., & O'Sullivan, K.K. (1991). Children and pain: Easing the hurt. *Orthopaedic Nursing*, *10*, 33-42.

Mc Cullough, L. B., Wilson, N., Teasdale, T., Kolpatechi, A., & Skelly, J. (1993). Mapping personal, family and professional values in log-term care decision. *The Gerontologist*, *33*, 324-332.

Melzack, R. & Wall, P. D. (1965). Pain mechanisms: A new theory. *Science*, *150*, 971-979.

Moos, R. H., & Lemke, S. (1980). Assessing the physical and architectural features of sheltered care settings. *Journal of Gerontology, 35*, 571-583.

Morris DB. (1991). *The culture of pain.* California: University of California Press.

National Board of Health and Welfare. (2002). *Nationell handlingsplan för äldrepolitiken – slutrapport.* Stockhom: Socialstyrelsen. (In Swedish).

Nettleman, M. D. (1998). Patient satisfaction- What is new? *Clinical Performance in Health Care, 6*, 33-37.

Nygren, P. (1978). *Den sociala grammatiken. Mot en kritisk social psykologi.* Lund, Sweden: Esselte studium. (In Swedish).

Orlando, I. J. (1990). *The dynamic nurse-patient relationship. Functions, process and principles.* New York: National League for Nursing.

Parasuraman, A., Zeithalm, V. A., & Berry, L. L. (1985). A conceptual model of service quality and its implications for research. *Journal of Marketing, 49*, 41-50.

Peterson, E.A. (1985). The physical..the spiritual..can you meet all of your patient's needs? *Journal of Gerontological Nursing, 11*, 23-27.

Puntillo, K.A. (1990). Pain experiences of intensive care unit patients. *Heart & Lung, 19*, 526-533.

Pålsson, M-B., Hallberg, IR., Norberg, A. & Björvell, H. (1996). Burnout, empathy and sense of coherence among Swedish district nurses before and after systematic clinical supervision. *Scandinavian Journal of Caring Sciences, 10*, 19-26.

Reerink, E. (1990). Defining quality of care: Mission impossible? *Quality Assurance in Health Care, 2*, 197-202.

Riggio, R. E., Singer, R. D., Hartman, K. (1982). Psychological issues in the care of critically-ill respirator patients: differential perceptions of patients, relatives, and staff. *Psychological Reports, 51*, 363-369.

Rombach, B. M. (1989). *Mätning av servicekvalitet i offentlig sektor. En kritisk granskning av attitydundersökningar i sjukvården* . Stockholm: Rapport från Handelshögskolan i Stockholm. Research Paper 6398. (In Swedish).

Rosenheck, M. D., Wilson, N. J., & Meterko, M. (1997). Influences of patient and hospital factors on consumer satisfaction with inpatient medicin health treatment. *Psychiatric Services, 48*, 1553-1556.

Ross, C. K., Steward, C. A., & Sincore, J. M. (1993). The importance of patient preferences in the measurement of health care satsifaction. *Medical Care, 31*, 1138-1149.

Ross, M. M. & Crook, J. (1998). Elderly recipients of home nursing services: pain, disability and functional competence. *Journal of Advanced Nursing,27*, 117-1126.

Roy, R. & Thomas, M .R. (1987). Elderly persons with and without pain: A comparative study. *The Clinical Journal of Pain, 3*, 102-106.

Rubin H. R., Ware, J. E., & Mayes, R. D. (1990). The PJHQ Questionnaire: exploratory factor analysis and empirical scale constructions. *Medical Care (Supplement), 28*, 22-29.

Samuelson, G., Invad, B., & Edebalk, P. G. (1993). *A method of ranking different quality attributes in home help services: In a consumer perspective. Multi-attributed utility technology.* Report VII:4, Lund, Sweden: Gerontologiskt Centrum.

Sarvimäki, A. & Ojala, S. (1994). De äldres livsbetingelser 2: Känslan av sammanhang. *Gerontologia, 8*: 140-149. (In Swedish).

SCB. (2000). *Äldres levnadsförhållanden 1980-1998*. (In Swedish).

Schmidt, I. & Fastbom, J. (2000). Quality of drug use in Swedish nursing homes. A follow-up study. *Clinical Drug Investigation, 20*, 433-446.

Selye, H. (1985). *The stress of life*. Second edition. New York: McGraw-Hill Book Co..

Seers, K. (1987). Perceptions of pain. *Nursing Times, 83*, 37-39.

Setterlind, S. & Larsson, G. (1995). The stress profile: a psychosocial approach to measuring stress. *Stress Medicine, 11*, 85-92.

Sitza, J., Wood, N. (1997). Patient satisfaction: A review of issues and concepts. *Social Science & Medicine, 45*, 1829-1843.

Sjöström, B. (1995). *Assessing acute postoperative pain*. Doctoral thesis. Göteborg studies in educational sciences. Göteborg: Acta Universitatis Gothoburgensis.

Smith, R. (1992). The unending pursuit. *Quality in Health Care, 1*, 45-47.

Sonn, U. (1995). *Longitudinal studies of dependence in daily life activities among the elderly*. Doctoral thesis. Department of Rehabilitation Medicine and Department of Geriatric Medicine, Göteborg: Göteborg University.

Staniszewska, S., & Ahmed. L. (1999). The concept of expectation and satisfaction: Do they capture the way patients evaluate their care? *Journal of Advanced Nursing, 29*, 364-372.

Stanton, D. J. (1991). The psychological impact of intensive therapy: The role of nurses. *Intensive Care Nursing, 7*, 230-235.

Starrin, B., Dahlgren, L., Larsson, G., & Styrborn, S. (1997). *Along the Path of Discovery: Quality methods and Grounded Theory*. Lund, Sweden; Studentlitteratur.

Statistical Yearbook of Sweden. (2003).

Steen, B. (2000). Preventive nutrition in old age - a review. *Journal of Nutrition Health Aging, 4*, 114-19.

Sternbach, R. (1987). *Leva med smärta*. Stockholm, Sweden: Bonnier Fakta Bokförlag AB. (In Swedish).

Swedish institute. (2003). The Swedish population. Internet: *www.si.se*

Thomas, L. H., & Bond, S. (1991). Outcomes of nursing care: The case of primary nursing: International *Journal of Nursing Studies, 28*, 291-314.

Thomas, L. H., MacMillan, J., McColl, E., Priest, J., Hale, C., & Bond, S. (1995). Obtaining patient's views of nursing care to inform the development of a patient satisfaction scale. *International Journal of Quality in Health Care, 7*, 153-163.

Tillich, P. (1952). *The courage to be*. Yale University Press, New Haven.

Tittle, M.B., Long, C. M., & McMillan S. C. (1992). Measurement of pain in postoperative abdominal surgery patients. *Applied Nursing Research*, 5, 26-31.

Travelbee, J. (1971). *Interpersonal aspects of nursing*. F.A. Davis Company, Philadelphia.

Turner, J. S., Briggs, S. J., Springhorn, H. E., & Potgieter, P. D. (1990). Patients' recollection of intensive care unit experience. *Critical Care Medicine, 18*, 966-968.

Törnkvist, L., Gardulf, A. & Strender, L-E. (2000). Patients' satisfaction with the care given by district nurses at home and at primary health care centres. *Scandinavian Journal of Caring Sciences, 14*, 67-74.

van Campen, C., Sixman, H., Friele, R. D., Kerssens, J. J., & Peters L. (1995). Quality of care and patient satisfaction: A review of measuring instruments. *Medical Care Research & Review, 52*, 109-133.

Verbrugge L. M. (1982). Sex differences in legal drug use. *Journal of Social Issues, 38*, 59-76.

Verbrugge, L. M. (1985). Gender and health. An update hypotheses and evidence. *Journal of Health and Social Behaviour, 26*, 156-182.

von Essen, L. (1994). *What is good caring?* Doctoral thesis. Uppsala: Acta universitalis upsaliensis.

von Essen, L., & Sjödén, P. O. (1991a). The importance of nurse caring behaviour as perceived by Swedish hospital patients and nursing staff. *International Journal of Nursing Studies, 28*, 267-281.

von Essen, L., & Sjödén, P. O. (1991b). Patient and staff perceptions of caring: review and replication. *Journal of Advanced Nursing, 16*, 1363-1374.

Vuori, H. (1982). *Quality assurance of health services.* Copenhagen, Denmark: World Health Organization, Regional Office for Europe.

Vuori, H. (1991). Patient satisfaction: Does it matter? *Quality Assurance in Health Care, 3*, 183-189.

Waldron, I. (1983a). Sex differences in health incidence, prognosis, and mortality. *Social Science and Medicine, 17*, 1107-1123.

Waldron, I. (1983b). Sex differences in human mortality: The role of generic factors. *Social Sciences and Medicine, 17*, 321-333.

Walker, J. (1994). Caring for elderly people with persistent pain in the community: A qualitative perspective on the attitudes of patients and nurses. *Health & Social Care, 2*, 221-228.

Walker, J. M., Akinsanya, J. A., Davis, B. D., & Marcer, D. (1990). The nursing management of elderly patients with pain in the community: study and recommendations. *Journal of Advanced Nursing, 15*, 1154-1161.

Walker, J. & Soafer, B. (1998). Predictors of psychological distress in chronic pain patients. *Journal of Advanced Nursing, 27*, 320-326.

Ware, Jr. J. E., & Snyder, M. K. (1975). Dimensions of patient attitudes regarding doctors and medical care services. *Medical Care, 13*, 669-682.

Ware, J. E., Davies. A. A., & Stewart, A. C. (1978). The measurement and meaning of patient satisfaction: a review of the literature. *Health and Medicine Care Services Review, 1*, 1-15.

Watson, J. (1985). *Nursing. The philosophy and science of caring.* Colorado: Colorado Associated University Press.

Watson, D., & Pennebaker, W. (1989) Health complaints, stress and distress: Exploring the central role of negative affectivity. *Psychological Review, 87*, 34-54.

Weber, M. (1922). *Wirtschaft and Gessellschaft.* Grundriss der verstehenden. Tubingen: Soziologie. S. C. B. Mohr (Paul Siebech, 1956).

Windle. C., & Paschall, N. (1981). Client participation in CMCH program evaluation: Increasing incidence, inadequate involvement. *Community Mental Health Journal, 17*, 66-75.

Wilde, B. (1994). *Quality of Care: Models, instruments and empirical results among elderly.* Doktoral thesis. Institutionen för Geriatrik, Vasa sjukhus, Göteborg: Göteborgs Universitet.

Wilde Larsson, B. (1999). Patients' views on quality of care: Age effects and identification of patient profiles. *International Journal of Clinical Nursing*. 8, 693-700.

Wilde Larsson, B., & Larsson, G. (2000). Quality of Care from the Patient's Perspective questionnaire . In I. Maltby, C. A., Lewis & A. Hills. (Eds.), *Commissioned Reviews on 250 psychological tests*. Lamper, Wales: Edwin Mellen Press.

Wilde Larsson, B., & Larsson, G. (2002). Development of a short form of the Quality from the Patient's Perspective (QPP) questionnaire. *Journal of Clinical Nursing, 11*, 681-687.

Wilde, B., Larsson, G., & Bredberg, L. (1994). *Äldre- och handdikappomsorgen i Hammarö kommun: Kartläggning av vård- och omsorgtagares, anhörigas och personals uppfattning om vårdkvalitet.* (Utredningsrapport nr 2). Karlstad: Centre for Public Health Research. (In Swedish).

Wilde Larsson, B., Larsson, G., & Carlson Rizell, S. (2004). Advanced home Care: Patients' and Family members' perceptions of quality of care. *Journal of Clinical Nursing, 13*, 226-233.

Wilde, B., Larsson, G., Larsson, M., & Starrin, B. (1994). Quality of care: development of a patient-centred questionnaire based on a grounded theory model. *Scandinavian Journal of Caring Sciences, 8*, 39-48.

Wilde, B., Larsson, G., Larsson, M., & Starrin, B. (1995). Quality of care from the elderly person's perspective: Subjective importance and perceived reality. *Aging. Clinical and Experimental Research, 7*, 140-149.

Wilde Larsson, B., Larsson, G., & Starrin, B. (1999). Patients'views on quality of care of care: A comparison of men and women. *Journal of Nursing Management, 7*, 133-139.

Wilde Larsson, B., Larsson, G., Larsson, M., & Starrin B. (2001*). KUPP-boken: Kvalitet Ur Patientens Perspektiv.* Fjärde upplagan. Stockholm: Vårdförbundet. (The Swedish Association of Health Professionals). (In Swedish).

Wilde, B., Starrin, B., Larsson, G., & Larsson, M. (1993). Quality of care from a patient perspective: A grounded theory study. *Scandinavian Journal of Caring Sciences, 7*, 113-120.

Williams B. (1994). Patient satisfaction: A valid concept? *Social Science & Medicine, 38*, 509-516.

Williams, S. J., & Calnan, M. (1991). Convergence and divergence: Assessing criteria of consumer satisfaction across general practice, dental and hospital care setting. *Social Science & Medicine, 33*, 707-716.

Williamson, J. W. (1978). *Assessing and improving health care outcomes. The health accounting approach to quality assurance.* Cambridge: MA., Ballinger.

World Health Organisation. (1988). *Quality assurance of health services.* Copenhagen: World Health Organisation, Regional Committee for Europe: Thirty-eight sessions.

Wyke, S., Hunt, K., & Ford, G. (1998). Gender differences in consulting a general practitioner for common symptoms of minor illness. *Social Sciences & Medicine, 46*, 901-906.

Yates, P., Dewar, A., & Fentiman, B. (1995). Pain: The views of elderly people living in long-term residential care settings. *Journal of Advanced Nursing, 21*, 667-674.

Zalon, M. (1993). Nurses' assessment of postoperative patients' pain. *Pain, 54*, 329-334.

Øvretveit, J. (1992). *Health service quality: An introduction to quality methods for health services*. Cambridge: University Press.

Øvretveit, J. (1993). *Measuring service quality: practical guidelines*. Letchworth, England: Technical Communications (Publishing) Ltd.

INDEX

B

C

D

E

F

T

U

V

W

Y